Dentofacial Deformities

INTEGRATED ORTHODONTIC AND SURGICAL CORRECTION

DENTOFACIAL DEFORMITIES

Integrated Orthodontic and Surgical Correction

VOLUME I
Edition 2

BRUCE N. EPKER, D.D.S, Ph.D
Center for the Correction of Facial Deformities
John Peter Smith Hospital
Fort Worth, Texas

JOHN P. STELLA, D.D.S.
Co-Director, Center for the Correction of Facial Deformities
Chairman, Department of Oral and Maxillofacial Surgery
John Peter Smith Hospital
Fort Worth, Texas

LEWARD C. FISH, D.D.S., M.S.
Center for the Correction of Facial Deformities
John Peter Smith Hospital
Fort Worth, Texas
In Private Practice, Hurst, Texas

With 629 illustrations and two-color line drawings

All illustrations new to the 2nd edition by
CHRIS GATES

Additional illustrations from 1st edition by
STEVEN WATSON, D.D.S., M.D.,
and KENT BOUGHTON

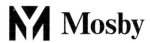 Mosby

St. Louis Baltimore Boston Carlsbad Chicago Naples New York Philadelphia Portland
London Madrid Mexico City Singapore Sydney Tokyo Toronto Wiesbaden

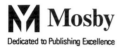

Mosby
Dedicated to Publishing Excellence

A Times Mirror
Company

Executive Editor: Linda L. Duncan
Developmental Editor: Melba Steube
Project Manager: Patricia Tannian
Production: York Production Services
Senior Book Designer: Gail Morey Hudson
Manufacturing Supervisor: Betty Richmond

SECOND EDITION

Printed in the United States of America
Composition by York Production Services
Printing/binding by Walsworth Publishing Co.

Mosby–Year Book, Inc.
11830 Westline Industrial Drive
St. Louis, Missouri 63146

Library of Congress Cataloging in Publication Data
Epker, Bruce N.
   Dentofacial deformities : integrated orthodontic and surgical correction / Bruce N. Epker,
John Paul Stella, Leward C. Fish; all illustrations new to the 2nd edition by Chris Gates; ad-
ditional illustrations from 1st edition by Steven Watson and Kent Boughton. — Ed. 2.
      p. cm.
   Includes bibliographical references and index.
   ISBN 0-8016-7729-7(v. 1)
   1. Teeth—Abnormalities—Surgery.   2. Jaws—Abnormalities—Surgery.   3. Face—
Abnormalities—Surgery.   4. Orthodontics, Corrective.   I. Stella, John Paul.   II. Fish,
Leward C.   III. Title.
   [DNLM: 1. Stomatognathic System—abnormalities.   2. Stomatognathic System—
surgery.   3. Orthodontics, Corrective.   WU 101.5 E64d 1994]
RK529.E63   1994
617.6'43—dc20
DNLM/DLC
for Library of Congress   94-23766
                                                                              CIP

94 95 96 97 98 / 9 8 7 6 5 4 3 2 1

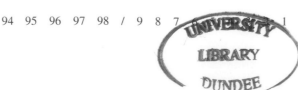

This work is dedicated to those very special individuals who have long and steadfastly encouraged, stimulated, guided, supported, and most of all trusted in me. These individuals have given to me selflessly and without concern for parity.

My parents, Dorothy and Arthur Epker, and my children, Justin and Jason, for their devotion, love, principles, and strength.

My mentors, Fred A. Henny, D.D.S., the surgeon's surgeon, and Harold M. Frost, M.D., the scientist's surgeon, for teaching me how to operate and think independently.

My professional orthodontic colleagues, Leward C. Fish, D.D.S., M.S., and Charles Sullivan, D.D.S., for their very special concern for the highest standard of patient care.

Finally, each and every former Oral and Maxillofacial Surgery Resident has given me much; but none has devoted their principles and energies in this area as have George Wessberg, D.D.S., Felice O'Ryan, D.D.S., Stephen Schendel, M.D., D.D.S., John Labanc, D.D.S., Roger A. West, D.D.S., and John Paul Stella, D.D.S. Their past and future works in the area of facial deformities will continue to be milestones.

Bruce N. Epker, D.D.S., Ph.D.

My part in composing this book has been one of the most fulfilling professional experiences of my life. For my wife and three boys, this book has truly been a test of their love for me. As a humble expression of my appreciation for their love, I dedicate this book to them. So, to my wife Anne, and our sons, Torre, Joshua, and John Mark, I offer my eternal love and apologies for late dinners and missed bedtime stories.

To my great mentors for whose contribution to my education I will always be indebted: my thanks to Drs. Melvin Moss, William Bell, Robert V. Walker, and Bruce Epker for their tireless dedication to the academic community.

John Paul Stella, D.D.S.

This work is dedicated to Iris S. and Leward F. Fish, my mother and father, who provided me with the opportunity to receive my education and who instilled in me a profound respect for the continuing pursuit of knowledge and the worth of sharing such acquired knowledge with others. To all those patients who have entrusted me with their care and from whom I have learned so much. To all those professional colleagues whose wisdom has furthered my knowledge and love of orthodontics. And especially to Michele, my wife, who has supported me in all ways during the two plus years required to prepare this manuscript. God bless them all.

Leward C. Fish, D.D.S., M.S.

Preface

During the past two decades continuous scientific study and critical evaluation of treatment methods and results has greatly increased our understanding of the integrated orthodontic and surgical correction of dentofacial deformities. This cumulative experience in conjunction with improved technology has resulted in significant improvements in the quality of patient care. In this second edition, we present the essential details of our integrated orthodontic and surgical treatment approach to each of the various dentofacial deformities in a clear and succinct manner using the aforementioned experience and technologic improvements. No attempt is made to present a detailed historical perspective of the topic, as this is not intended as a comprehensive reference source on the topic of dentofacial deformities. It is rather a textbook that presents the details of treatment planning and techniques that we have found to be important for the successful integrated orthodontic-surgical correction of dentofacial deformities.

The book is now published in three volumes because of major revisions. The first volume includes sections on evaluation and treatment planning and describes the orthodontic-surgical correction of the Class II deformities. The second volume includes the correction of Class III, Class I, and bimaxillary protrusion deformities. The third volume contains sections on the treatment of secondary cleft lip palate facial deformities and facial asymmetries. Bone graft harvesting techniques and adjunctive esthetic procedures complete the book.

Section I deals with evaluation and treatment planning. This section is of practical value and omits much of the philosophic and theoretical verbosity often associated with this topic. Our method of systematically examining the patient with a dentofacial deformity is described. Forms we have developed to aid in recording the examination results are included. In Chapter 2 the results of this systematic evaluation are then used to plan the patient's treatment in a clinically practical and applicable manner. Unique to a book of this nature, Chapter 3 discusses in a logical, succinct, and practical manner appropriate orthodontic and surgical consultations. The last two chapters of Section I present care common to all dentofacial deformity patients and a meaningful scheme for collecting records, monitoring treatment progress, and identifying and managing complications throughout the entire course of orthodontic-surgical treatment.

Each of the sections in this text discusses the treatment of a basic group of deformities—Class II, Class III, Class I, bimaxillary protrusion, cleft lip-palate, and asymmetries. Each section is divided into a number of chapters essential to cover each of the variants. Most of the chapters are divided into three parts. The first describes the most common or "usual" orthodontic and surgical treatment of the deformity in question. The second part presents adjunctive surgical techniques that are frequently helpful in the treatment of select individuals when added to the "usual" approach. The third section presents alternative treatment approaches, describing treatment of less common variations of the deformity. In each chapter a step-by-step approach to presurgical orthodontic treatment, immediate presurgical planning, surgical techniques, and postsurgical orthodontic treatment are succinctly and sequentially described. While the orthodontic mechanics illustrated are essentially the bioprogressive technique, the orthodontic principles discussed are applicable to any technique. The individual clinician must determine how best to apply the principles presented within the scope of the technique with which he or she is familiar. Both orthodontic and surgical aspects of treatment that are important with regard to predictably obtaining a stable result are discussed, including consideration for the acceptable age at which to correct the various deformities. Finally, the result of each approach is illustrated by an example patient.

The last two sections of Volume III sequentially describe techniques for harvesting bone from the illiac crest, cranium, chest, tibia, and chin, and adjunctive esthetic procedures including mandibular angle augmentation, skeletal nasal base augmentation, forehead resculpting, and rhinoplasty integration with orthognathic surgery.

This textbook is a practical, state-of-the-art guide to the essential elements of the combined orthodontic-surgical correction of dentofacial deformities. It is presented in such a way that the clinician can readily use it as a guide to the treatment of patients with all types of dentofacial deformities. Our ultimate objective in writing this book is to improve the quality of care delivered to individuals with dentofacial deformities.

Bruce N. Epker, D.D.S., Ph.D.
John Paul Stella, D.D.S.
Leward C. Fish, D.D.S., M.S.

Acknowledgments

The authors would like to thank the following clinicians for their participation in the treatment of some of the patients illustrated in this book:

O. Lynn Duren, D.D.S., Longview, Texas; Robert J. Isaacson, M.S., D.D.S., West Long Branch, New Jersey; Haruo Ishjkawa, D.D.S., M.S.D., Tokyo, Japan; Jerry Mills, D.D.S., Bedford, Texas; Steven Potter, D.D.S., M.S., Fort Worth, Texas; Carroll Sherman, D.D.S., M.S., Longview, Texas; and Charles R. Sullivan, D.D.S., Fort Worth, Texas.

Also, we would like to acknowledge the generous contributions from the following companies who supported the artwork developed for this book:

Techmedica; Porex Surgical, Inc.; Leibinger; Walter Lorenz Instrument Company; Synthes Maxillofacial; Stryker Corporation; and Integra LifeScience Surgical Projects.

Contents

Dentofacial Deformities

INTEGRATED ORTHODONTIC AND SURGICAL CORRECTION

SECTION I   *EVALUATION AND TREATMENT PLANNING*

INTRODUCTION

Section 1 is composed of five chapters: Chapter 1, Systematic Patient Evaluation; Chapter 2, Essentials of Treatment Planning; Chapter 3, The Patient Consultations; Chapter 4, Treatment Considerations and Monitoring Common to All Dentofacial Deformity Patients; and Chapter 5, Etiology, Identification, and Management of Complications. The material presented in these chapters is the basis for diagnosis and treatment of every dentofacial deformity presented in the remainder of this book. As such, the time spent reading and, more importantly, *understanding* the information presented in this section is of great importance.

The first chapter presents a comprehensive, step-by-step method of evaluating a patient with a dentofacial deformity. Soft-tissue, skeletal, and dental components are sequentially examined to determine the contribution of each to the patient's esthetic and functional anomaly. Evaluation forms are included that serve as a checklist to ensure completeness of the examination and that facilitate documentation of the clinical findings. A clinically relevant method to assess the patient's social-psychologic attitude is included, as is a method to assess the health of the temporomandibular joints. Adjunctive procedures beneficial for the evaluation of specific, less common conditions are described, with an explanation of when and how they are useful.

Chapter 2 presents a method for developing the comprehensive orthodontic-surgical treatment plan based on the data accumulated from the clinical evaluation. Basic surgical and orthodontic treatment decisions are made, then an efficient sequence for executing this treatment is devised.

While every practitioner has his or her own unique style of consulting with the patient regarding the various aspects of treatment, Chapter 3 presents a method of patient-doctor dialogue that has proven successful for the authors. During this consultation the details of the patient's treatment are discussed, any specific concerns of the patient are addressed, and *written information is given to the patient* summarizing both the care common to the treatment of all dentofacial deformity patients and the specific treatment plan for the patient.

As the title implies, Chapter 4—Treatment Considerations and Monitoring Common to All Dentofacial Deformity Patients—describes orthodontic treatment, perioperative care, and progress records common to all patients being treated for the correction of dentofacial deformities. The various protocols set forth provide the practitioner both a means of establishing clinical habits that are reliable and reproducible and a means of objectively evaluating the results of treatment. By following the record-gathering protocol described, a means to evaluate, diagnose, and manage complications critically is available. In addition, the long-term esthetic and functional results can be critically evaluated and treatment improved.

The etiology, identification, and management of complications is discussed in Chapter 5. Simply stated, a complication exists when the achieved result is significantly different from the expected result. When complete records are available the clinician is able to diagnose the specific nature of the complication, inform the patient of the complication and its recommended management, treat the complication, and evaluate the outcome.

It is recommended that each clinician take time to become thoroughly familiar with the principles and protocols set forth in Section I. Doing so will allow the clinician to make better treatment decisions, thus making the orthodontic-surgical correction of dentofacial deformities a pleasant experience for both the patient and the practitioner.

CHAPTER 1

Systematic patient evaluation

ESSENTIAL PATIENT EVALUATIONS

To do an adequate evaluation of individuals with dentofacial deformities and subsequently plan treatment for them, certain examinations are necessary. In routine cases these evaluations include the following:

A. General patient evaluation
   1. Medical history
   2. Dental evaluation
      a. Dental history
      b. Dental health
B. Social-psychologic evaluation
C. Esthetic facial evaluation
   1. Front-face analysis
   2. Profile analysis
D. Cephalometric evaluation
   1. Soft tissue
   2. Skeletal relations
   3. Dental relations
E. Panoramic or full-mouth periapical evaluations
F. Occlusal evaluation
   1. Functional
   2. Static
G. Masticatory muscle and temporomandibular joint evaluation
   1. Masticatory muscle
   2. Mandibular movements
   3. Temporomandibular joint symptoms
   4. Temporomandibular joint signs

The first part of this chapter will sequentially discuss the details of these essential evaluations. Additional or adjunctive evaluations are often indicated either as the result of unusual findings discovered during these essential evaluations or because of special patient problems. These are discussed in the second part of this chapter.

Medical history

The patient population seeking treatment for correction of dentofacial deformities is widely varied in age and generally has no serious coexisting medical conditions. However, certain medical conditions must be considered before instituting orthodontic-surgical correction of a dentofacial deformity. Particular attention must be given to cardiopulmonary, endocrine, hematologic, neurologic, and allergic problems in the medical history. Medical problems in these areas can potentially complicate the general anesthesia or reconstructive surgery and must be further evaluated by use of appropriate laboratory studies, discussion with the patient's physician, or consultation with appropriate medical specialists. Direct communication with the patient's physician is essential to relate precisely what the surgical phase of treatment will entail so that specific recommendations regarding medical management are based on accurate information. Following discussion with the patient's physician and/or other consultants, risk management and realistic potentials for related complications must be carefully documented and discussed with the patient and his/her family. With proper consultation and preparation most patients with coexisting medical conditions who desire correction of their facial deformities can undergo orthodontic-surgical correction without life-threatening risks. In unusual instances the magnitude of the medical risk may be a contraindication to treatment.

Dental evaluation

After the medical history is obtained, consideration is given to the dental history, dental health, and periodontal status. It is important to consider not only what dental procedures will be necessary but also at what time in the overall treatment these procedures are best done. *The timing of indicated restorative and periodontal procedures is critical to achieving optimal overall results.*

Dental history

Patient commitment is essential to successful treatment. The dental history is an important barometer of the patient's probable commitment to integrated orthodontic-surgical treatment. All previous restorative, orthodontic, periodontal, and facial pain control therapy needs to be reviewed. When these have been previously performed, the patient's response to treatment and his/her perception of the success or failure of these treatments are ascertained. This information is important to allow accurate estimation of the patient's biologic and psychologic response to the correction of his/her facial deformity. The following two examples will help illustrate this.

A 41-year-old woman had comprehensive periodontal therapy 5 years previously. She relates that the surgery was quite unpleasant; however, she is pleased that she underwent treatment since she places a high priority on maintaining her natural dentition. Further, she has maintained excellent oral hygiene since therapy, and her periodontist reports that she has had a stable result following treatment. This patient is likely to respond favorably to orthodontic-surgical treatment, both biologically and psychologically.

In contrast to the above example, a 26-year-old man is being evaluated for correction of his facial deformity; he states that he had undergone orthodontics 7 years previously to correct "bucked teeth." He reports that the 2 years of orthodontic treatment resulted in essentially no change in his condition, and several times during and since treatment he has had to be treated for "gum disease." The records of the previous orthodontist and periodontist revealed a major, although incomplete, improvement in his occlusion and constant neglect of his oral hygiene with progressive periodontal disease. In view of this history, before orthodontic-surgical correction of his dentofacial deformity is instituted, critical attention must be paid to both his current periodontal status by referral to a periodontist and his social-psychologic profile. Whether to institute orthodontic-surgical treatment in this patient must be predicated on a clear understanding of his psychologic makeup; specifically, his motivation for seeking correction of the existing dentofacial deformity needs to be known. This is best determined by a more comprehensive professional psychologic examination. (See section on "Social-Psychologic Evaluation" below.)

Dental health

The basic consideration herein is the overall health of the patient's dentition. If the teeth have been poorly cared for and/or oral hygiene is poor, the first phase of treatment, *before making orthodontic-surgical records,* is to establish a healthy dentition by dental prophylaxis and proper home care. The patient who will not establish good oral hygiene habits is a poor candidate for orthodontic-surgical treatment, and intervention is most often best deferred or refused.

Once the patient demonstrates good home care and a clean and healthy dentition, orthodontic-surgical records are taken and a tentative treatment plan is adopted. The orthodontist must then inform the general dentist which teeth if any will need to be extracted for orthodontic reasons. This avoids the unnecessary restoration of these teeth. Making this decision for the patient with a healthy mouth is predicated on surgical and orthodontic consideration alone. However, for the patient with caries or periodontal or periapical pathology, which teeth to extract may be predicated, in part, on the health of individual teeth and/or the prognosis for restoring the teeth to a healthy condition. In some instances it is preferable to remove a badly broken down tooth or a periodontally involved tooth, while perhaps making the orthodontic treatment or surgery more difficult, *so long as there is no compromise in the overall treatment result.* When the patient has missing teeth, the general dentist is informed whether the ultimate restoration of the spaces will be necessary or if these spaces will be closed by the proposed surgery and/or orthodontic treatment.

Next, the general dentist must evaluate periapical pathology or carious lesions in any teeth not to be extracted pursuant to the orthodontic-surgical treatment. These are appropriately restored at this time. If a tooth cannot be saved, the orthodontist and surgeon must be informed so that they can review the tentative treatment plan and decide what changes can be made to accommodate the loss of the tooth or teeth.

All indicated restorations are done before orthodontic-surgical treatment except inlays, crowns, bridges, or partial dentures, which are deferred until the completion of the orthodontic-surgical treatment. Teeth that require a crown or inlay are restored with a good temporary restoration before orthodontic-surgical treatment, with plans made to do the definitive restorations after completion of orthodontic-surgical treatment.

Finally, teeth with over-contoured and poorly shaped restorations are properly restored before any orthodontic-surgical intervention. This may involve recontouring the existing restoration, replacing the restoration, or placing temporary crowns or inlays. Osseointegrated dental implants may be employed to restore missing teeth and/or provide anchorage for orthodontic purposes. If orthodontic anchorage is lacking from existing natural dentition, it may be prudent to place osseointegrated dental implants early in the treatment course to facilitate the necessary or indicated orthodontic tooth movement. Conversely, if adequate anchorage exists but a tooth or teeth are missing, osseointegrated dental implant(s) may be placed at the time of the orthognathic surgical procedure when doing so will not interfere with the necessary postsurgical orthodontics, or they may be placed following completion of the orthodontic-surgical treatment.

Periodontal status

The specific pretreatment periodontal needs are determined on a case-by-case basis in consultation with the patient's general dentist and/or periodontist. Both acute periodontal disease and inadequate attached gingiva must be managed before orthodontic-surgical treatment. Much of the acute disease process—gingivitis or periodontitis—is eliminated by the process of performing prophylaxis, instituting proper home care, restoring the teeth, and recontouring poorly done restorations. Root planing and/or curettage may be necessary to resolve the acute phase of periodontal disease, arrest a chronic disease process, or prevent further bone destruction in select cases. Definitive periodontal surgery—gingivectomy, gingivoplasty, and/or bone recontouring—is usually best deferred until completion of orthodontic-surgical treatment because the orthodontics and surgery alter the existing anatomy and the appropriate periodontal procedures cannot be determined until the final anatomy has been produced.

Treating inadequate attached gingiva, a problem that most commonly exists in the anterior mandibular area, is best done *before* orthodontics and surgery. When teeth are to be orthodontically moved into a more normal relationship with the underlying bone and its overlying soft tissues, an increase in the amount of attached gingiva can occur. Thus, when such movements are a part of the planned treatment, it may be prudent to observe carefully the questionable areas of attached gingiva in anticipation that they will improve. However, it is generally recommended that moderate to severe deficiencies in attached gingiva be resolved by placement of a free gingival graft before any orthodontic tooth movement.

Social-psychologic evaluation

The social-psychologic makeup of patients is often neglected when correction of facial deformities is considered. Yet the psychologic makeup of the patients is important because, despite an objectively favorable treatment result, certain patients will express dissatisfaction with their results. This can occur for two basic reasons: (1) unrealistic patient expectations regarding the results of treatment, or (2) failure of the clinician to inform the patient realistically of the probable treatment result (especially esthetic). The second reason is not addressed here, but it is discussed in Chapter 3—The Patient Consultations.

Unrealistic expectations are most likely to occur in two types of patients—those with acquired deformities and those with external motivations. Patients possessing a facial deformity acquired by surgery, trauma, or disease must be care-

SOCIAL-PSYCHOLOGIC EVALUATION

1. Nature of the dentofacial deformity:
   Congenital   Specific nature————
   Developmental   When recognized————
   Acquired   When acquired————

2. Duration of concern about the dentofacial deformity:
   1 - 2 - 3 - 4 - 5 - 6 - 7 - 8 - 9 - 10

   Weeks   **Months**   **Years**

3. Esthetic severity of dentofacial deformity:
   1 - 2 - 3 - 4 - 5 - 6 - 7 - 8 - 9 - 10

   Slight   **Moderate**   **Marked**

4. Functional severity of dentofacial deformity:
   1 - 2 - 3 - 4 - 5 - 6 - 7 - 8 - 9 - 10

   Slight   **Moderate**   **Marked**

5. Patient ability to define dentofacial deformity:
   1 - 2 - 3 - 4 - 5 - 6 - 7 - 8 - 9 - 10

   Defined   **Defined**   **Defined**
   with   **with**   **with**
   difficulty   **assistance**   **ease**

6. Patient's perspective of the effect of the dentofacial deformity on social adjustment:
   1 - 2 - 3 - 4 - 5 - 6 - 7 - 8 - 9 - 10

   Severe   **Some**   **No**
   effect   **effect**   **effect**

7. Patient's perspective of the effect of the dentofacial deformity on vocational aspira-
   tions:
   1 - 2 - 3 - 4 - 5 - 6 - 7 - 8 - 9 - 10

   Marked   **Moderate**   **Minimal**

8. Patient's expectations from orthodontic-surgical treatment:
   1 - 2 - 3 - 4 - 5 - 6 - 7 - 8 - 9 - 10

   Unrealistic   **Not clear**   **Realistic**

   Motivational assessment

   External   Ambiguous   Internal

fully counseled regarding realistic treatment results. They must be made aware of and accept the fact that even with the most skillful therapy they will probably never look exactly like they did before their misfortune. If they are unable to accept this fact, treatment is best delayed until they can cope with treatment realities often psychological counseling may be required.

Unrealistic expectations also are seen in patients who are externally motivated to seek improvement of their facial appearance. The individual who is experiencing difficulties—either personal or professional—and believes that these problems will be rectified by improving his/her facial appearance is an excellent and not uncommon example. Treatment of such patients must be entered into only after careful consideration and psychologic consultation. *Frequently it is best not to treat these patients, since they are generally unhappy with the results achieved.* If it is decided to treat such a patient, it is best done in conjunction with psychologic counseling, and even then, preferably on the recommendation of a psychologist or psychiatrist.

Conversely, internal motivations are those that exist in individuals who desire improvement for themselves, not for others. Those with internal motivations generally make excellent patients, who have a realistic attitude toward their overall treatment.

Thus, distinguishing between external and internal motivations is important. A deliberate social-psychologic evaluation will help to assess the motivation of patients reasonably. The evaluation form below is useful in this regard. This form is not filled out by the patient. Rather, these issues are discussed during the examination and consultation conversations with the patient and the form is subsequently completed by the clinician. Responses judged 6 to 10 are generally indicative of an internally motivated patient, whereas a predominance of 1 to 4 responses is indicative of a patient who would benefit from additional expert psychologic consultation before initiating treatment. All 1 to 4 responses must be individually weighed. For example, a low-level response on items 3 and 4 may not necessarily be indicative of external motivations, whereas low-level responses on items 6, 7, and 8 definitely indicate external motivation. When the results of this assessment are believed to be either ambiguous or indicative of external motivations, it is generally preferable to have the individual undergo a more comprehensive psychologic evaluation by a qualified individual.

Esthetic facial evaluation

The esthetic facial evaluation is done directly on the patient, with the patient standing or seated comfortably. The observer must help the patient maintain a head posture with the Frankfort horizontal and interpupillary lines parallel to the floor, because patients with facial deformities commonly exhibit compensatory head posturing that masks their deformity and may result in erroneous esthetic measurements. It is important that this examination be done in a systematic manner so that no detail is overlooked. The major emphasis is placed on front face esthetics because that is how individuals most often view themselves and one another.

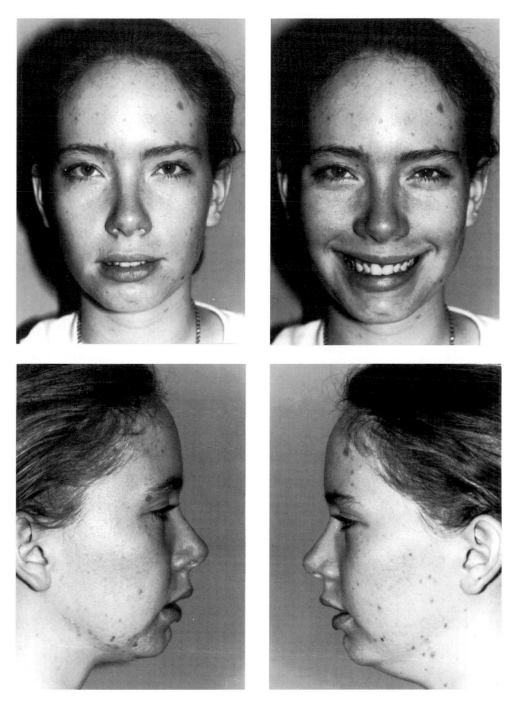

FIG. 1-1

Although the actual details of the esthetic facial evaluation are recorded directly from the patient, facial photographs are essential to document the pretreatment condition. The minimum recommended facial photographs are: (1) front face with teeth lightly together and lips in repose, (2) front face smiling, and (3) right and left profile with teeth lightly together and lips in repose. In addition, submental and 3/4 oblique views are taken of patients who have associated deformities of the neck, nose, and/or cheeks who may undergo simultaneous adjunctive esthetic surgery (Fig. 1-1). The frontal and profile photographs are also taken in

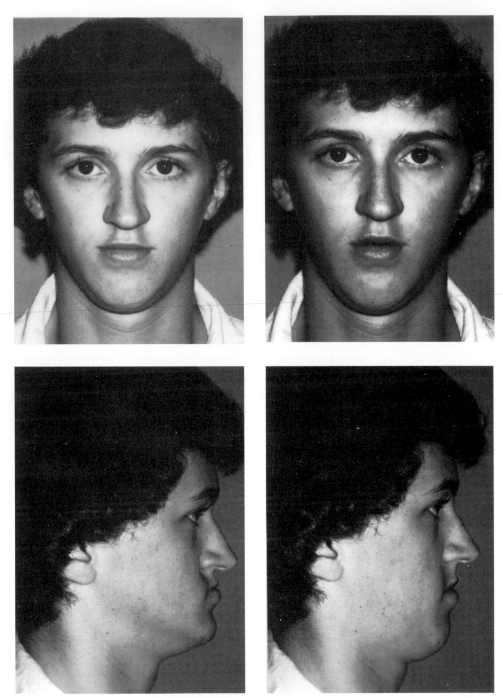

FIG. 1-2

mandibular rest position for any "overclosed" individual to permit more accurate assessment of facial esthetics and upper tooth-to-lip relations. (Fig. 1-2) All photographs are taken with the Frankfort horizontal and interpupillary lines parallel to the floor. Patients with long hair should place it behind their ears and shoulders to aid the clinician in photographing the head in the aforementioned position.

The reader is referred to the accompanying Esthetic Facial Evaluation Forms while reading this section. These forms are both a sequential checklist for performing the evaluation and the means of recording essential data. The equipment required for this evaluation is a millimeter ruler and/or large, anthropometric caliper. *Only abnormal findings need be recorded.* These findings will subsequently serve as the primary means for making the basic decision regarding what type of surgery will be most esthetically beneficial for the patient. A computerized version of this esthetic evaluation of patients is being developed and will be available soon.

Front face analysis

Determinations are first made regarding the total face. Detailed evaluations of the facial thirds are then sequentially performed.

GENERAL FACIAL CHARACTERISTICS

Symmetry, balance, and morphology are the three major elements that are important in the production of good front face esthetics.

SYMMETRY

Right-left symmetry is studied first. While no face is perfectly symmetric, the absence of obvious asymmetry is necessary for good esthetics. When a facial asymmetry is identified, a varied approach to evaluation is taken as described in Section VII on facial asymmetries.

BALANCE

The total face height is defined by the distance from points trichion (Tr) to gnathion (Gn) and may be divided into facial thirds by the points glabella (G) and subnasale (Sn) (Fig. 1-3).

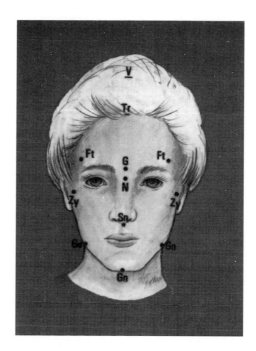

FIG. 1-3

FACIAL ESTHETIC EVALUATION

Front face esthetics

General facial characteristics

Symmetry _____

Balance

Upper third_____ mm ÷ Total _____ mm = _____ (0.30 ± 0.0)
Middle third_____ mm ÷ Total _____ mm = _____ (0.35 ± 0.0)
Lower third_____ mm ÷ Total _____ mm = _____ (0.35 ± 0.0)

Morphology

Bitemporal _____ mm ÷ Total _____ mm = _____ (0.65 ± 0.0)
Bizygomatic_____ mm ÷ Total _____ mm = _____ (0.75 ± 0.0)
Bigonial _____ mm ÷ Total _____ mm = _____ (0.55 ± 0.0)

The upper, middle, and lower facial thirds may be defined as the distance from trichion to glabella, glabella to subnasale, and subnasale to gnathion, respectively. The ratio of the upper, middle, and lower facial thirds to the total facial height in a normal attractive person is 0.30, 0.35, and 0.35, respectively. Values outside the range of normal are noted on the esthetic evaluation forms.

That part of the head traditionally called "the face" lies between glabella and gnathion. The face is divided into two equal halves by the point subnasale such that the distance from glabella to subnasale, and that from subnasale to gnathion are equal (Fig. 1-3).

MORPHOLOGY

All facial thirds—upper, middle, and lower—*are optimally of the same basic morphologic configuration* in any individual. Rather than having one facial third appear short and square and the other two appear long and narrow, all should have the same basic morphology for facial harmony to exist. The morphology of any given facial third is determined by dividing the width of each facial third by the total facial height.

The widths of the facial thirds are measured between three pairs of points bilaterally. The forehead width is defined by the distance between the points frontotemporale (Ft)—the slight elevation of the linea temporalis on either side of the forehead. The width of the middle third of the face is defined by the distance between the points zygion (Zy)—the most lateral point of the zygomatic arch. The distance between gonion (Go) bilaterally determines the width of the lower third of the face (Fig. 1-3). These horizontal measurements (bitemporal, bizygomatic, and bigonial) when divided by the total facial height (Tr-Gn) produce ratios of 0.65, 0.75, and 0.66, respectively. Ratios larger than the norm indicate a short and/or wide tendency, while those smaller than the norm indicate a long and/or narrow tendency for the specific facial third being assessed. An attractive face will have all facial thirds presenting with the same basic morphology—long/narrow, normal, or short/wide.

FACIAL ESTHETIC EVALUATION

Front face esthetics

Upper third face
Morphology

Width _____ mm ÷ height _____ mm = _____ (2.20 ± 0.0)

Shape and symmetry of: Calvarium _____

Temporal areas _____

Frontal area _____

Eyebrows _____

Supraorbital rims _____

UPPER THIRD FACE—HAIRLINE TO EYEBROWS (Tr-G)

The upper third face is perhaps the most variable, since it is affected by the hairline and hairstyle. Nevertheless, the general morphology, shape, and symmetry of the calvarium are noted.

MORPHOLOGY. The morphology of the upper third face may be quantified by calculating the ratio of the bitemporal width (Ft-Ft) to the height of the upper third face (Tr-G) (Fig. 1-3). This ratio in an attractive individual is approximately 2.20. Values less than 2.20 indicate a long/narrow third; greater than 2.20 a short/wide third.

SHAPE AND SYMMETRY. The temporal areas, frontal areas, eyebrows, and supraorbital rims are specifically observed for abnormalities, which are often associated with various craniofacial syndromes. These areas are usually within normal limits in individuals with dentofacial deformities.

MIDDLE THIRD FACE—EYEBROWS TO SUBNASALE

The general morphology of the middle third face, orbits, nose, cheeks, and ears are systematically evaluated.

MORPHOLOGY. The morphology of the middle third face is quantified by calculating the ratio of the bizygomatic width (Zy-Zy) to the height of the middle third face (G-Sn) (Fig. 1-3). This ratio in an attractive female is approximately 2.20; in a handsome male it is approximately 2.30. Values less than these norms tend to be classified as long/narrow and greater than these norms as more short/wide.

EYES AND ORBITS. Examination of the eyes and orbits begins with measurements of intercanthal and interpupillary distances. Increased intercanthal distance is telecanthus; increased interocular distance is ocular hypertelorism. The mean values and standard deviations for Caucasian adults are listed on the accompanying Facial Esthetic Evaluation Form. (The norms are slightly larger for dark-skinned people.) These values are established by 6 to 8 years of age and do not change significantly after this time.

FACIAL ESTHETIC EVALUATION

Front face esthetics

Middle third face
Morphology

Width _____ mm ÷ height _____ mm = _____   (F)(2.20 ± 0.5)
                                                                (M)(2.30 ± 0.5)

Eyes and orbits

Intercanthal distance (34 ± 4 mm) _____ mm
Interoccular distance (65 ± 4 mm) _____ mm
Inner–outer canthal symmetry _____
Upper eye lid symmetry _____
Lower eye lid symmetry _____
          Ptosis   Ectropion   Entropion
Other (Muscles, Sclera, etc.) _____

Nose

Form and symmetry of: Glabella_____
                      Dorsum_____
                      Tip_____
                      Alar bases_____
Alar base width _____ mm ÷ Nose length _____ mm = _____ (0.60 ± 0.0)

Cheeks

Symmetry of: Malar eminences_____
             Infraorbital rims_____
             Paranasal areas_____
Projection of malar eminences (relative to lateral canthus):
Right: _____ mm lateral   Left: _____ mm lateral
       _____ mm inferior   _____ mm inferior

Ears

Symmetry _____
Level _____
Projection _____
Deformation _____ Partial agenesis _____

The vertical symmetry of the inner and outer canthi is recorded. Generally a true horizontal line will bisect the inner and outer canthi of both eyes. This is perhaps the most meaningful method of evaluating true ocular-orbital symmetry. A common malrelation, lateral canthal dystopia, occurs when the outer canthi are inferiorly positioned. The upper and lower eyelids are evaluated for right-to-left symmetry and specifically for the presence of ptosis, ectropion, or entropion. When these exist and are important to the patient, their precise etiology must be determined. Finally, ocular muscle imbalance, sclera discoloration, and the presence of sclera showing between the lower eyelid and pupil are assessed. The latter is commonly associated with skeletal deficiency in the midfacial area.

NOSE. The nose is studied for form and symmetry. When deformities exist in the nose, their specific anatomic location—glabella, dorsum, tip, or alar bases—is noted. Normal alar base width is generally several millimeters wider than the intercanthal distance (34 ± 4 mm). Finally, proportions of the alar base width (A1-A1) to the nasal length (N-Prn) are determined. An attractive proportional nose has an alar width to length of 0.60 (Fig. 1-4).

When the nose is found to be significantly unesthetic, a more detailed evaluation is performed as described in Appendix II at the end of this chapter.

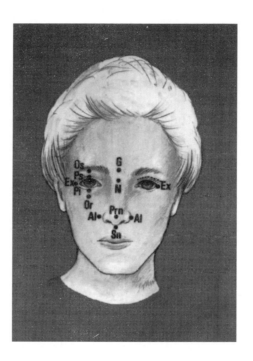

FIG. 1-4

CHEEKS. Evaluation of the cheeks consists of sequential assessment of the malar eminences, infraorbital rims, and paranasal areas for symmetry and normal projection. The malar eminences are normally present 10 ± 2 mm lateral and 15 ± 5 mm inferior to the lateral canthus (Fig. 1-5). These measurements are taken

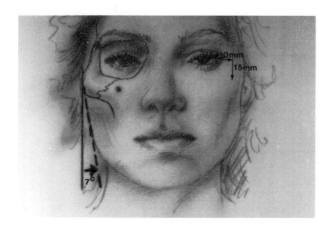

FIG. 1-5

using an imaginary *x,y*-coordinate system originating at the lateral canthus. The lateral most projection of the malar eminence may also be related to the mandibular angle. Normally, a 7° angle is formed by the intersect of a malar eminence/mandibular angle tangent and a true venticle originating at the malar promience (Fig. 1-5). The examiner should not be deceived by optical illusions that are created by the lower jaw or nose being abnormal in size.

Evaluation of these areas can be supplemented by viewing the patient from both the submental and the superior aspects. Further, palpation is useful in evaluating these areas, especially in detecting fullness in the region of the buccal fat pad. Excessive fullness of the buccal fat pad may obscure a normal projecting malar prominence and therefore should be noted (see "Adjunctive Esthetic Maxillofacial Procedures, Buccal Lipectomy," in Chapter 7).

EARS. The ears are observed for symmetry, level, and projection. Any notable asymmetry is first recorded. Normal vertical level is present when the upper third of the ear projects above a horizontal line passed through the inner and outer canthi of the eyes. Finally, any abnormality in projection and any deformation or partial agenesis is noted.

When the ear is found to exhibit significant abnormalities or esthetic alterations, a more detailed evaluation is performed as described in Appendix III at the end of this chapter.

LOWER THIRD FACE—SUBNASALE TO MENTON

MORPHOLOGY. The morphology and balance are first evaluated, followed by the teeth, chin, and mandibular angles. The morphology of the lower facial third may be quantified by calculating the ratio of the bigonial width (Go-Go) to the height of the lower facial third (Sn-Gn) (Fig. 1-6). The normal ratio is 1.30. Ratios less than the norm indicate a facial third that is long and/or narrow; values greater than the norm indicate that the lower third is short and/or wide.

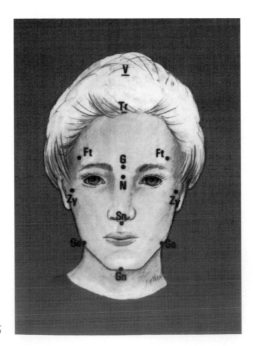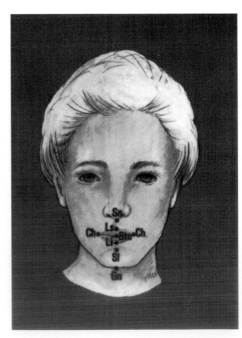

FIG. 1-6

FACIAL ESTHETIC EVALUATION

Front face esthetics

Lower third face
Morphology

Width _____ mm ÷ height _____ m = _____ (1.40 ± 0.25)

Balance

Subnasale-stomion:Stomion-gnathion (1:2)_____
Subnasale-vermilion:Vermilion-gnathion (1:1) _____

Lips

Symmetry at rest _____ smiling _____
    Intrinsic   —   Nerve   —   Dentoskeletal
Upper:lower vermilion (1:1.25) _____
Interlabial distance (0-3 mm) _____ mm
Commissure width (55 mm) _____ mm and symmetry _____

Teeth

Exposure of upper teeth at rest_____ mm; smiling _____ mm
    Symmetry _____
Exposure of lower teeth at rest_____ mm; smiling _____ mm
    Symmetry _____
Dental symmetry _____
Dental midlines_____

Chin

Symmetry: right_____ mm; left _____ mm _____
Shape_____

Mandibular angles

Symmetry _____
Projection: deficient–hyperplastic _____

Mandibular border   *Poorly defined*   –   *Average*   –   *Well defined*

Submental and neck area

Skin:	*Tight*	–	*Normal*	–	*Lax*
Lipomatosis:	*None*	–	*Some*	–	*Severe*
Hyoid bone level:	*Low*	–	*Normal*	–	*High*

BALANCE. The normal vertical length of the lower third face is approximately equal to that of the middle third face when good esthetics exist. The ratio of the vertical distance from subnasale (Sn) to upper lip stomion and that from upper lip stomion to soft-tissue gnathion (Gn) is about 1:2. The ratio of the vertical distance from subnasale to the vermilion cutaneous margin of the lower lip (Li) and that from the vermilion cutaneous margin of the lower lip to soft-tissue menton is about 1:1. Disparities in these relations define the precise nature of existing lower third face imbalances. These measurements must be made with the facial musculature at rest.

The significance of these vertical relationships is of clinical importance as variations in them are characteristic of several types of facial deformities (Table 1-1).

TABLE 1-1.   *VERTICAL RELATIONS IN DENTOFACIAL DEFORMITIES*

Value measured	Normal	Vertical maxillary excess*	Vertical maxillary deficiency†	Vertically long chin	Vertically short chin
Middle third face	1				
Lower third face	1	Excessive	Deficient	Excessive	Deficient
Subnasale to stomion	1				
Stomion to menton	2	Excessive	Deficient	Excessive	Deficient
Subnasale to lower lip vermilion border	1	Excessive	Deficient		
Lower lip vermilion border to menton	1			Excessive	Deficient

No entry is indicative of normalcy.

†The listed abnormalities exist when the patient is evaluated in centric occlusion and will all become close to normal when the patient is evaluated in mandibular rest position.

LIPS. The lips are extremely important in the overall esthetics of the face and are evaluated both in repose and during animation. At rest, the symmetry of the lips relative to the face and the dentition is noted. If asymmetry exists, one must determine if the existing asymmetry is primarily the result of (1) an intrinsic lip deformity, as exists in many patients with clefts, (2) facial nerve dysfunction, or (3) an underlying dental-skeletal asymmetry. Each of these conditions requires different treatment considerations.

The lower lip generally has about 25% more vermilion exposed than the upper lip in repose. This ratio of exposed vermilion is more important than absolute values. Further, when good esthetics exist, an interlabial separation of up to 3 mm exists in repose. The width of the lips from commissure to commissure is normally about equal to the interpupillary distance (55 mm).

The upper teeth are normally exposed beneath the upper lip up to 3 mm with the lips relaxed. Generally there is less exposure in males than in females. When recording upper tooth exposure, it is important to consider the shape of the patient's upper lip. Normally the upper lip tubercle hangs slightly inferior to the vermilion on either side of it, however, the tubercle may be superior to the adjacent vermilion or entirely absent. Such a deformity has been called a "gull-wing" upper lip. Recognition of this condition is important because "gull-wing" lip deformity may be confused with vertical maxillary excess and lead to inaccurate treatment decisions. When the upper anterior teeth are relatively level, "gull-wing" lip deformity is clinically demonstrated by measuring and recording the exposure of each tooth as it relates to the upper lip as illustrated below.

NORMAL LIP PATIENT   "GULL-WING" PATIENT

3 3 3 | 3 3 3   2 4 6 | 6 4 2

The numbers as recorded represent individual tooth exposure. The most medial numbers represent exposure of the upper central incisors, the next numbers the lateral incisors, and the most lateral numbers show the exposure of the canines. Patients with true vertical maxillary excess usually show excessive tooth exposure from embrasure to embrasure, while those with "gull-wing" deformity exhibit excessive exposure of the central incisors with progressively less tooth exposure laterally. (Care must be taken when looking at interlabial distance in lateral photographs and/or lateral cephalometric projections as the two aforementioned conditions are easily confused in those projections.)

Additional helpful values for assessing anthropometric esthetic relationships in the perioral area are in Appendix IV and illustrated in its associated figure. When abnormalities are identified in the perioral area it is helpful to use these additional evaluations.

TEETH. Symmetry is the single most important factor in producing an esthetic smile. This includes the symmetry of both lip movement and tooth exposure. If the smile is asymmetric, the clinician must determine if the asymmetry is due to the lip or the teeth. It is important to differentiate between an asymmetry caused by facial muscle dysfunction, an intrinsic lip deformity, or an underlying skeletal–dental–soft-tissue asymmetry such as hemifacial microsomia.

When a dental-skeletal asymmetry is noted—a cant of the maxillary occlusal plane relative to the globes—it is important to determine the magnitude of the cant and which side, if either, is at the correct vertical level. When clinically determining cant of the maxilla, it is helpful to have the patient bite on a tongue blade and measure each tooth as it relates to the lower eyelid margins while the patient is staring in a neutral gaze (Fig. 1-7). Careful evaluation of the tooth to lip relations, as previously described, is imperative to determine the most appropriate surgical procedure for correction of the canted maxilla—superior versus inferior repositioning, or some of each.

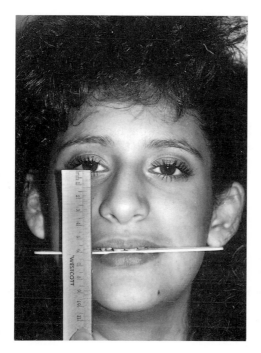 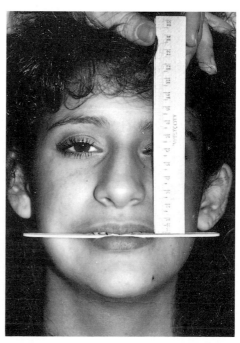

FIG. 1-7

Tooth exposure during smiling is highly variable depending on which facial muscles are activated. Some individuals activate only the risorius muscles, which results in only a slight lateral and superior movement of the commissures. The other extreme is represented by the individual who activates all the perioral elevator-retractor-depressor muscles. In this instance the lips are drawn centrifugally in all directions, exposing both the upper and lower teeth. Importantly, the least esthetic condition exists when no exposure of the upper teeth occurs during smiling because the teeth are so superiorly located that, despite normal lip movement, they never become visible.

The lower teeth are seldom exposed at rest. When they are, it generally indicates (1) poor support of the lower lip because of an anteroposterior chin deficiency, (2) severe mandibular dentoalveolar protrusion, or (3) hypotonicity of the lower lip.

The dental midlines should be coincident with one another and with the facial midline. When such is not the case, it is essential to specify which midline is deviated relative to the facial midline—maxillary, mandibular, or both—in which direction the discrepancy exists, and by how much.

CHIN. The chin is evaluated for symmetry, vertical relations, and morphology and its relationship to the mandibular angles and inferior border of the mandible. The latter is compared with that of the rest of the face. Often the chin may be more tapered or more square than the rest of the face. When such is the case it must be noted because, though minimal before treatment, such inconsistency in morphology may become more noticeable with certain types of treatment (genioplasty), and must be corrected to achieve optimal facial esthetics.

MANDIBULAR ANGLES-INFERIOR BORDERS

The mandibular angles are assessed with regard to both their symmetry and fullness as being deficient, normal or excessive. The definition of the mandibular angles and inferior borders of the mandible is an important consideration in neck esthetics as this prominence (or lack thereof) defines the breaking point between the face and neck. The neck relative to the mandible borders takes on a subtle hourglass appearance with its superior aspect being well defined by the concavity immediately below the inferior mandibular borders. The soft tissues of the neck are normally closely adherent to the structures underlying them. The mandibular borders become less well defined when tissue laxity, lipomatosis, chin deficiency, and/or hyoid bone sag become progressively worse.

Patients with a long lower third face height exhibit a greater confluence of the lower face and neck that may be confused with lipomatosis, soft-tissue laxity, or both. The converse is true for a patient with a short lower third face height.

SUBMENTAL AND NECK AREA. When examining the submental and neck area, the patient is evaluated in repose with the head in a natural position. This is perhaps most easily achieved by having the examiner's and patient's heads at the same level looking directly into one another's eyes. Significant deviations from this position can produce important changes in neck esthetics, especially if the patient extends or positions the head forward.

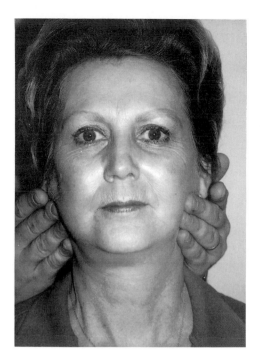 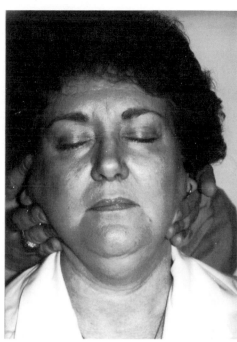

FIG. 1-8

SKIN. The skin of the submental and neck region may be judged as tight, normal, or lax. Skin laxity is best diagnosed by the clinician gently pulling the soft tissues upward just inferior and anterior to the ear, simulating a neck lift (Fig. 1-8). Tissues that are easily displaced upward are generally redundant. Residual fullness during this maneuver usually is indicative of lipomatosis. The patient on the left in Fig. 1-8 has submental fullness primarily due to redundant skin. The patient on the right has submental fullness due to redundant skin and cervical facial lipomatosis.

When skin laxity is present and the patient also has mandibular retrognathia or microgenia, it is helpful to have the patient protrude the lower jaw to a more normal anteroposterior chin position. While the patient maintains this posture, the clinician can reassess, both visually and by palpation, the soft-tissue laxity or lack thereof. In this manner, the clinician is able to determine the relative contributions of skin laxity, lipomatosis, and mandibular (chin) retrusion to the appearance of the neck. Importantly, the correction of various dentofacial deformities can either improve or worsen the neck-chin appearance (Table 1-2). If the planned orthognathic surgical procedure may worsen neck esthetics, a cosmetic surgical procedure on the neck must be considered to offset the untoward effects.

TABLE 1-2.   *EFFECTS OF ORTHOGNATHIC PROCEDURES ON NECK ESTHETICS IN PRESENCE OF FULLNESS OR LIPOMATOSIS*

Procedure	Improve	Worsen	No effect
Mandibular advancement	X		
Advancement genioplasty	X		
Maxillary superior repositioning	X		
Combinations of three above procedures	X		
Mandibular set-back		X	
Reduction genioplasty		X	
Maxillary inferior repositioning		X	
Combinations of preceding three procedures		X	
Maxillary advancement			X
Mandibular total subapical osteotomy			X

LIPOMATOSIS. Localized neck lipomatosis often exists independently of generalized body fat. In the younger population, the fat usually appears in the tissue plane between the skin and the platysma muscle. In older patients, localized lipomatosis is commonly found both deep and superficial to the platysma muscle in the midline.

The clinician can make a semiquantitative estimate of the amount of subcutaneous fat present by grasping the submental tissues between the thumb and forefinger—the pinch test. This is best done with the patient in both natural head position and while the patient is extending the head and contracting the platysma muscle (Fig. 1-9). Performing the pinch test in this manner allows the clinician to

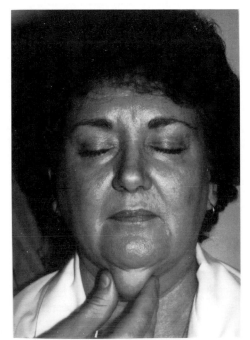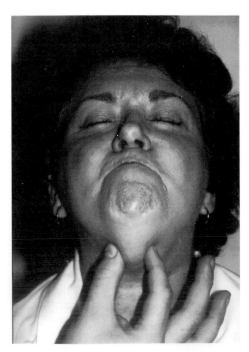

FIG. 1-9

determine better whether the cervical facial fat is predominantly supraplatysmal or subplatysmal.

HYOID BONE LEVEL. The position of the hyoid bone is best assessed by grasping it gently between the thumb and index finger. Once the hyoid bone is grasped, its relation to the mandibular inferior border is noted. Normally, the hyoid is no more than 20 mm below this border. The position of the hyoid bone can also be noted cephalometrically as discussed later in this chapter. When the hyoid bone is located more anterior and/or inferior than the norm, isolated soft-tissue cosmetic procedures in the neck will have limited results.

Profile analysis

The sequential analysis of the upper, middle, and lower third face in profile is next carried out and abnormal findings are recorded.

PROFILE ESTHETICS

Upper third face

Frontal bossing_____

Supraorbital rim projection (5–10 mm)_____ mm

Glabellar angle: Excessive   –   Normal   –   Deficient

UPPER THIRD FACE

The forehead is normally shaped such that it has an anterior slope from superior to inferior with an accentuation or projection of the supraorbital rims. As with all periorbital structures, the projection of the supraorbital rims are primarily evaluated as they relate to the globes. Normally the supraorbital rims will project 5 to 10 mm beyond the most anterior projection of the globe. When variations in the shape of the forehead and position of the supraorbital rims exist, the distinction is made between frontal bossing and supraorbital hypoplasia. Frontal bossing exists when the projection of the supraorbital rims is normal and a reverse slope of the forehead is present. Supraorbital rim hypoplasia exists when the supraorbital rims do not project adequately in relation to the globes.

The glabellar angle is next evaluated. This is the angle formed by the intersection of the lines glabella–nasion and nasion–pronasale (Fig. 1-10). Normally this angle is 132 ± 15 degrees. This angle may be judged as excessive, normal, or deficient. An excessive glabellar angle implies frontal bossing and/or a depressed nasal dorsum. A deficient glabellar angle implies the converse.

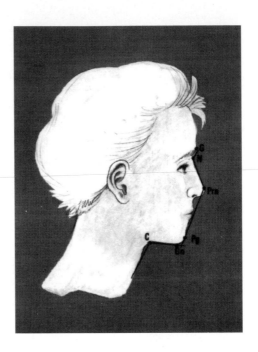

FIG. 1-10

MIDDLE THIRD FACE

NOSE. Profile examination of the middle third face begins with a general assessment of the nose. The nasal bridge projects 5 to 8 mm anteriorly to the globes. The nasal dorsum is described as normal, convex, or concave in appearance. The appearance of the nasal tip is evaluated for both the presence or absence of a supratip break and the direction of nasal tip rotation, either turned up or down. Differentiation is made between a dorsal hump and a downturned nasal tip because, while these two conditions are similar in appearance on casual examination, their implications for treatment are different.

The skeletal nasal base furnishes support to the alar base of the nose. The ratio of the linear distance in the horizontal plane from the nasal tip (Prn) to subnasale (Sn) and from subnasale to the alar base crease (Ac) is normally 2:1 (Fig. 1-11). Values approaching 1:1 are suggestive of lack of nasoskeletal support for the alar base and imply maxillary and/or middle third face deficiencies.

The nasolabial angle is now assessed; it is normally between 90 and 110 degrees. This angle is often defined as that formed between imaginary lines tangent to the columella (C) and the upper lip vermilion (Ls) and intersecting at subnasale (Sn) (Fig. 1-12). When this angle is abnormal, care must be used to distinguish between an upper lip posture problem and an abnormal columella angula-

PROFILE ESTHETICS

Middle third face
Nose

Nasal bridge projection (5–8 mm) _____ mm
Dorsum prominence:	Convex	–	Straight	–	Concave
Supratip break:	Absent	–	Normal	–	Excessive
Nasal tip:	Upturned	–	Normal	–	Downturned
Collumella:	Angled upward	–	Horizontal	–	Angled downward

Tip to subnasale:subnasale to alar base (2:1) _____
Nasolabial angle (90–110 degrees) _____ degrees

Eyes

Lateral orbital rim projection (− 12 to − 8 mm) _____ mm
Infraorbital rim projection (0 to 2 mm) _____ mm

Cheeks

Malar prominence:	Convex	–	Flat	–	Concave
Infraorbital prominence:	Convex	–	Flat	–	Concave
Paranasal prominence:	Convex	–	Flat	–	Concave

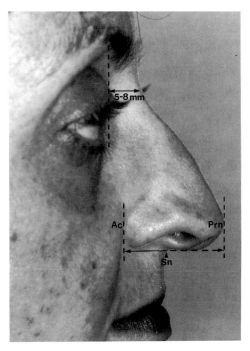

FIG. 1-11

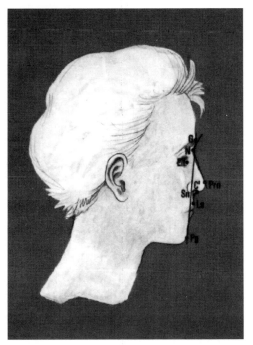

FIG. 1-12

tion. For this reason it is best also to use the relations of the upper lip to the subnasale perpendicular as a guide in determining protrusion or retrusion of the upper lip and dentition. (See lower third face evaluation of the lips and the following part of this chapter on cephalometric evaluation.) Appendix II and its associated illustration presents more specific parameters for nasal esthetics that are useful when a rhinoplasty is specifically planned as part of the orthognathic surgery.

EYES. The skeletal rim of the eye is examined in profile relative to the most anterior projection of the globe. The lateral orbital rims normally lie 8 to 12 mm behind the most anterior projection of the globe while the infraorbital rim is normally 0 to 2 mm anterior to the globe. Values greater than these in the posterior direction are indicative of midface deficiency. When significant esthetic abnormalities exist in the periorbital area, Appendix I and its accompanying illustration can help provide a more detailed evaluation of this area.

CHEEKS. The esthetic unit known as the cheek is composed of three basic subunits: malar prominence, infraorbital prominence, and paranasal prominence. The malar prominence is normally a distinct convexity located 15 mm directly inferior to the lateral canthus of the eye. If abnormal it is judged as being either flat or concave.

The infraorbital prominence is that part of the cheek located on a line directly below the pupil of the eye at the horizontal level of the infraorbital rim. The infraorbital prominence is normally flat to convex.

The paranasal prominence is normally convex. Flat to concave appearance is suggestive of maxillary and/or midface deficiency. Importantly, when the paranasal areas are viewed, an abnormal chin projection that may produce an optical illusion or actually influence the soft-tissue drape in this area must be disregarded. The patient with mandibular prognathism who is "overclosed" will appear to be concave in this area. When the patient is "overclosed," these areas are best evaluated with the mandible in rest position to eliminate these soft-tissue posturing effects.

LOWER THIRD FACE

Sequential observation in the lower third face includes the lips, labiomental fold, and chin projection.

LIPS. The protrusion or retrusion of the upper lip is described as it relates to subnasale perpendicular, an imaginary line through subnasale and perpendicular

PROFILE ESTHETICS

Lower third face
Lips

Upper (protrusive–normal–retrusive) relative to subnasale perpendicular
Lower (protrusive–normal–retrusive) relative to the upper lip

| *Labiomental fold:* | Deficient | – | Excessive |
| *Chin projection:* | Retrusive | – | Protrusive |

Submental and neck area
Mandibular angles

| Right: | Well defined | – | Average | – | Poorly defined |
| Left: | Well defined | – | Average | – | Poorly defined |

Neck-chin angle (110 degrees) _____ degrees
Neck-chin length (50 mm) _____ mm

---

to the Frankfort horizontal. The most prominent portion of the vermilion of the upper lip should lie not more than 2 mm ahead or behind subnasale perpendicular. Ideally, the upper lip vermilion should just touch this line. Normally the upper lip projects slightly (2 mm) anterior to the lower lip in repose. Protrusion or retrusion of each lip is independently noted because this relates to the underlying dental support.

LABIOMENTAL FOLD. A discernible labiomental fold gives definition to the lower half of the lower third face. The lack of a noticeable labiomental fold or an excessively deep fold detracts from this pleasant definition.

CHIN PROJECTION. Chin projection is primarily related to the nose and subnasale perpendicular in the middle third face and the lips in the lower third face. Numerically its most prominent aspect should lie 2 to 6 mm behind an imaginary subnasale perpendicular line assuming normal nasal and maxillarly prominence. Importantly, the chin projection must be related to the entire profile to determine if it is adequately balanced with the forehead, cheeks, paranasal areas, and neck.

SUBMENTAL AND NECK AREA. The submental and neck area esthetic exam can be subdivided into three areas: mandibular angle definition, neck-chin angle, and neck-chin length.

The mandibular angle in profile is normally well defined, with a subtle but definite submandibular depression inferior to the inferior border component of the mandibular angle. The posterior border of the mandibular angle should also be easily identified and generally is most easily detected inferior to the ear lobe extending down to the inferior border of the mandible. Skin laxity, cervical facial lipomatosis, parotid hypertrophy, and an excessively high mandibular plane angle will all obscure the outline of the mandibular angles.

The neck-chin area normally exhibits an obtuse angle (110 degrees), and the distance from pogonion to the neck-chin angle is about 50 mm (Fig. 1-13). The

FIG. 1-13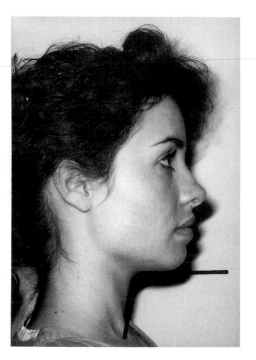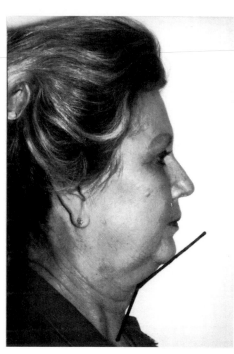

presence of these relations give definition to the chin and submental area. The excessively obtuse neck-chin angle or deficient neck-chin length decreases this definition. The same factors that predictably obscure the mandibular angle also unfavorably affect the definition of the neck-chin angle.

Cephalometric evaluation

Cephalometry is an excellent tool for quantifying classifying, and communicating patient data. It is useful as a treatment planning tool through the construction of prediction tracings to study profile changes and to allow the planning of both extractions and orthodontic mechanics to meet specific treatment objectives. It is critical in monitoring progress during treatment and in studying changes specifically produced by treatment. *Cephalometric evaluation is not the primary diagnostic device to determine surgical treatment.* The primary objective of treatment is to make the facial appearance more normal, *not* to make the patient's cephalometric measurements "normal." While in most instances improving the facial appearance makes the cephalometric measurements *more* normal, in some instances this may not be true.

It is recommended that cephalometric radiographs be taken with the teeth in centric occlusion and the lips in repose. This centric occlusion radiograph is obtained for all patients. A second cephalometric radiograph is made: (1) to document centric relation, when there is a clinically significant difference between centric occlusion and centric relation, and (2) to study the freeway space, permit assessment of the upper tooth to lip relations, and study the "true" relations of the maxilla and mandible to one another. This lateral rest position cephalometric radiograph is discussed in greater detail later in this chapter.

Posteroanterior cephalometric radiographs are most helpful in patients with soft tissue and/or skeletal facial asymmetries and in select individuals with vertical maxillary excess. Such radiographs are best enhanced with barium markers to better define soft-tissue contours. The indications and use of posteroanterior cephalometric radiographs are presented later in this chapter.

Standard lateral cephalometric radiographs

The following cephalometric analysis is a compilation of measurements from a number of different analyses and contains relationships that have been found to be most clinically useful in developing a treatment plan. It is divided into soft-tissue relations, skeletal relations, and dental relations for ease of presentation and understanding.

Soft-tissue relations

The first requirement for the cephalometric study of soft-tissue relations is that the radiograph be taken with the lips in repose. Measurements taken from a radiograph made with the lips tightly pulled together will mask true soft-tissue–skeletal–dental relations, especially in vertical excess conditions. A soft-tissue screen is used to allow easy visualization of the soft tissues. The radiograph cassette is placed as low as possible to include the neck-chin area and far enough forward to include the entire nose. In this analysis the Frankfort horizontal plane is determined by using anatomic porion, not mechanical porion (cephalostat ear rod). Mechanical porion is highly variable, whereas anatomic porion—the most superior aspect of the *bony* external auditory canal—is highly reproducible.

VERTICAL RELATIONS (MEASURED PERPENDICULAR TO FRANKFORT HORIZONTAL PLANE)

MIDDLE THIRD FACE HEIGHT: LOWER THIRD FACE HEIGHT (G-SN:SN-ME)

The ratio of the distance from glabella to subnasale and from subnasale to soft-tissue menton (Fig. 1-14, *A* and *B*). The actual numerical values for these relations vary greatly with age, sex, and race. However, in Caucasians the ratio of middle to lower third face is about equal.

Clinical norm: 1:1

Interpretation: These values are approximately equal when good facial balance exists. Major imbalances must be noted and are best interpreted as either deficient or excessive after the subsequent parameters are recorded.

UPPER LIP LENGTH (SN-ST)

The length of the upper lip from subnasale to stomion (Fig. 1-14, *C*). The lowest point of the upper lip in the midline is defined as stomion.

Clinical norm: Males 22 ± 2 mm

Females 20 ± 2 mm.

Interpretation: Excesses and deficiencies can exist in the length of the upper lip. To make the definitive diagnosis of either a short or long upper lip, such diagnosis must be made relative to the remainder of the vertical facial dimensions.

SUBNASALE-STOMION:STOMION MENTON (SN-ST:ST-ME)

The ratio of the distance from subnasale to upper lip stomion compared to the distance from upper lip stomion to soft-tissue menton (Fig. 1-14, *C* and *D*).

Clinical norm: 1:2

Interpretation: This measurement assesses one of the important vertical relationships in the lower third of the face. This ratio is 1:2 when good balance exists. Increases in the upper portion of this ratio (Sn-St) are most often indicative of a short lower two-thirds of the lower face or, rarely, a long upper lip. A ratio approaching 1:1 is often a good indication for a rest-position lateral cephalometric radiograph. Increases in the lower portion of this ratio (St-Me) are most often indicative of vertical maxillary excess or, rarely, a short upper lip.

SUBNASALE-LOWER LIP VERMILION: LOWER LIP VERMILION-MENTON (SN-LLV:LLV-ME)

The ratio of the distance from subnasale to the mucocutaneous junction of the lower lip compared to the distance and from that point to soft-tissue menton (Fig. 1-14, *E* and *F*).

Clinical norm: 1:0.9

Interpretation: Increases in the upper portion of this ratio (Sn-LLV) are generally indicative of vertical maxillary excess or eversion of the lower lip due to ei-

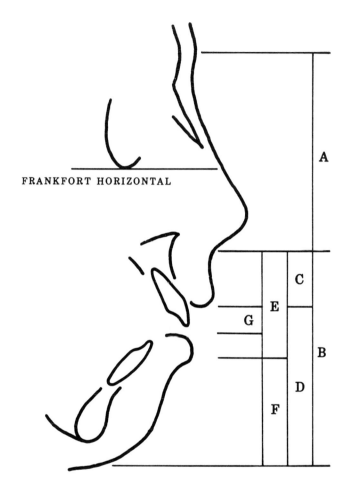

FRANKFORT HORIZONTAL

FIG. 1-14

ther poor lower lip support or posture. Increases in the lower portion of this ratio (LLV-Me) are indicative of a vertically excessive chin or vertical maxillary deficiency.

INTERLABIAL DISTANCE

The distance between the upper lip stomion and the lower lip stomion with the lips in repose (Fig. 1-14, *G*).

Clinical norm: 0 to 3 mm

Interpretation: Excessive interlabial distance indicates lip incompetence—the inability to close the lips without hyperfunction of the perioral musculature.

HORIZONTAL RELATIONS (MEASURED PARALLEL TO FRANKFORT HORIZONTAL PLANE)

The first step before making these horizontal measurements is to construct a reference line called the subnasale perpendicular. This is done by passing a line through subnasale and perpendicular to the *anatomic Frankfort horizontal plane.*

SUBNASALE PERPENDICULAR TO UPPER LIP

The horizontal distance from subnasale perpendicular to the most anterior portion of the upper lip vermilion (Fig. 1-15, *A*).

Clinical norm: 0 ± 2 mm

Interpretation: This is a measurement of the relative prominence of the upper lip. When the lip lies anterior to this line, the lip support is excessive. When the lip lies posterior to this line, upper lip support is insufficient.

SUBNASALE PERPENDICULAR TO LOWER LIP

The horizontal distance from the subnasale perpendicular to the most anterior projection of the lower lip vermilion (Fig. 1-15, *B*).

Clinical norm: -2 ± 2

Interpretation: A measurement of the relative prominence of the lower lip. Increased negative values indicate recession of the lower lip and positive values indicate protrusion of the lower lip.

SUBNASALE PERPENDICULAR TO CHIN

The horizontal distance from subnasale perpendicular to the soft tissue chin at the level of pogonion (Fig. 1-15, *C*).

Clinical norm: -4 ± 2 mm

Interpretation: A measurement of the relative prominence of the soft-tissue chin. This value, in conjunction with the preceding values, permits decisions to be made regarding the profile esthetic balance between the lips and chin.

Skeletal relations

There are literally hundreds of measurements that have been proposed to evaluate the facial skeletal relations. Indeed, some clinicians are unable to extract meaningful information due to the sheer volume of such data, while others use one or two angular values that may have little clinical relevance. The six skeletal measurements illustrated herein have been chosen because, when used together, they become a powerful analysis that allows the clinician to assess the features that are clinically meaningful and necessary in a skeletal analysis. The objectives of the skeletal analysis are (1) to locate the chin in space both vertically and anteroposteriorly (facial axis, facial depth, and mandibular plane), (2) to locate the maxilla anteroposteriorly (convexity and maxillary depth), and (3) to relate the effective length of the maxilla to the mandible (maxillary length:mandibular length). Integration of these skeletal parameters is essential in making meaning-

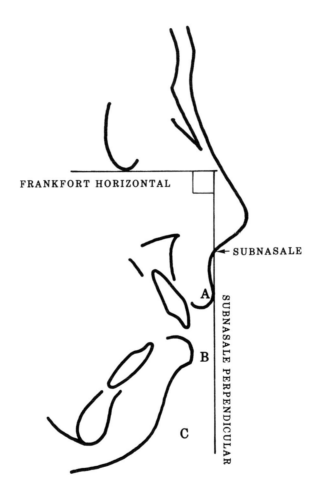

FRANKFORT HORIZONTAL

SUBNASALE

SUBNASALE PERPENDICULAR

A

B

C

FIG. 1-15

ful treatment decisions. Isolated use of one or two is fraught with a high probability of error and indeed is probably meaningless. Additional measurements may
be of value in specific deformities and are discussed with the deformity to which
they apply.

FACIAL AXIS ANGLE

The posteroinferior angle formed by the intersection of the basion-nasion
line and the facial axis (a line from the most posterosuperior point to the ptery-
gomaxillary fissure to gnathion) (Fig. 1-16, *A*).

Clinical norm: 90 ± 3 degrees

Interpretation: This measurement indicates the direction of growth of the
chin and the maxillary first molars. A small value is indicative of a recessive chin
or a vertically long face. A large value indicates a prominent chin or a vertically
short face.

FACIAL DEPTH ANGLE

The posteroinferior angle formed by the intersection of the anatomic
Frankfort horizontal plane and the facial plane (Na-Po) (Fig. 1-16, *B*).

Clinical norm: 87 ± 3 degrees at age 9 years
                 (increases 1 degree every 3 years)
                 89 ± 3 degrees in adult females
                 90 ± 3 degrees in adult males

Interpretation: This measurement defines the anteroposterior position of the
bony chin. Small values indicate a recessive chin, and large values indicate a
prominent chin.

MANDIBULAR PLANE ANGLE

The anteroinferior angle between the anatomic Frankfort horizontal plane
and the mandibular plane (a line tangent to the symphysis and the gonial portion
of the mandible) (Fig. 1-16, *C*).

Clinical norm: 26 ± 4 degrees at age 9
                 (decreases 1 degree every 3 years)
                 24 ± 4 degrees in adults

Interpretation: This angle relates the posterior facial height to the anterior facial height, thus expressing the vertical relation of the mandible. Patients with
high angles tend to have weak masticatory musculature, vertical excesses, and
open bites. Patients with low angles tend to have strong musculature, vertical deficiencies, and deep bites.

A. FACIAL AXIS ANGLE

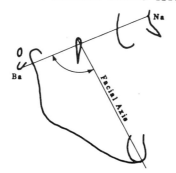

B. FACIAL DEPTH

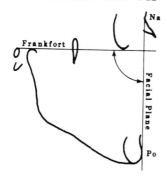

C. MANDIBULAR PLANE ANGLE

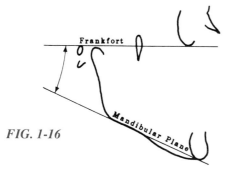

FIG. 1-16

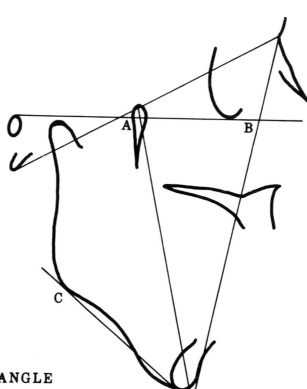

MAXILLARY DEPTH ANGLE

The posteroinferior angle formed by the intersection of the anatomic Frankfort horizontal plane and a line from nasion to point A (Na-A) (Fig. 1-17, *A*).

Clinical norm: 90 ± 3 degrees
                     Constant with age

Interpretation: Indicates the anteroposterior position of the maxilla. Used to help determine if a Class II or Class III problem is caused by the position of the maxilla. In true midface deformities in which nasion is recessive, this value will not reflect the true degree of retrusion of the maxilla.

FACIAL CONVEXITY

The distance between point A and the facial plane (Na-Po) (Fig. 1-17, *B*).

Clinical norm: 1 ± 2 mm

Interpretation: Values greater than 3 mm indicate a Class II skeletal pattern. Values less than −2 mm indicate a Class III skeletal pattern. This measurement does not indicate which jaw is primarily responsible for the anteroposterior discrepancy but simply indicates how the maxilla and mandible *relate to each other in space*.

MAXILLARY LENGTH:MANDIBULAR LENGTH

A ratio of the distance from condylion to point A and from condylion to gnathion (Co-A:Co-Gn) (Fig. 1-17, *C*).

Clinical norm: 1:1.3

Interpretation: This ratio is used to assess the relative length of each jaw independent of any vertical discrepancy that might be present. The ratio does not determine which jaw is incorrect, only that a discrepancy in length does or does not exist.

A. MAXILLARY DEPTH

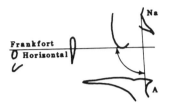

B. CONVEXITY

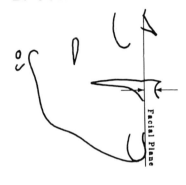

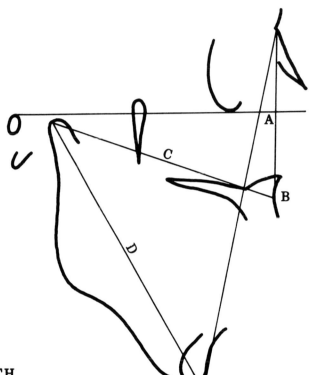

C. MAXILLARY and
D. MANDIBULAR LENGTH

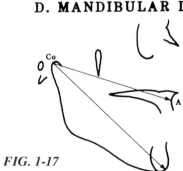

FIG. 1-17

Dental Relations

Once again, many possible measurements have been described. The four that follow are the most clinically meaningful. Those that are most accurately determined from analysis of the dental models have been eliminated from the cephalometric analysis (i.e., class of malocclusion, overbite, overjet, etc.) and are recorded as part of the occlusal analysis.

UPPER MOLAR POSITION

The horizontal distance from pterygoid vertical to the distal surface of the upper first molar (Fig. 1-18, *A*)

Clinical norm: (Age of the patient in years +3) $\pm$ 3 mm
Adult female 18 $\pm$ 3 mm
Adult male 21 $\pm$ 3 mm

Interpretation: Helps to determine if the malocclusion is caused by the position of the upper molar. May aid in decisions about headgear, extractions, and maxillary position. Small values indicate that the molar is too far distal and may also be indicative of a posteriorly placed maxilla. Thus, headgear or other methods of distalizing molars should be avoided in such a patient. Large values tend to indicate the opposite. This value may be misleading when maxillary teeth have been extracted, especially when such was done for orthodontic reasons.

LOWER INCISOR PROTRUSION

The distance from the tip of the most prominent lower incisor to the A-pogonion (A-Po) line measured perpendicular to the A-Po line (Fig. 1-18, *B*).

Clinical norm: 1 $\pm$ 2 mm

Interpretation: Defines the protrusion of the lower arch and the position of the dentition between the jaws, a key esthetic and functional objective.

LOWER INCISOR INCLINATION

The angle between the long axis of the most prominent lower incisor and the A-Po line (Fig. 1-18, *C*).

Clinical norm: 22 $\pm$ 4 degrees

Interpretation: Indicates the amount of tipping involved in producing the observed anteroposterior position of the lower incisors.

INTERINCISAL ANGLE

The angle formed by the long axis of the most prominent upper and lower central incisors (Fig. 1-18, *D*).

Clinical norm: 130 $\pm$ 6 degrees

Interpretation: Low angles indicate protrusion of the incisors. High angles are most frequently associated with Class II division II deep bites.

A. UPPER MOLAR POSITION

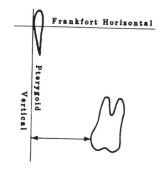

B. LOWER INCISOR
PROTRUSION

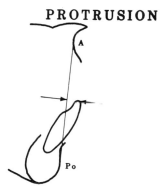

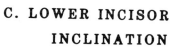

C. LOWER INCISOR
INCLINATION

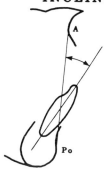

FIG. 1-18

D. INTERINCISAL ANGLE

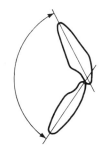

When a majority of these cephalometric relationships are illustrated together, the result appears as shown in Fig. 1-19. Maxillary depth is shown in the position of its reciprocal angle for ease of illustration. Measurements not included because of space limitations are (1) upper lip and lower lip to subnasale perpendicular and (2) lower incisor and interincisal angulation.

This format has been adopted as the standard cephalometric representation for this book. The reader is encouraged to become familiar with it. The form on page 41 is used to record the cephalometric measurements.

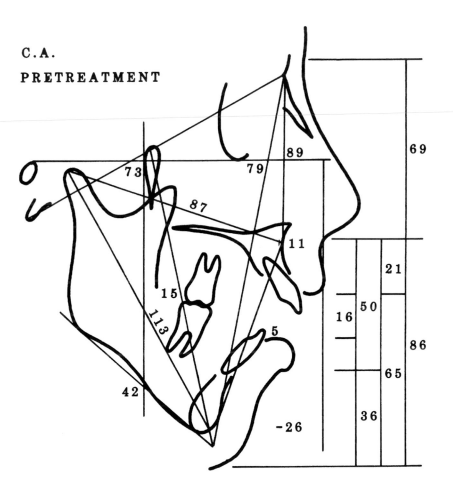

FIG. 1-19

CEPHALOMETRIC EVALUATION FORM

Soft-tissue relations

	Normal	Patient
Vertical		
G-Sn:Sn-Me	1:1	_____
Upper lip length (Sn-St)	20 ± 2 mm	_____
Sn-St:St-Me	1:2	_____
Sn-LLV:LLV-Me	1:0.9	_____
Interlabial distance	0 to 3 mm	_____
Horizontal		
Subnasale perpendicular to:		
Upper lip	0 ± 2mm	_____
Lower lip	−2 ± 2 mm	_____
Chin	−4 ± 2 mm	_____
Skeletal relations		
Facial axis angle	90 ± 3 degrees	_____
Facial depth angle	89 ± 3 degrees	_____
Mandibular plane angle	24 ± 3 degrees	_____
Maxillary depth angle	90 ± 3 degrees	_____
Convexity	1 ± 2 mm	_____
Maxillary length:mandibular length	1:1.3	_____
Dental relations		
Upper molar to PTV Male	21 ± 3 mm	_____
Female	18 ± 3 mm	_____
Lower incisor to A-Po	1 ± 2 mm	_____
	22 ± 4 degrees	_____
Interincisal angle	130 ± 6 degrees	_____

Panoramic or full-mouth periapical radiographic evaluations

A panoramic radiograph is evaluated for overt sinus, intranasal (septum and turbinates), bony, temporomandibular joint, periapical, periodontal and dental pathology. If any of the latter three are suspected, appropriate periapical or bite-wing radiographs are indicated. The existence of sinus or temporomandibular joint disease must be pursued with additional appropriate studies as discussed later in this chapter in the section on "Adjunctive Evaluations." It is generally preferable not to make a definitive diagnosis of general dental problems or perio-dontal disease when such problems are suspected as a result of the panoramic radiographic examination, but to refer patients to their general dentist. If periodontal disease exists, consultation with a periodontist is indicated, preferably on referral from the patient's general dentist. The form below may be used to record the findings from the panoramic radiographic evaluation.

RADIOGRAPHIC EVALUATION

Maxillary sinus pathology   Right   Left

Describe: _____

Bony pathology

Mandible: _____

Maxilla: _____

Nasal septum: _____

Temporomandibular joint pathology   Right   Left

Describe: _____

Impacted teeth numbers: _____

PERIAPICAL PATHOLOGY:

(R) 8 7 6 5 4 3 2 1 | 1 2 3 4 5 6 7 8 (L)

8 7 6 5 4 3 2 1 | 1 2 3 4 5 6 7 8

PERIODONTAL PATHOLOGY:

(R) 8 7 6 5 4 3 2 1 | 1 2 3 4 5 6 7 8 (L)

8 7 6 5 4 3 2 1 | 1 2 3 4 5 6 7 8

DENTAL CARIES:

(R) 8 7 6 5 4 3 2 1 | 1 2 3 4 5 6 7 8 (L)

8 7 6 5 4 3 2 1 | 1 2 3 4 5 6 7 8

Miscellaneous: _____

Occlusal evaluation

There are two phases of the occlusal evaluation: functional and static. The former is completed by evaluation of the patient, the latter by analysis of the dental models. The results of this evaluation are recorded on the occlusal evaluation form that appears later in this chapter.

Functional evaluation

The functional evaluation is done to determine the compatibility between centric occlusion (CO) and centric relation (CR) and to assess tooth wear. Since many Class II and asymmetric individuals have "habitual occlusions," the compatibility between CO and CR must be carefully evaluated. This can often be best done with a leaf gauge. Failure to appreciate meaningful inconsistency in CO and CR may result in significant errors in both treatment planning and in surgery. In addition, tooth attrition is assessed as being absent (0) to severe (5). Severe indicates exposure of the dentin and suggests either severely disturbed masticatory function or significant parafunctional habits, both of which may affect postoperative skeletal stability.

Static evaluation

The static evaluation is performed on anatomically oriented models and is begun by doing an intraarch analysis, followed by interarch analysis and a tooth mass evaluation.

INTRAARCH RELATIONS

The intraarch analysis is done for both the maxillary and mandibular arches. The midline of the arch relative to the skeleton and soft tissues of the face must be noted. Arch form, symmetry, undererupted, supraerupted, and missing teeth are noted. Any anomalies of the occlusal plane—steep angle, flat angle, canted—are noted and recorded, and the curve of Spee is studied. Finally, the amount of crowding is measured to aid in determining the need for extractions.

INTERARCH RELATIONS

Interarch relations are the arch relations that exist in all three planes of space. Anteroposteriorly, the angle classification is observed for both molar and canine, and the incisor overjet is examined. The incisor overbite is noted in addition to any vertical dysplasia in the buccal segments. Transverse relations, including coordination of upper and lower midlines and buccal or lingual crossbites, are evaluated. When a Class II or III malocclusion exists, it is important to note the existing transverse relations when the models are held together in a Class I occlussal relation. This is indicative of the true nature of any transverse abnormality. If there exists a transverse discrepancy of the teeth, it is important to note if this is the result of abnormally shaped (pegged laterals, over or undersized premolar and/ or molars) teeth, or due to an actual skeletal discrepancy, as these two problems have very different treatment implications.

TOOTH MASS RELATION

The evaluation of tooth mass is critical, since many patients exhibit discrepancies of such a magnitude that they must be taken into consideration to achieve a good occlusion with normal overbite-overjet relations. The use of Bolton's analysis is not recommended as the primary method of assessing tooth mass relations because of its potential for inaccuracy. The use of occlusograms or carefully done occlusal plaster and wax setups are more reliable. This topic is covered in detail in Chapter 2.

OCCLUSAL EVALUATION FORM

Functional evaluation

CO-CR: *Compatible*   *Incompatible*   *Describe:* _____

_____

Tooth attrition

Posterior Teeth

UR 0   1   2   3   4   5   UL 0   1   2   3   4   5
LR 0   1   2   3   4   5   LL 0   1   2   3   4   5

Anterior teeth

U   0   1   2   3   4   5   L   0   1   2   3   4   5

Static evaluation

Intraarch relations

Midline to face: Upper   R   L   _____ mm

                            Lower   R   L   _____ mm

Arch form: Upper _____   Lower _____

Arch symmetry: Upper _____   Lower _____

Missing teeth   (M)   R   8 7 6 5 4 3 2 1 | 1 2 3 4 5 6 7 8   L
Overerupted teeth (O)   _____
Unerupted teeth   (U)   8 7 6 5 4 3 2 1 | 1 2 3 4 5 6 7 8

Occlusal plane cant: _____

Curve of Spee: Excessive   Reverse

Crowding: Upper _____   Lower _____ mm

Interarch relations

Molar   right: I   II   III   left: I   II   III
Canine   right: I   II   III   left: I   II   III
Overjet: _____ mm

Overbite: _____ mm   Open bite: _____ mm

Upper to lower midline: _____

Crossbite:_____   Where: R 8 7 6 5 4 3 2 1   1 2 3 4 5 6 7 8 9 L

Transverse discrepancy in Class I relation: Molars _____ mm

                                                 Premolars _____ mm

                                                 Canines _____ mm

Tooth mass relation

Relative to the upper tooth mass, the lower tooth mass is:
Normal

Excessive _____ mm

Deficient _____ mm

Masticatory muscle and temporomandibular joint evaluation

It is important diagnostically and prognostically to evaluate and record problems related to the masticatory muscles and the temporomandibular joints. While true temporomandibular joint disease is not common in patients with dentofacial deformities, noting signs or symptoms prior to orthodontic-surgical treatment avoids conflicts regarding whether problems were preexisting or arose during treatment. A basic masticatory muscle and temporomandibular joint examination is done in four parts: (1) masticatory muscles, (2) mandibular movements, (3) temporomandibular joint symptoms, and (4) temporomandibular joint signs. If significant abnormalities are disclosed in this evaluation, it is important that the muscles and joint(s) be further evaluated and an accurate diagnosis made before instituting definitive orthodontic-surgical treatment of the existing dentofacial deformity. It is beyond the scope of this book to discuss the detailed differential diagnosis of temporomandibular joint dysfunctional disorders. The following comments are intended to aid the clinician in making the initial examination and to determine if a more detailed examination is necessary. Some aspects of a more detailed examination of the masticatory muscles and temporomandibular joint are discussed in the second section of this chapter.

Masticatory muscle

The masticatory muscle examination has two primary functions. First, to identify any painful muscles and/or trigger points. Second, to identify the deficient masticatory muscle mass that often exists in patients who have sustained trauma to this area or who have undergone previous orthognathic surgery.

Patients who either report or have clinically apparent pain in the muscles of mastication should have this muscle pain resolved prior to instituting any treatment. Myofascial pain of the masticatory muscles is best resolved using a simple physical therapy protocol that includes: (1) massage perpendicular to the muscle fibers while the mandible is gently opening and closing, (2) warm moist heat, (3) a soft, nonchew diet, and (4) nonsteroidal antiinflammatory agents. The massage should be done for 5 minutes five times a day. This includes massage upon awakening, after each meal, and 30 minutes prior to bedtime. Warm, moist heat is best applied twice daily—in the morning and prior to bedtime—for 20 minutes each time.

This simple protocol will resolve the myofascial pain of the masticatory muscles within 2 weeks in the majority of patients. When the myofascial pain is resolved and the mandibular excursions are normal, orthodontic-surgical correction of the patient's deformity may begin.

Patients who have either undergone previous orthognathic surgery or sustained trauma to the masticatory muscles often exhibit deficient masticatory muscle mass and/or strength. They frequently complain of difficulty eating due to decreased bite force, fatigue, and/or pain on chewing. Masticatory muscle mass is evaluated by palpation of the muscles at rest and during clenching. The clinician can easily discern deficiencies or asymmetries in masticatory muscle mass while palpating bilaterally during clenching. To help increase masticatory muscle mass and strength, an extensive physical therapy regimen is outlined for the patient. This regiment consists of exercising 5 to 10 minutes five times daily in all five extreme jaw excursions—maximum opening, right lateral, left lateral, maximum protrusive, and clenching. Nonsteroidal antiinflammatory agents may be prescribed as needed. Typically, this regimen continues for 2 to 4 weeks or until the patient reports adequate bite force and resolution of fatigue when chewing.

MASTICATORY MUSCLE AND TEMPOROMANDIBULAR JOINT EVALUATION

Masticatory muscles

	Right		Left	
	Rest	**Loading**	**Rest**	**Loading**
Masseter	_____	_____	_____	_____
Medial pterygoid	_____	_____	_____	_____
Temporalis	_____	_____	_____	_____
Digastrics	_____	_____	_____	_____
Sternocleidomastoid	_____	_____	_____	_____
Trapezius	_____	_____	_____	_____

Temporomandibular joint
Mandibular movements

Maximal opening: (50 mm) _____ mm   Deviation: Left _____ mm
                                                      Right _____ mm

Protrusive: (6 mm) _____ mm   Deviation: Left _____ mm
                                                      Right _____ mm

Excursive: (6 mm each)   Left _____ mm
                         Right _____ mm

Temporomandibular joint symptoms (pain)

Rest: Left _____
            Right _____
Movement: Left _____
            Right _____
Loading: Left _____
            Right: _____

Temporomandibular joint signs

Popping: Left   less than 10 mm   _____
                   10 to 20 mm   _____
                   greater than 20 mm   _____
            Right less than 10 mm   _____
                   10 to 20 mm   _____
                   greater than 20 mm   _____
            Functional or Anatomic
Crepitation: Left _____
             Right _____

Mandibular movements

Maximal interincisal opening, protrusive, and excursive movements are recorded in this evaluation. The normal interincisal opening is about 50 mm; minimum normal protrusive and excursive movements are approximately 6 mm. If deviations of greater than 2 to 4 mm occur during opening, they are noted and recorded. If opening is reduced or deviations exist, it is important to determine if this is caused by true temporomandibular joint abnormalities or masticatory muscle problems. This can often be simply accomplished by asking the patient to touch the specific area(s) of soreness or tightness that prevent(s) normal execution of these movements. *Far too often masticatory muscle pain or spasm is called temporomandibular joint dysfunction.* If muscle dysfunction exists, it can generally be eliminated by standard means (rest, heat, nonsteroidal analgesics). The patient's jaw movement is then reevaluated after all influences of muscle dysfunction have been eliminated.

Temporomandibular joint symptoms

Symptoms attributed to the temporomandibular joint include pain specifically localized in the preauricular and external auditory canal areas, as reported by the patient. When true temporomandibular joint pain exists, it is almost always accentuated by movement and by loading of the joint. Joint loading is achieved during this examination by having the patient bite hard on a tongue blade sequentially placed in one canine area, then the other, and finally between the incisors. Biting on the left canines will load the right joint; thus, biting on the left canines will accentuate pain in the right joint and vice versa. When the patient bites hard on the incisors, both joints are loaded. If the patient reports increased pain on the side on which he/she is biting, this response is almost pathognomonic for muscle or dental pain.

Temporomandibular joint signs

A large percentage (30% to 80%) of the total adult population who are asymptomatic have popping and/or clicking of one or both of their temporomandibular joints on auscultation with a stethoscope. The clinical significance of this is not agreed on in the absence of symptoms and limited mandibular movement. However, it is important to record if this occurs during the normal functional range of mandibular motion or only on extreme opening. Moreover, it is important to note that most patients who have early popping (before 20 mm of interincisal opening) exhibit an associated premature protrusive movement of the condyle(s) as the pop occurs. In these instances the question is whether the noise is secondary to an underlying muscle dysfunction or caused by a true anatomic internal derangement. This question can often be answered by having the patient undergo 2 to 4 weeks of specified jaw physiotherapy. This is done by demonstrating normal jaw movement to the patient and by instructing the patient to exercise for 10 minutes, five times a day, in front of a mirror in an attempt to eliminate the premature protrusive movement. The patient is instructed to open maximally and close while viewing themselves in a mirror. They are told to try to open symmetrically, without deviation or premature protrusive movements. When this regime is followed, the majority of patients (75% to 80%) readily eliminate the popping and any associated symptoms.

These patients have a functional pop and do not generally require other methods of treatment. Those who are not "cured" by this regimen may have a true anatomic internal derangement and may require surgical or other forms of treatment. The individual with an opening or closing lock with or without joint noise generally has a true anatomic internal derangement, and additional evaluations are indicated, as discussed later in this chapter.

Crepitation is very uncommon in asymptomatic joints and may be an early sign of true degenerative joint disease. When crepitation exists, it is best to obtain laminograms of the joints to evaluate them better for the presence of early degenerative joint disease.

Predicated on the findings in this examination, when possible or probable organic temporomandibular joint pathology exists—significant hypomobility, deviation on opening, locking, pain localized to the temporomandibular joint(s)—further detailed temporomandibular joint studies are indicated. Importantly, *the clinician must not confuse myofascial pain dysfunction with true temporomandibular joint problems.*

ADJUNCTIVE EVALUATIONS

A number of patients seeking consultation for correction of their facial deformity benefit from additional evaluation to ascertain more completely the true nature of their deformity or to plan better for treatment. The following is a list of adjunctive evaluations that have been found to be the most useful.

A. Comprehensive psychologic evaluation
B. Additional photographs
1. Symmetry view
2. Submental view
3. Superior view
4. Three-quarter face views
C. Computer-assisted analysis
1. Video manipulation
2. Three-dimensional CT scan reconstruction
D. Additional radiographs
1. Rest-position lateral cephalometric radiograph
2. Posteroanterior cephalometric radiograph
3. Temporomandibular joint laminograms
4. Sinus series
5. Computed tomographic scans
6. Radionucleotide scans
E. Diagnostic occlusal splint
F. Velopharyngeal evaluation
1. Speech evaluation
2. Nasoendoscopy
G. Tongue evaluation
1. Speech evaluation
2. Radiographic evaluation of tongue posture
3. Clinical evaluation of tongue posture
H. Masticatory muscle evaluation
1. Electromyography and bite force determinations
2. Masseter muscle biopsy

The discussion below covers basic comments regarding when, where, and how these adjunctive evaluations are used. Certainly, other studies may be indicated in select cases.

Comprehensive psychologic evaluation

When the social-psychologic profile of the patient obtained as part of the initial records suggests that the patient is unstable, externally motivated, or deeply affected by the existing deformity, referral to a competent clinical psychologist or psychiatrist is indicated. This is done after discussion with the patient during which he/she is informed that in addition to the standard concerns of surgery, his/her response to the proposed treatment is also a matter of concern. The result of this evaluation can help the clinician determine the advisability of instituting orthodontic-surgical correction of the deformity. These findings may lead to a decision to institute treatment, but only with appropriate support from the psychologist or psychiatrist.

Additional photographs
Symmetry view

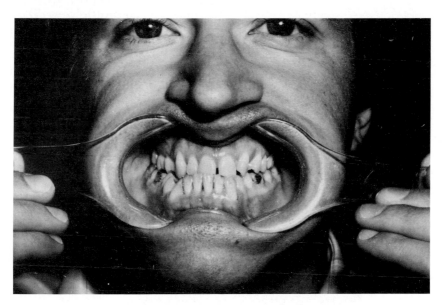

FIG. 1-20

The symmetry view is taken when the patient has an overt facial asymmetry, significant (2 to 3 mm) anterior dental midline asymmetry, or a significant cant of the occlusal plane (Fig. 1-20). It permits assessment and documentation of the relation of the dental midlines to the facial midline and the clinical relevance of any occlusal plane cant. This information is essential in both planning treatment and evaluating treatment results. This photo should be taken with the patient's interpupillar line and Frankfort horizontal parallel to the floor. The clinician may need to place the patients head in the desired position manually since the patients have commonly developed a compensatory head posture to minimize the cosmetic impact of their asymmetry. Photographing the patient with his/her interpupillary line and Frankfort horizontal parallel to the floor objectively illustrates the true direction and magnitude of the asymmetry. In some craniofacial anomalies and in severe hemifacial microsomia the orbital structures may be asymmetric. In such cases photographic records are best taken in natural head position.

Submental view

The submental view is taken with the patient's head hyperextended about 45 degrees. It is useful to assess symmetry and projection of the anterior cranial vault, orbital areas, and cheeks. Nasal deformities are also well documented and studied in this view.

Superior view

The superior view is taken with the patient's head hyperflexed about 45 degrees. Like the submental view, it is useful in assessing anterior cranial vault, orbital, cheek, and nasal deformities. It is often more useful than the submental view for demonstrating and diagnosing cheek deformities.

Three-quarter face views

Three-quarter face views are taken with the patient's head turned midway (45 degrees) between the front face and profile view. The interpupillary line and Frankfort horizontal are parallel to the floor and the head is turned so that the bridge of the nose is tangent to the medial canthus of the eye furthest from the camera (Fig. 1-21). The primary use of this view is to document and diagnose facial anomalies associated with the auricular and preauricular areas, the mandibular angle, the ascending ramus of the mandible, the nose, and the cheeks.

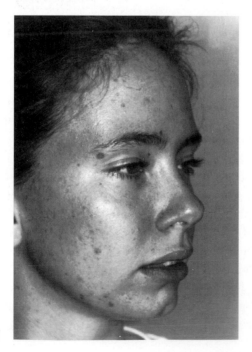 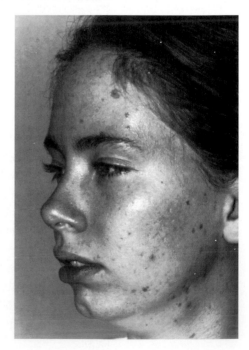

FIG. 1-21

Computer-assisted analysis
Video manipulation

Historically, photographic surgery was used to illustrate the anticipated soft-tissue changes due to proposed orthognathic surgery. This procedure, however, has several shortcomings. First, the lines where the photographs were cut are obvious and distracting. Second, subtle changes in upper lip and subnasale position are poorly represented on photographic cut-out surgery.

A newer and better method of showing the patient the predicted facial outcome of proposed skeletal surgery is computer-assisted video surgery. The equipment required to execute video surgery includes a computer with color monitor, a video camera, a digitizer board, and a software program that includes accurate ratios of soft- to hard-tissue changes for a given skeletal movement.

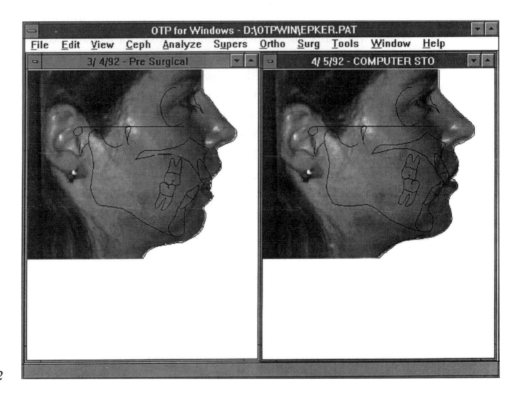

FIG. 1-22

Video surgery uses the technology of computer graphics and a video camera to provide visual treatment objectives and quality case presentation to patients and professional colleagues. It is relatively easy to use and involves three basic steps. Step 1, a lateral cephalogram is placed on a digitizing board and preselected hard- and soft-tissue landmarks are input. Step 2, the patient's video image is transferred to the computer, which subsequently displays it superimposed on and "frozen" to the lateral cephalometric landmarks entered in Step 1. Step 3, skeletal changes simulating the proposed surgery in direction and magnitude are made on the cephalometric tracing. The computer simultaneously appropriately manipulates the displayed video image by using the programmed ratios of soft- to hard-tissue change and displays the "new" profile appearance.

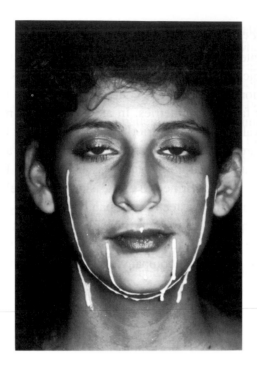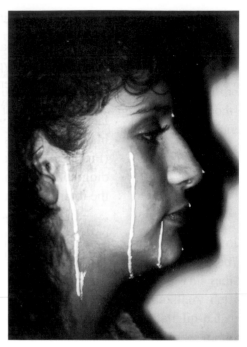

FIG. 1-25

cesses. By manipulating the tracing of these films, the clinician can make a "pre-diction tracing" (Section VII) to achieve more predictable results from both skeletal straightening and soft-tissue augmentation.

Before taking the PA cephalometric radiograph for an asymmetric patient, three parallel lines are placed on the patient's face with a barium cream as follows (Fig. 1-25):

1. A vertical line 1 cm anterior to the tragus, starting at Frankfort horizontal, and continuing inferiorly, perpendicular to Frankfort, to the level of the thyroid prominence.
2. A vertical line below the lateral canthus of the eye, starting at Frankfort horizontal and continuing inferiorly perpendicular to Frankfort. This second line continues around the submental region to join its counterpart from the opposite side.
3. A vertical line starting at the lip commissure, extending inferiorly parallel to the other lines, and continuing around the chin to the contralateral lip commissure.

These three parallel lines help determine the relative medial lateral symmetry of the soft tissues overlying the ramus, maxilla and mandibular body, and symphysis, respectively.

Three midline points are likewise marked with barium cream or nipple markers as follows (Fig. 1-25):

1. Glabella.
2. Tip of nose, as nose is viewed as an independent esthetic unit. This is best done by visually blocking out the surrounding soft tissues and placing a barium dot on the anatomic central tip of the nose.
3. Center of chin button as an independent esthetic unit.

Patients with facial asymmetries often have developed a compensatory head posture to offset the visual impact of their asymmetry. They may be so unconsciously skilled at this, that an unaware clinician could overlook asymmetries of various facial esthetic units. Thus, it is important to position these patients so that their Frankfort horizontal and interpupillary lines are parallel to the floor when placing the aforementioned barium lines and markers.

When a PA cephalometric radiograph is to be obtained with barium markers, the lateral cephalometric radiograph is likewise obtained with the barium markers (Fig. 1-26). This allows visualization of the location of the barium markers in the anteroposterior dimension and permits objective evaluation of the symmetry of placement of the barium line markers. Ideally, the barium lines appear as only three lines on the lateral cephalometric radiograph as the contralateral markers are superimposed. This seldom occurs, but the lines should approximate one another within a few millimeters. In procuring the films, it is suggested that the lateral film be made first. If the barium lines are seen to be sufficiently different as to be misleading, they are moved as necessary to produce a more accurate representation.

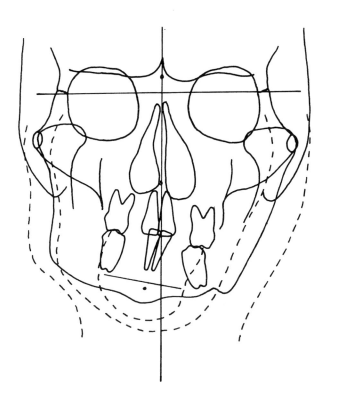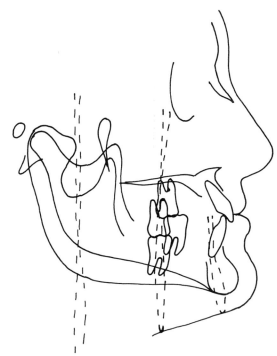

FIG. 1-26

Velopharyngeal evaluation

Speech examination

Recognition of the specific nature of speech abnormalities, especially velopharyngeal insufficiency (VPI), is difficult for the untrained ear. When the patient has speech difficulties, or when maxillary advancement surgery is planned for the patient with a secondary cleft dentofacial deformity, a speech evaluation is generally indicated. Although a consensus may not exist as to the optimal means of evaluating VPI, a clinical speech evaluation by a competent speech pathologist is generally indicated. On referral, it is important to request evaluation specifically of velopharyngeal function relative to its adequacy. If it is inadequate, it will usually require physical management in the form of a pharyngeal flap. In this instance maxillary advancement surgery can be done without being concerned that it will create the need for unnecessary additional surgery, since a pharyngeal flap is already indicated. If it is adequate, any benefits accrued from total maxillary surgery must be weighed against the fact that such surgery may worsen speech and require pharyngeal flap surgery. When maxillary advancement surgery is apt to result in the need for secondary corrective VPI surgery, this must be discussed with the patient (or parent). In either instance, nasoendoscopy is necessary to evaluate the velopharyngeal mechanism objectively and to provide important information to help with decisions regarding velopharyngeal function.

Nasoendoscopy

Nasoendoscopy is an excellent adjunct to speech evaluation, especially in secondary cleft deformities for which maxillary advancement surgery is contemplated. It allows evaluation of the existing status of the velopharyngeal mechanism under direct visualization, thus allowing a more precise determination of possible detrimental changes that may occur with maxillary advancement surgery. This examination is routinely done for all patients with secondary cleft dentofacial deformities who would optimally undergo maxillary advancement surgery for correction of their skeletal deformity. When the choice between maxillary advancement and mandibular set-back is esthetically equivocal or only slightly favors maxillary surgery, the result of the nasoendoscopic examination may make the choice more straightforward.

Tongue evaluation

Speech examination

A consultation with a speech pathologist is indicated if a reduction glossectomy is contemplated. This provides information regarding whether or not there are speech abnormalities compatible with an abnormally large tongue. When such speech abnormalities exist, a properly done reduction glossectomy will most often improve rather than worsen speech.

Radiographic evaluation of tongue posture

Radiographic evaluation of tongue posture may be done from a cephalometric radiograph taken in mandibular rest position. This permits assessment of the tongue placement at rest in the oral cavity (Fig. 1-30). This may help confirm an

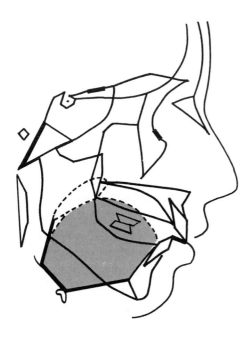

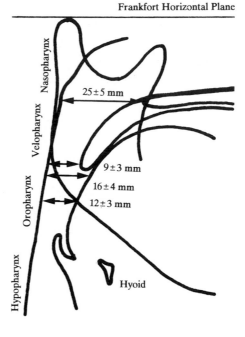

FIG. 1-30   FIG. 1-31

abnormal posture, such as when the tongue occupies the entire oral cavity, habitually protrudes from the oral cavity, or lies abnormally low relative to the palate. Caution is necessary regarding the interpretation of such a radiograph as the posture of the "normal" tongue is highly variable.

Clinically diagnosing the level of obstruction is critical to the ultimate success of planned corrective surgery for patients with confirmed sleep apnea. Evaluating the distance from the velum and tongue to the posterior pharyngeal wall will give the clinician some idea of the level and location of the obstruction. This is best done using a rest position lateral cephalometric radiograph. Normative values for these distances are presented in Fig. 1-31.

Clinical evaluation of tongue posture

There are no scientifically reliable methods to delineate abnormal tongue posture or macroglossia. However, if the tongue protrudes from the mouth when the patient is asleep, we consider it excessive relative to the confines of the oral cavity. This is perhaps the best available clinical evaluation for true macroglossia associated with dentofacial deformities. This condition is rare and, with few exceptions, orthodontic-surgical correction of the dentofacial deformity is done first, with consideration for secondary tongue reduction in individuals with a probability of tongue-induced relapse.

Patients with obstructive sleep apnea require objective clinical evaluation regarding the reason for the obstruction. Tests include sleep lab studies, nasopharyngoscopy, and lateral cephalometric radiographs. After reviewing the data thus accumulated, a predictable treatment plan can be initiated.

Masticatory muscle evaluation
Electromyography and bite-force determinations

These studies are used for patients with the chief complaint of (1) inability to bite forcefully enough to incise or masticate normal foods and/or (2) fatigue of the masticatory muscles during normal masticatory activities. This fatigue is usually accompanied by pain.

In these instances electromyography (EMG) is performed. With the electrodes placed over the masseter, muscle activity and bite force are measured simultaneously and the electromyographic data are compared with that obtained from a normal individual who generates the same bite force. Usually the patient exhibits several times the normal EMG activity to generate a given bite force. If the individual's relative EMG activity is excessive, it indicates muscle hyperfunction. If it is very low, it suggests possible motor nerve dysfunction.

Masseter muscle biopsy

Masseter muscle biopsy is done for select individuals to diagnose the existence of muscle pathology or the presence of a motor nerve/muscle-related dysfunction. A competent muscle pathologist can readily make these determinations with a properly obtained and prepared muscle biopsy.

SUMMARY: PATIENT EVALUATION AND DATA GATHERING

On completion of the evaluation of the dentofacial deformity patient, a clearly defined list of the existing problems can be made. The clinician may now develop a rational treatment plan that takes into consideration all the problems in a logical, sequential fashion. Chapter 2 will describe the essentials of treatment planning as schematically illustrated in Fig. 1-32.

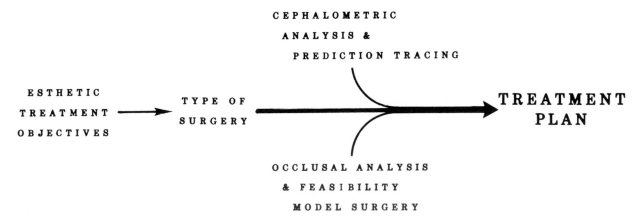

FIG. 1-32

Appendix I

EYES AND ORBITS

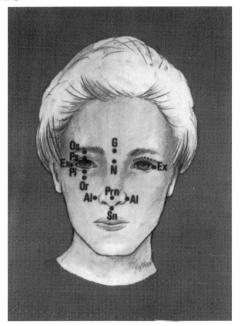

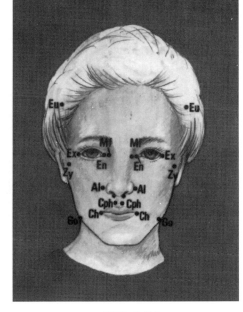

FIG. 1-33   *FIG. 1-34*

En:	Endocanthion	Os:	Orbitale superiorius
Eu:	Eurion	Pi:	Palpebrale inferius
Ex:	Exocanthion	Ps:	Palpebrale superius
G:	Glabella	Zy:	Zygion
Or:	Orbitale		

Vertical proportions

Orbit height/upper face height	Os-Or/G-Sn	50%
Upper lid height/orbit height	Os-Ps/Os-Or	40%
Lid sulcus/lid margin	Sulcus/Ps	10 mm
Eye fissure height/orbit height	Ps-Pi/Os-Or	35%
Upper lid/iris	Ps/Iris	2 mm
Lower lid/iris	Pi/Iris	2 mm
Lower lid height/orbit height	Pi-Or/Os-Or	25%

Horizontal proportions

Biocular width/head width	Ex-Ex/Eu-Eu	60%
Intercanthal width/biocular width	En-En/Ex-Ex	34%
Intercanthal width/zygomatic width	En-En/Zy-Zy	25%
Fissure width/intercanthal width	En-Ex/En-En	95%
Fissure width/biocular width	En-Ex/Ex-Ex	33%
Interpupillary width/biocular width	Mid Pupil/Ex-Ex	70%
Eye fissure cant/horizon	En-Ex/horizon	5%

Vertical/horizontal proportions

Orbit height/biocular width	Os-Or/Ex-Ex	35%
Orbit height/fissure width	Os-Or/En-Ex	95%
Fissure height/fissure width	Ps-Pi/En-Ex	35%

Appendix II

NOSE
Frontal

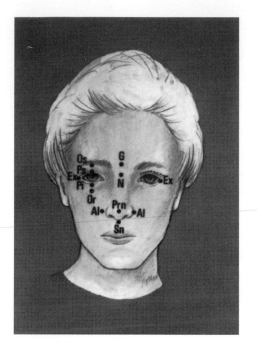

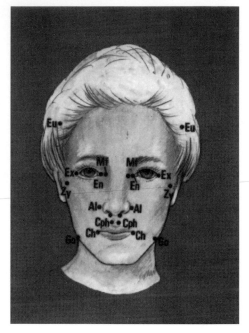

FIG. 1-35   FIG. 1-36

Ac:	Alar curviture point
Al:	Alare
C:	Anterior most point of columella
En:	Endocanthion
G:	Glabella
Ls:	Labiale superius
Mf:	Maxillofrontale
N:	Nasion
Prn:	Pronasale
Pg:	Pogonion
Sn:	Subnasale

Vertical proportions

Nose length/middle third height	N-Sn/G-Sn	90%
Dorsum length/middle third height	N-Prn/G-Sn	80%
Dorsum length/nose length	N-Prn/N-Sn	90%

Horizontal proportions

Nasal root width/alar width	Mf-Mf/Al-Al	50%
Nasal root width/intercanthal width	Mf-Mf/En-En	50%
Alar width/intercanthal width	Al-Al/En-En	100%
Columella width/alar width	Columella/Al-Al	25%

Profile

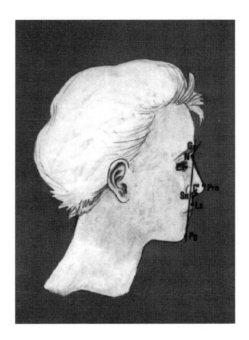

FIG. 1-37

Nasal root/nasal protrusion	En-Dorsum/Sn-Prn	75%
Nasal protrusion/nasal length	Sn-Prn/N-Sn	40%
Nasofrontal angle	N-Prn/N-G	135°
Nasofacial angle	G-Pg/N-Prn	35°
Nasolabial angle	Sn-C/Sn-Ls	100°

Nasal base

Tip length/nasal protrusion	Prn-C/Prn-Sn	45%
Columella length/nasal protrusion	C-Sn/Prn-Sn	55%
Columella length/alar length	Sn-C/Ac-Prn	35%
Nasal tip width/alar width	Tip Width/Al-Al	75%
Nasal protrusion/alar width	Prn-Sn/Al-Al	60%
Nasal protrusion/alar length	Prn-Sn/Ac-Prn	60%
Alar thickness	Ala	5 mm
Columella thickness	Columella	8 mm

Appendix III

EARS

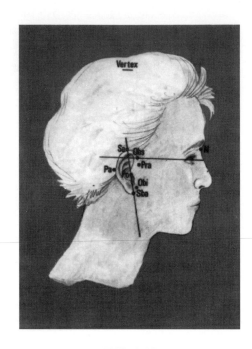

FIG. 1-38

N:	Nasion
Obs:	Otobasion superius
Obi:	Otobasion inferius
Pa:	Postaurale
Pra:	Preaurale
Po:	Porion
Sa:	Superaurale
Sba:	Subaurale
V:	Vertex

Location

Vertical	V-Po	130 mm
Horizontal	N-Obs	115 mm
Lateral protrusion from malar bone		25%

Proportions

Width to length	Pra-Pa/Sa-Sba	55%
Attachment length/vertical length	Obs-Obi/Sa-Sba	85%

Angles

Medial long axis to horizontal	Sa-Sba/Horizontal	100%

Appendix IV

PERIORAL AREA

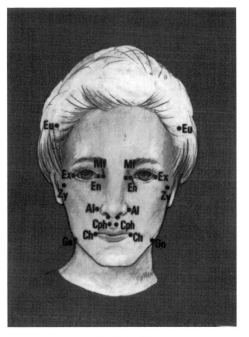

FIG. 1-39

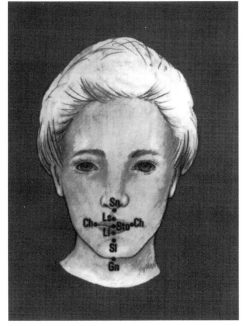

FIG. 1-40

Al:	Alare	Li:	Labiale inferius
Ch:	Cheilion	Ls:	Labiale superius
Cph:	Crista philti	Sl:	Sublabiale
Ex:	Exocanthion	Sn:	Subnasal
Gn:	Gnathion	Sto:	Stomion
Go:	Gonion		

Vertical proportions

Lower face	Sn-Gn	100%
Upper lip	Sn-Sto	30%
Lower lip	Sto-Sl	25%
Chin	Sl-Gn	45%

Lips

Upper lip/lower lip	Sn-Sto/Sto-Sl	120%
Skin upper/upper lip	Sn-Ls/Sn-Sto	70%
Skin lower/lower lip	Li-Sl/Sto-Sl	60%
Vermilion upper/lower	Ls-Sto/Sto-Li	85%

Horizontal proportions

Mouth width/biogonial width	Ch-Ch/Go-Go	55%
Mouth width/zygoma width	Ch-Ch/Zy-Zy	40%
Mouth width/biocular width	Ch-Ch/Ex-Ex	60%
Alar base width/mouth width	Al-Al/Ch-Ch	65%
Philtrum width/mouth width	Chp-Chp/Ch-Ch	20%
Columella width/philtrum width	Columella/Chp-Chp	75%

Vertical/horizontal proportions

Upper lip height/mouth width	Sn-Sto/Ch-Ch	40%
Lower face height/mouth width	Sn-Gn/Ch-Ch	130%

Esthetic changes accompanying mandibular advancement

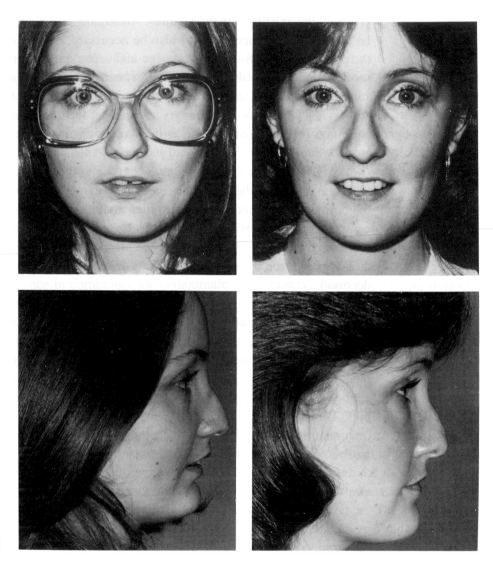

FIG. 2-1

FRONT FACE

Variable increase in lower third face
  height
Reduces lower lip eversion
Reduces prominent labiomental fold
Increases neck-chin definition

PROFILE

Increases chin prominence
Reduces lower lip eversion
Increases lower lip protrusion
Decreaes chin-neck angle
Improves neck-chin definition

Esthetic changes accompanying maxillary superior repositioning

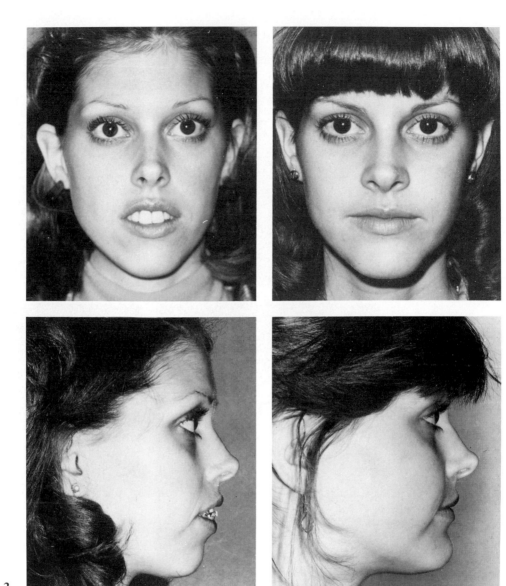

FIG. 2-2

FRONT FACE	PROFILE
Widens alar bases (controllable—see Chapter 7)	Accentuates paranasal areas
Reduces exposure of maxillary anterior teeth	Elevates nasal tip (controllable—see Chapter 7)
Reduces interlabial distance	Reduces interlabial distance
Reduces lower third face vertically	Increases chin prominence
Shortens distance from upper lip stomion to menton	Reduces lower third face vertically
Decreases distance from subnasale to mucocutaneous junction of lower lip	

Esthetic changes accompanying mandibular setback

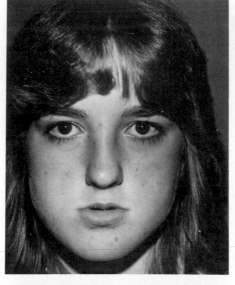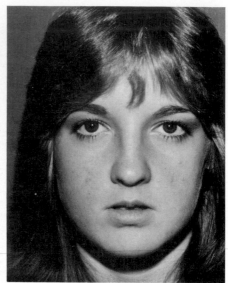

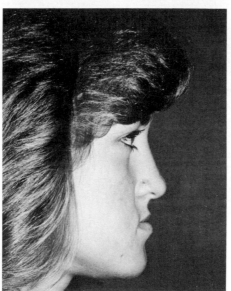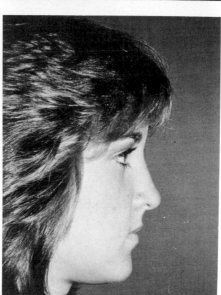

FIG. 2-3

FRONT FACE	PROFILE
Decreases chin prominence	Reduces chin prominence
Increases exposure of upper lip ver-milion	Reduces lower lip eversion
Decreases lower third face height (slight)	Shortens neck-chin line
Increases squareness of face	Increases paranasal fullness (postural)

Esthetic changes accompanying total maxillary advancement

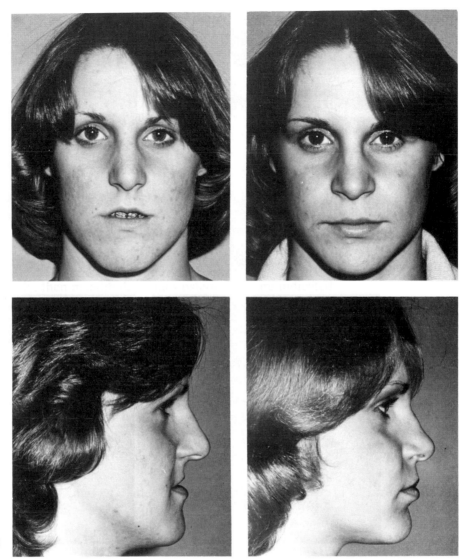

FIG. 2-4

FRONT FACE

Widens alar bases (controllable—see
    Chapter 7)
Increases prominence of upper lip
Increases exposure of upper lip ver-
    milion
Reduces chin prominence (relative)

PROFILE

Accentuates paranasal areas
Reduces prominence of nose
Elevates nasal tip
Accentuates upper lip
Deaccentuates chin

If the result is satisfactory then nothing else need be done. However, if the chin remains too recessive, or the orthodontic treatment is not possible, the prediction is redone with a genioplasty. If the upper jaw is moved so far back that facial esthetics will be compromised, a prediction tracing is done with a simultaneous mandibular advancement. If this still produces a deficient chin, another tracing is done with superior repositioning, mandibular advancement, and genioplasty. Each prediction involves progressively more surgery.

On occasion several predictions are done, each employing different surgical and orthodontic options, and critical esthetic analysis is used to determine the best possible result. If two predictions produce equivocal results, the one involving the simplest surgery is the treatment of choice. If both the esthetic result and surgical difficulty are equivocal, the one involving the simplest orthodontic treatment is selected. Note that while profile esthetics is important, great care is taken to understand the front face effect of all procedures that are evaluated. *No procedure that improves profile esthetics is considered if it will compromise the patient's front face esthetics.*

MAKING THE BASIC ORTHODONTIC DECISIONS

Once the surgical procedure(s) has been decided on, the basic orthodontic decisions must be made. *These decisions are predicated on the surgical procedure to be done and cannot be made before deciding on the surgical procedures(s).* The orthodontic decisions that must be made are: (1) What tooth movement is indicated? (2) What are the anchorage requirements for this movement? (3) Do teeth need to be extracted? (4) If so, which teeth are to be extracted? (5) Are there tooth mass problems? and (6) Is there sufficient alveolar bone? The first four questions are answered by doing an orthodontic-surgical prediction tracing. The tooth mass question is best answered by doing an orthodontic setup of the teeth. The sufficiency of alveolar bone is determined by analysis of the dental casts and radiographs. Each of these are discussed below in more detail.

What tooth movement is necessary?

Once a cephalometric prediction tracing has been done, the tooth movement in both the anteroposterior and vertical planes can be easily visualized. (See description of cephalometric prediction technique later in this chapter.) If the original mandible is superimposed on the prediction tracing mandible, the dental changes are apparent (Fig. 2-6). The same, of course, applies to the maxilla (Fig. 2-7). Importantly, which of the changes will be produced at surgery and which are produced by orthodontics alone must be understood. For instance, both the vertical and anteroposterior changes in the maxilla that are shown in a prediction tracing for correction of vertical maxillary excess are primarily accomplished by the surgery; thus, the orthodontic considerations in the maxilla consist only of aligning the teeth and positioning the roots within the alveolar bone.

The orthodontist must pay particular attention to the tooth movements necessary in relation to the ability to produce them. In some instances the tooth movements called for by a particular cephalometric prediction tracing cannot be

Dental Changes in the Mandible

Pretreatment Position ──────

Desired Posttreatment Position ── ── ── ──

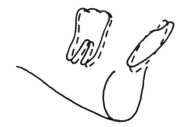

FIG. 2-6

Dental Changes in the Maxilla

Pretreatment Position ──────

Desired Posttreatment Position ── ── ── ──

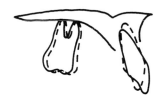

FIG. 2-7

accomplished or would require such extreme orthodontic treatment as to be considered unacceptable. In this case the prediction tracing must be redone, usually with an adjunctive surgical procedure such as a genioplasty or some other surgical modification, to produce a similar esthetic and occlusal result without requiring impossible or unadvisable orthodontic treatment. For example, the cephalometric prediction tracing reveals that an individual with 6 mm of crowding in the lower arch will require 8 mm of retraction of the lower incisors to allow an optimal correction of the chin position by mandibular advancement. Such treatment is clearly unreasonable even with extractions because to do so would require 22 mm of arch length. One possible solution is to add an augmentation genioplasty so that the lower incisors can be left somewhat more protrusive and a similar facial result will still be achieved. Not only must the tooth movements be attainable, but care must be taken in judging the potential stability of the desired movements. *The addition of surgery to a treatment plan does not decrease the potential for orthodontic relapse.* Orthodontic movements that, by themselves, are potentially unstable remain so, and are to be avoided in combined orthodontic-surgical correction of a dentofacial deformity.

Thus, while the maxillary arch with an open bite due to an extreme curve at Spee can be leveled by orthodontically extruding the anterior teeth, doing so is best avoided because of the potential for relapse of such extrusion. The alternative is to avoid extrusion by aligning the maxillary teeth segmentally and leveling the arch surgically.

INCREASED OVERJET

Due to:

Excessive

Attrition   Labiolingual

Thickness

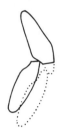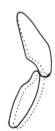

FIG. 2-14

quire more overjet—thus more tooth mass—for the same amount of overbite) (Fig. 2-14), and (3) Both methods assume normal axial inclination of the teeth depending on their anatomy, some (incisor teeth take up more arch length when they are tipped labially because the contact points are further gingivally) (Fig. 2-15).

UPRIGHT LOWER ANTERIORS

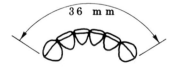

36 mm

Contacts

Near Incisal Edge

FLARED LOWER ANTERIORS

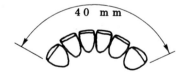

40 mm

Contacts

More Gingivally

FIG. 2-15

To overcome the inherent inaccuracy in previous methods of tooth mass discrepancies, White proposed the use of occlusograms. This method is a great improvement and works well in the majority of cases. Its only weakness is that it again fails to take into account the axial inclination of the teeth, which is important in cases in which the incisors will be proclined more than the ideal. In view of this, it is perhaps best to do an orthodontic setup by carefully removing the teeth from the model and waxing them into the best possible occlusion to assess most accurately the tooth mass problems and the solution to these problems (Fig. 2-16).

Anterior tooth mass discrepancies of up to 4 mm can usually be corrected by interproximal recontouring of the five interproximal areas from canine to canine. If the discrepancy is 4 mm or greater, the removal of a lower incisor will probably be necessary along with some recontouring of the upper incisors unless the width of the lower incisor is equal to the discrepancy. One word of caution must be expressed regarding recontouring. For the patient with very square lower incisor crowns, major recontouring may be impossible because of root width. (The

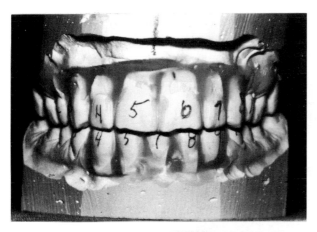

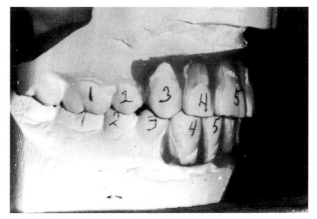

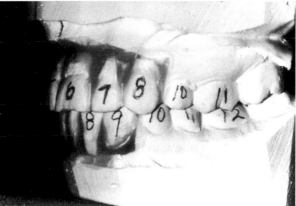

FIG. 2-16

same problem can arise in the upper arch but it is less common.) There must always be enough room between the roots to permit a normal interproximal gingival contour. When the gingiva may be compromised by the amount of recontouring necessary, either extracting a lower incisor and recontouring the upper incisors, or crowning, placing facings, or bonding the upper anteriors to widen them, or leaving space distal to the upper lateral incisors should be considered.

Segmental maxillary feasibility model surgery

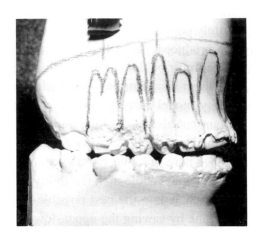

FIG. 2-21

Step 1. The models are duplicated, trimmed to simulate the anatomy, and arbitrarily mounted on an articulator using a wax bite to ensure proper occlusion. The roots of the teeth adjacent to planned interdental osteotomies or ostectomies are drawn on the cast (Fig. 2-21).

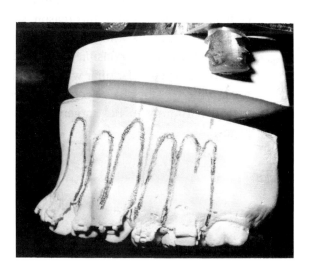

FIG. 2-22

Step 2. The teeth and alveolus are sectioned from the upper model base along a reference line made approximately 5 mm above the tooth root apices (Fig. 2-22).

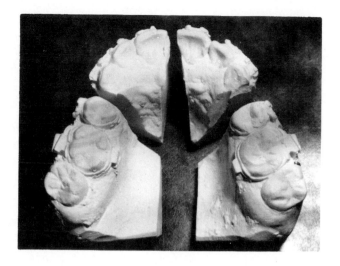

FIG. 2-23

Step 3. The maxilla is sectioned into the appropriate segments taking care not to cut through the tooth roots (Fig. 2-23).

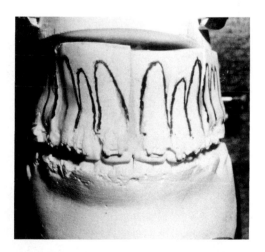

FIG. 2-24

Step 4. The anterior segment(s) is placed into its best occlusal relationship with the lower teeth and held in this position with soft wax (Fig. 2-24). The object is to establish a Class I canine occlusion with normal overbite and overjet. In some instances it may be necessary to section this anterior segment between the central incisors to increase or decrease intercanine width, close a midline diastema, etc.

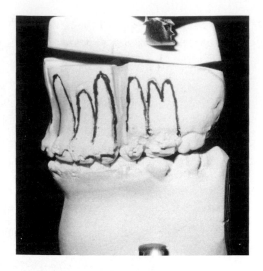

FIG. 2-25

Step 5. Each posterior segment is placed into its best occlusal relationship and held into position with soft wax. Using soft wax permits easy adjustment of the segments during the initial positioning (Fig. 2-25).

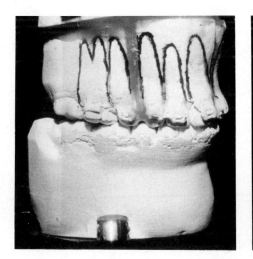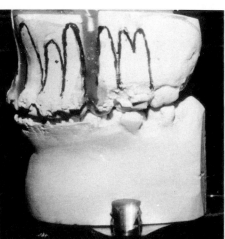

FIG. 2-26

Step 6. Once the best possible occlusion is achieved, the segments are joined to one another and to the base with sufficient sticky wax to prevent them from moving (Fig. 2-26).

Segmental maxillary ostectomy with an anterior mandibular subapical ostectomy and midline ostectomy feasibility model surgery

When a lower subapical procedure is planned in conjunction with other maxillary or mandibular surgery, the lower subapical ostectomy is almost always completed first. The objective is to produce as ideal a lower arch as possible. Thus, the lower curve of Spee is leveled, the midline maintained or corrected to the facial midline, and any spaces where interdental osteotomies have been done are as small as possible, consistent with good surgical technique.

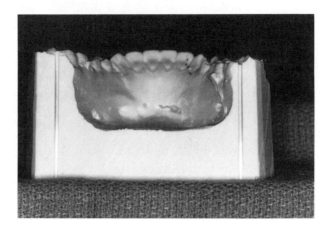

FIG. 2-27

When the mandibular arch shape is to be altered (i.e., lower subapical with midline split of the mandible, or any other procedure designed to narrow or widen the mandibular dental arch) it is best to place "condylar grooves" on the back of the mandibular model (Fig. 2-27). When performing the model surgery for an anterior mandibular subapical ostectomy with midline ostectomy, the condylar groove should still be aligned at the completion of the feasibility model surgery (Fig. 2-28).

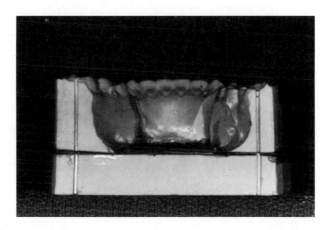

FIG. 2-28

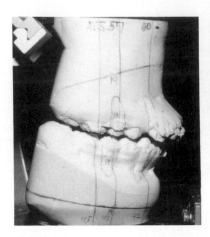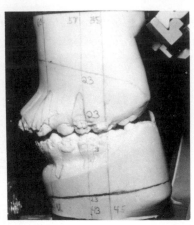

FIG. 2-29

Step 1. The models are duplicated, trimmed to simulate the anatomy and arbitrarily mounted on an articulator using a wax bite to ensure proper occlusion. The roots of the teeth adjacent to planned interdental osteotomies or ostectomies are drawn on the casts (Fig. 2-29). Finally, "condylar grooves" are placed on the back of the mandibular model to ensure that intercondylar distance remains constant and that only rotational changes occur when the mandibular arch is narrowed (Fig. 2-27).

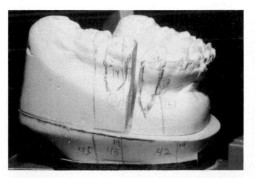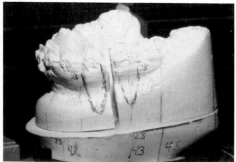

FIG. 2-30

Step 2. The illustrated model surgery is for correction of a bimaxillary protrusion. The entire lower dentoalveolar segment is sectioned from the lower cast at a level safely below the tooth root apices. This is done to allow the necessary constriction of the premolars (see Chapter 6). To allow repositioning of the lower segments into their desired positions, appropriate plaster is removed from both the interdental sites and the base while carefully avoiding the tooth roots (Fig. 2-30). The reference grooves are checked frequently during the model surgery and are maintained straight with minimal disruption to ensure maintenance of the presurgical condylar position (Fig. 2-28).

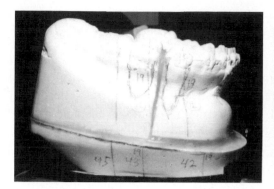
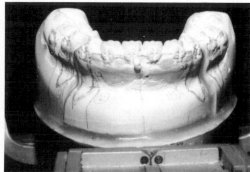

FIG. 2-31

Step 3. The anterior mandibular subapical segment is positioned to achieve the best possible arch form and curve of Spee and held with soft wax (Fig. 2-31).

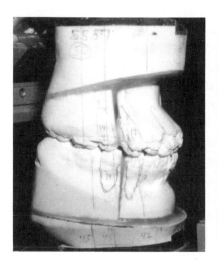
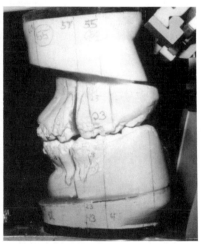

FIG. 2-32

Step 4. After the lower subapical ostectomy is completed, the upper arch is sectioned and reassembled on the newly constructed lower arch as described in the previous section (Fig. 2-32).

Once the feasibility model surgery is done, it is evaluated by the orthodontist who will be responsible for finishing the occlusion. *The orthodontist is responsible for the decision to proceed with the orthognathic surgery or to delay same.* If the occlusion produced by the feasibility model surgery produces a situation that is difficult, unpredictable, or impossible to correct orthodontically, then surgery is delayed until the orthodontist moves the teeth into a position from which these specific problems are no longer encountered. When the orthodontist again believes he has achieved the presurgical goals, new models are made, the feasibility model surgery is redone, and the results are again examined. Once the occlusion that can be produced by surgery is acceptable to the orthodontist, the patient is ready for surgery.

ORTHODONTIC-SURGICAL CEPHALOMETRIC PREDICTION TRACING

One of the most important treatment planning tools is the cephalometric prediction tracing. There are two different types of prediction tracing—orthodontic-surgical and surgical. The first, described in this chapter, is used for overall treatment planning and illustrates the effect of both orthodontic tooth movement and surgical skeletal changes. The surgical prediction tracing is done as part of the two-patient concept presented earlier in this chapter and immediately before surgery to plan the specific surgical movements. It includes no dental changes other than those to be produced by surgery. The reasons for doing orthodontic-surgical cephalometric predictions are: (1) to assess accurately the profile esthetic results of the proposed surgery and orthodontics, (2) to determine the desirability of adjunctive surgical procedures such as genioplasty, (3) to help determine the sequencing of surgery and orthodontics, (4) to help decide if extractions are necessary, (5) to determine which teeth to extract if extraction treatment is required, and (6) to determine the anchorage requirements.

Because of the extreme diversity of orthodontic and surgical procedures employed in the orthodontic-surgical correction of dentofacial deformities, it is impossible to illustrate the method of developing a cephalometric prediction tracing for every possible dentofacial deformity. The method employed for mandibular advancement, maxillary superior repositioning, and combined maxillary superior repositioning and mandibular advancement surgery will be discussed and illustrated. With the exception of those methods employed in treatment planning for the correction of asymmetries (Volume III, Section VII), all orthodontic-surgical corrections are basically the same as, the reverse of, or a combination of these procedures. Thus, once the clinician is thoroughly familiar with the techniques involved for doing the predictions illustrated, the principles are easily applied to all other dentofacial deformities. There is no easy method for learning to do cephalometric prediction tracings. Only by doing them through trial and error and by careful observation of the actually achieved results can the prediction tracing technique be perfected.

Mandibular advancement

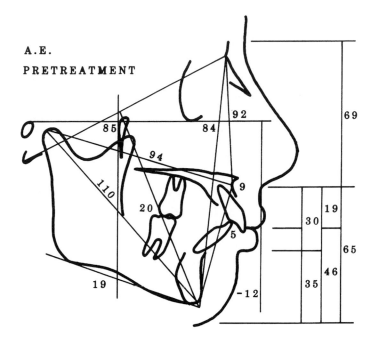

FIG. 2-33

The pretreatment cephalometric tracing of a patient who would benefit from a mandibular advancement is seen in Fig. 2-33. Throughout this discussion this pretreatment tracing will be called the ***tracing*** (black), and the prediction tracing that is being constructed will be called the ***prediction*** (red).

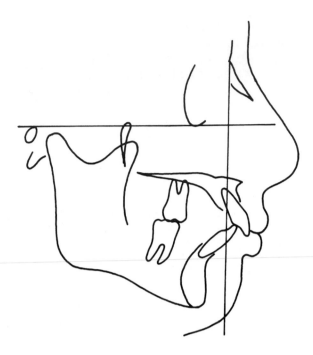

FIG. 2-34

Step 1. Indicate the desired facial depth on the ***tracing*** (Fig. 2-34). In many patients with mandibular deficiency this is done by passing a line from nasion through Point A and extending it inferiorly, as Point A is frequently in its normal relation (90 degree maxillary depth). When this is not so, as illustrated by this patient, it is suggested that the clinician begin by doing an initial prediction at the ideal facial depth (males, 90 degrees; females, 89 degrees) and studying these results. If the chin appears too prominent, the prediction is redone with a decreased facial depth. Conversely, if the chin is still deficient, the prediction is redone with an increased facial depth until the desired result is achieved.

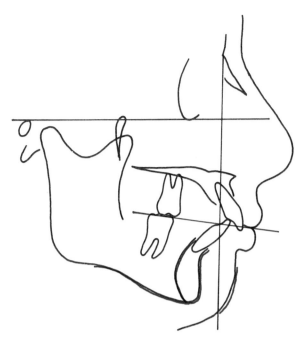

FIG. 2-35

Step 2. Begin the *prediction* by tracing the distal portion of the mandible, the soft-tissue chin, and the occlusal plane on a clean piece of acetate (Fig. 2-35). At this time it is frequently best to use a lightly dotted line for the soft-tissue chin and the corresponding part of the mandible, as doing so makes it easier to add a genioplasty (if needed) at a later time. (The subsequent addition of a genioplasty will require alteration of this area and a lightly dotted line is easier to erase or ignore). This is a straightforward procedure, except for the occlusal plane in the patient with a deep bite, for whom a choice must be made between the functional occlusal plane and the molar-incisor occlusal planes (Fig. 2-36). This choice is not made casually as it will eventually affect the facial esthetics, the amount and direction of advancement, and the necessary orthodontic treatment.

OCCLUSAL PLANES

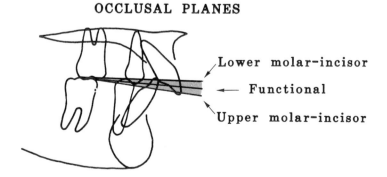

FIG. 2-36

1. Choosing the functional occlusal plane. Because the patient with deep bite frequently has both an excessive curve of Spee in the lower arch and a reverse curve of Spee in the upper arch, choosing to advance the mandible along the functional occlusal plane will mean that the orthodontist will have to level both the upper and lower arches by intrusion of the anterior teeth. The advantages of such a choice are that (1) pogonion will be advanced the same distance as the teeth (little, if any, clockwise rotation of the distal segment), (2) the vertical dimension of the lower face will be increased only slightly, (3) less retraction of the lower anterior teeth will be necessary to produce the desired chin projection, and (4) when a genioplasty is necessary, augmentation will be smaller. The only disadvantage arises in the patient who has a short lower face height, for whom increased vertical dimension is desirable.

2. Choosing the molar-incisor occlusal planes. Clearly, the patient with deep bite has two divergent molar-incisor occlusal planes: one from maxillary molar to maxillary incisor and one from mandibular molar to mandibular incisor (Fig. 2-36). If the mandible is to be advanced along these divergent planes, the distal mandible must first be rotated clockwise so that the planes: coincide before advancing. When this is done, the teeth are advanced more than pogonion and the lower face height is increased by the amount of the excess overbite. Thus, *this occlusal plane is chosen when is it desired to intentionally increase the lower face height (when it is short) or when minimal advancement of pogonion is desired.* Otherwise, a large genioplasty or excessive retraction of lower anterior teeth will be necessary. The differences in these two techniques are illustrated in Fig. 2-37.

MANDIBLE ADVANCED ALONG:
Functional occlusal plane ————
Molar-incisor occlusal plane - - - - - -

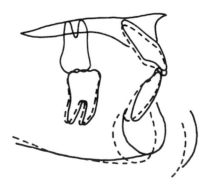

FIG. 2-37

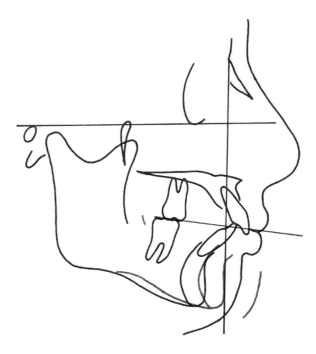

FIG. 2-38

Step 3. Slide the *prediction* forward along the chosen occlusal plane until bony pogonion lies on the line indicating the desired facial depth (Fig. 2-38).

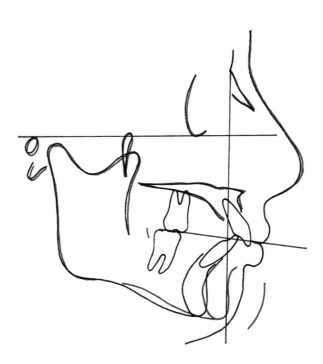

FIG. 2-39

Step 4. Trace the fixed structures (Fig. 2-39).

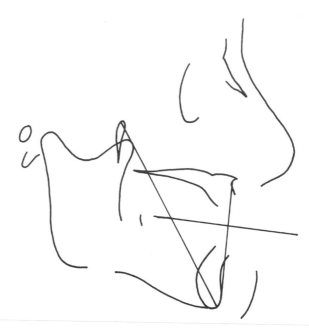

FIG. 2-40

Step 5. Draw the A-Po line and the facial axis on the *prediction* (Fig. 2-40). These lines are used to place the teeth in their ideal positions.

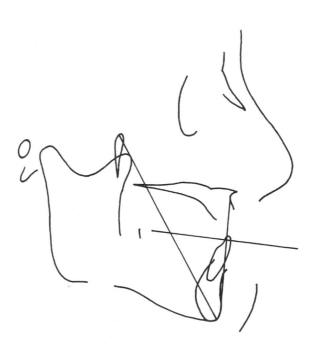

FIG. 2-41

Step 6. Place the lower incisor in its ideal position (Fig. 2-41). This position, as determined by Rickets, is with the incisal edge 1 mm ahead of the A-Po line and the long axis at 22 degrees to the A-Po line. It is not unusual that the 22 degrees will have to be compromised to keep the apex of the tooth within the symphysis. Once the lower incisor has been placed, the clinician must determine where the lower molar should be placed.

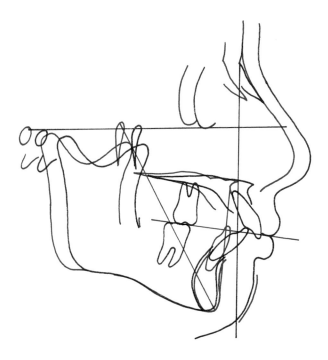

FIG. 2-42

Step 7. Superimpose the distal mandible of the ***prediction*** on that of the ***tracing*** (Fig. 2-42). The change in lower incisor position is carefully studied at this time. Most frequently the lower incisor will have been retracted and uprighted in the Class II patient. The amount of this retraction must be noted and the space required to effect this retraction (2 mm of arch length for each 1 mm of incisor retraction) must be added to the existing lower arch crowding and any planned lower arch expansion to determine the total arch length discrepancy.

Planned expansion of the lower arch must be taken into account in determining total arch length discrepancy. Rickets' data shows that there is approximately a 1-mm increase in total arch length for every 1-mm increase in intercanine width, every 2-mm increase in interpremolar width, and every 4-mm increase in intermolar width.

While other factors are ultimately taken into account before deciding the extraction question (see extraction discussion earlier in this chapter), for purposes of doing this prediction tracing only total arch length discrepancy is considered. The following calculation is made (using the appropriate numbers from the patient) to determine where to place the lower molar in an anteroposterior direction:

Lower arch crowding (measured on the models)	-1 mm
Lower incisor movement x 2 (from the above superimposition) (-8mm x 2)	-16 mm
Arch length gained (from planned lower arch expansion, if any)	+0 mm
Total arch length discrepancy	-17 mm

The single most common problem encountered in doing a cephalometric prediction tracing for mandibular advancement is the inability to produce the desired lower incisor tooth movement because the total arch length discrepancy is greater than the width of two premolars. When this situation exists, as it does in the example patient, the clinician must remember that there exists a normal range (-1 to +3 mm) for placement of the lower incisor relative to the A-Po line. Thus, one may leave the incisor slightly more prominent than the ideal. If the total arch length discrepancy is still greater than the width of two premolars even when considering the above range of normal, the clinician must alter the prediction tracing by addition of an augmentation genioplasty before Step 2 (doing so will advance pogonion; thus, the A-Po line will be farther forward, and less retraction of the incisors will be necessary).

For the example patient, placing the lower incisors at +3 mm to the A-Po line produces the following acceptable calculation:

Lower arch crowding (measured on the models)	-1 mm
Lower incisor movement x 2 (from superimposition) (-6 mm x 2)	-12 mm
Arch length gained (from planned lower arch expansion, if any)	+0 mm
Total arch length discrepancy	-13 mm
Extract lower premolars (width measured on the models)	+15 mm
Lower molar forward half of	2 mm = **1 mm**

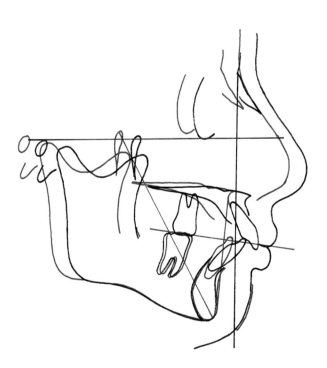

FIG. 2-43

Step 8. Once the total arch length discrepancy has been determined, subtract this amount from the width of the tooth or teeth to be extracted; the remainder of the space is closed by bringing the lower molars forward. Since only one molar is illustrated and the same change will occur on each side, the molar is placed on the occlusal plane and advanced half the amount of the extra space, if any, produced by extraction (Fig. 2-43).

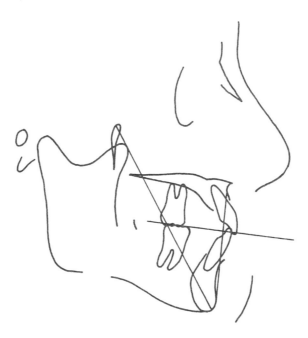

FIG. 2-44

Step 9. Once the lower molar has been placed, place the upper molar in an ideal Class I occlusion. (*Note*: Occasionally the clinician may elect to produce a Class III molar relationship. When this is so, one must remember to include this decision in the prediction tracing by placing the upper molar in the desired occlusal relation.) The upper incisor is placed in an ideal overbite-overjet relationship with the long axis of the tooth 5 degrees more upright than the new facial axis (Fig. 2-44). Once the teeth have been placed in their ideal position, the soft-tissue profile is completed.

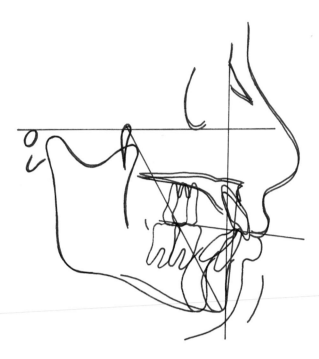

FIG. 2-45

Step 10. Superimpose the ***prediction*** on the fixed structures of the ***tracing*** and note the change in the upper incisor position. Anteroposteriorly the upper lip vermilion will change in the same direction as the upper incisor movement but only by about half as much. Subnasale is not affected by dental changes; thus, draw the new lip in the appropriate position and connect it to subnasale by a smooth curve (Fig. 2-45). (*Note*: Subnasale may change with maxillary surgery. The specifics of those changes are discussed in subsequent chapters.)

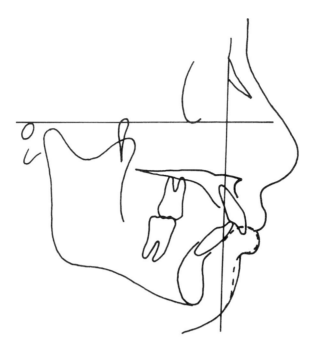

FIG. 2-46

Step 11. The determination of lower lip placement is more difficult than that of the upper lip since frequently it is not only supported by the lower incisor but also everted by the upper incisors. When this is the case, draw a dashed line on the tracing to indicate the approximate lip thickness that would be present if there were no upper incisor impingement (the lower lip is generally of equal thickness from Point B superiorly and is usually the same thickness as the upper lip) (Fig. 2-46).

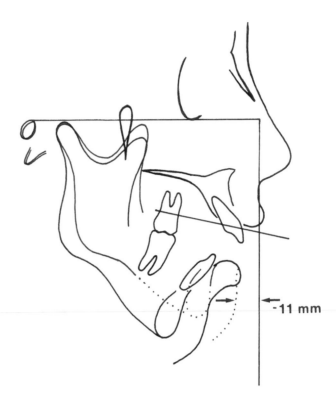

-11 mm

FIG. 2-54

Step 4. After tracing the fixed structures and while maintaining this orientation of the *prediction* relative to the *tracing* observe the anteroposterior position of the chin. The soft-tissue chin optimally lies 2 to 6 mm behind the subnasale perpendicular originally drawn on the *tracing*. Factors such as the size of the nose, the length of the neck-chin line, and the size of the neck-chin angle will play a role in individual chin assessment. If the chin is clearly deficient at this point, an augmentation genioplasty is indicated (Fig. 2-54).

When an osseous augmentation genioplasty is done, there is a soft-tissue effect in a ratio of 1:0.7. (The authors prefer an osseous augmentation genioplasty whenever possible, with only limited application of alloplastic chin implant materials.) Thus, if the patient ideally needs 7 mm more soft-tissue chin, an osseous genioplasty of about 10 mm will be necessary. (Simultaneous mandibular advancement will be discussed subsequently. While simultaneous mandibular advancement will certainly increase the chin projection, it is important to understand that *the need for simultaneous mandibular advancement is predicated on the upper lip and nose esthetics* as discussed in Chapters 7 and 8, *not* on the anteroposterior deficiency of the chin, which is more easily corrected by a genioplasty).

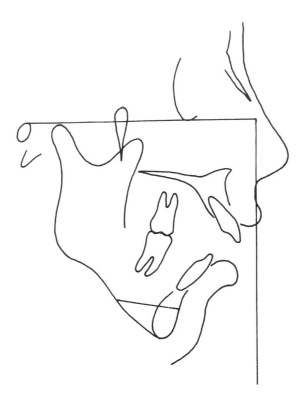

FIG. 2-55

Step 5. Add the indicated augmentation genioplasty if it is required. To do so, the following steps are done:

Step 5A. Draw a horizontal line on the symphysis of the *tracing* at least 30 mm below the occlusal plane to indicate the desired position of the osteotomy (Fig. 2-55). This line is drawn parallel to Frankfort horizontal when no vertical change is desired. It may be angled upward anteriorly relative to Frankfort when it is desired to shorten the chin vertically, or (rarely) angled downward when the opposite is true.

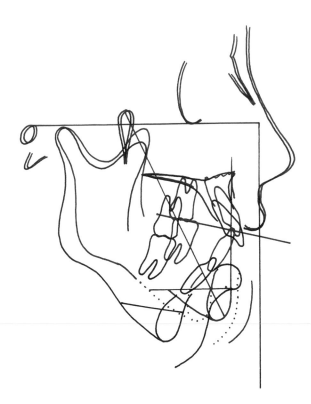

FIG. 2-63

Step 9. Superimpose the ***prediction*** on the ***tracing*** registering on the fixed structures (Fig. 2-63). Carefully study the change in Point A and the upper incisor in relation to the upper lip before beginning the completion of the soft tissue. While this superimposition is held, the nose and upper lip are completed.

DRAWING A NEW NOSE. The upper two thirds of the nose are usually not affected by superiorly repositioning the maxilla. The effect on the nasal tip is to elevate and protrude it by varying amounts. This variation is dependent on the surgical method of dealing with the anterior nasal spine and the nasal septum (Chapter 7). On the average the nasal tip elevates approximately 1 mm and moves forward approximately 0.5 mm for every 10 mm of superior movement. This effect is greater when the maxilla (Point A) moves forward and superiorly and is less pronounced if the maxilla moves posteriorly. (With regard to maxillary advancement, published data suggest that the nasal tip elevates 2 mm with 7 mm of maxillary advancement as measured by change in Point A. Because nasal effects are directly related to surgical techniques, the surgeon must study his or her own surgical results to become proficient in predicting nasal changes.)

The columella and subnasale are remarkably unaffected by superior and/or posterior repositioning and in most instances are drawn exactly as they were before surgery. The only exception is when the maxilla is moved anteriorly and the anterior nasal spine is left intact. Change in subnasale with maxillary advancement is not only dependent on magnitude of maxillary advancement but also lip thickness as measured from Point A to soft-tissue subnasale. Lips measuring 17 mm or less have approximately 50% advancement of soft-tissue subnasale relative to advancement of Point A and only 30% change in subnasale in individuals with lip thicknesses greater than 17 mm. Subnasale and nasal tip appear to remain quite stable with posterior maxillary repositioning regardless of the magnitude of change of Point A.

DRAWING THE UPPER LIP. Before surgery, the upper lip support for patients with vertical maxillary excess is generally formed by the alveolus below Point A with the upper incisor forming part of this support only in the more mild cases of vertical excess and in those with open bite. After surgery, upper lip support will be both alveolar and dental. To predict the new upper lip position the change in the upper lip support is studied. When the maxilla and incisor are moved up and slightly back, paralleling a line from original Point A to original labial surface of upper incisor, the lip support is not changed, and thus there will be no effect on anteroposterior position of the lip.

Vertically the lip may shorten slightly. (The amount of this shortening is directly dependent on the surgeon's closure of the vestibular incision as discussed in Chapter 7.) When Point A and the incisors move anteriorly and superiorly, the lip support will be increased. The amount of anterior change in the upper lip is somewhat dependent on the amount the support is increased, but is generally 50% of the amount that the lip support is increased. Thus, if the lip support moves anteriorly 6 mm, the upper lip will move 3 mm anteriorly. Likewise when the lip support is moved posteriorly, the lip will move posteriorly approximately 50% of the change. Thus, 6 mm of posterior movement of the lip support will produce a 3-mm reduction in lip prominence. (There obviously are limits to the above statements because a lip will only thicken or thin a limited amount in response to orthodontic and surgical movements. Nevertheless, the 50% rule will apply to the vast majority of patients.)

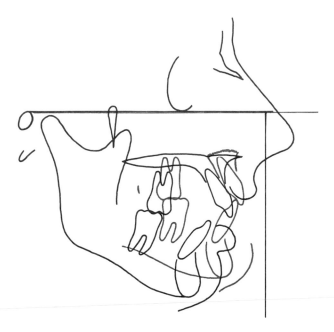

FIG. 2-71

Step 4. Place *prediction 2* on the *tracing* referenced on the Frankfort horizontal and slide *prediction 2* along the Frankfort horizontal plane until the upper incisor is in its desired anteroposterior position relative to the upper lip on the *tracing* (Fig. 2-71). Remember, the upper lip that is 17 mm or less in thickness will move approximately 50% of the dentoalveolar support behind it. Thicker lips (greater than 17 mm) will move about 30% of the dentoalveolar anterior movement. (*Note*: If the chin is still deficient after the upper incisor has been advanced to its desired anteroposterior position, the chin projection is corrected with a genioplasty.)

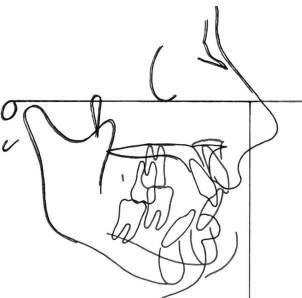

FIG. 2-72

Step 5. Holding *prediction 2* in its desired anteroposterior position and maintaining the vertical changes referenced by the Frankfort horizontal, trace the fixed structures, that is, basion, pogonion, orbit, nasion, proximal segment of mandible, forehead, and upper two-thirds of the nose (Fig. 2-72).

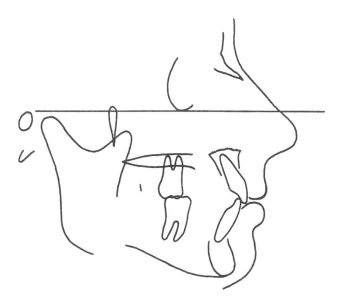

FIG. 2-73

Step 6. Complete the soft tissue. This is done exactly as in Steps 9 through 12 for superior repositioning (Fig. 2-73). This completes this prediction tracing.

DEVELOPING THE DEFINITIVE TREATMENT PLAN

The definitive treatment plan is developed as a result of the interaction of the proposed solutions to all the problems that have been identified (Fig. 2-74). This definitive treatment plan most often involves a preliminary phase and then the actual orthodontic-surgical phase. The preliminary phase consists of dealing with factors such as potential medical risks, existing general dental conditions, periodontal problems, psychologic considerations, impacted teeth in the path of elective osteotomies, and temporomandibular joint problems. After this, the patient is ready for the definitive orthodontic-surgical phase of treatment. The following discussion is primarily concerned with the definitive orthodontic-surgical phase of treatment. A brief discussion of temporomandibular joint considerations in the patient with a dentofacial deformity is presented first as the specific nature of a coexisting joint problem may have direct bearing on the optimal time to treat the joint—before, during, or after treatment of the dentofacial deformity.

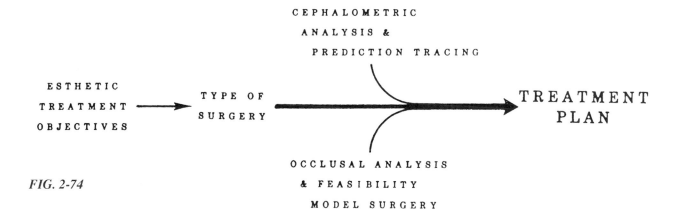

CEPHALOMETRIC

ANALYSIS &

PREDICTION TRACING

ESTHETIC
TREATMENT → TYPE OF → TREATMENT
OBJECTIVES   SURGERY   PLAN

OCCLUSAL ANALYSIS

& FEASIBILITY

MODEL SURGERY

FIG. 2-74

Such fixation holds the skeletal components firmly in place while the initial adaptive changes occur within the soft tissues surrounding the surgically repositioned skeleton. As such, the larger the skeletal movement achieved at surgery, the longer the period of maxillomandibular fixation. At release of fixation, sufficient adaptation has taken place so that the neuromuscular matrix is no longer a factor responsible for relapse. If skeletal maxillomandibular fixation is not employed in such cases, the stretched neuromuscular matrix will predictably cause relapse of the surgically corrected dentoskeletal components toward their original position and tend to reestablish the original dentofacial deformity.

Two caveats apply to stabilization procedures for all dentofacial deformity patients regardless of whether they are excess or deficiency states. First, it is best to avoid the use of rigid fixation in mandibular asymmetry cases since the three-dimensional change in condylar position can be dramatically unpredictable. Second, when employing rigid fixation, it is best to have a preoperative occlusion requiring minimal postsurgical orthodontic finishing and to place the dentoosseous segments *very precisely* into the desired position. Rigid fixation is quite unforgiving, and postsurgical orthodontic treatment will be unduly time-consuming and result in unfavorable dental compensations if the surgeon fails to achieve the intended occlusal result. Contrast this to the more forgiving skeletal fixation that allows postsurgical orthodontic and orthopedic manipulations whereby entire segments may be rapidly moved to expedite postsurgical orthodontic finishing.

Finally, *no patient should be unconditionally promised a surgical treatment exclusive of skeletal maxillomandibular fixation*. Untoward intraoperative events may compel a surgeon to employ skeletal maxillomandibular fixation with the patient's jaws wired together in order to secure the dentoosseous segments appropriately.

Postsurgical orthodontic treatment

This portion of the treatment plan will list the orthodontic procedures anticipated to complete the occlusion following surgery. When surgery is done first, this will be an orthodontic treatment plan with a sequence of mechanics designed to correct the malocclusion produced at surgery. When surgery follows some preparatory orthodontics, this portion will usually involve routine finishing procedures (such as root paralleling, marginal ridge leveling, and perfecting interdigitation) followed by the proposed method of retention.

REFERENCES

Bolton, W.A.,: Disharmony in tooth size and its relation to the analysis and treatment of malocclusion, Angle Orthod. **28:**113, 1958.

Ellis, E. III., Tharanon, W., and Gambrell, K.: Accuracy of face-bow transfer: effect on surgical prediction and postsurgical result, J. Oral Maxillofac Surg. **50**(6):562, 1992.

Ewing, M., and Ross, R.B.: Soft tissue response to mandibular advancement and genioplasty, Am. J. Orthod. Dentofac. Orthop. **101**(6):550, 1992.

Fish, L.C., and Epker, B.N.: Diagnosis and treatment planning for the correction of dentafacial deformities, Fort Worth, Texas, 1981, the authors.

Heartwell, C.M., and Rahn, A.O.: Articulators: classification. In Syllabus of complete dentures, ed 2. Philadelphia, 1974, Lea & Febiger.

Kerr, W.J., Miller, S., and Dawber, J.E.: Class III Malocclusion: surgery or orthodontics:? Br. J. Orthod. **19**(1):21, 1992.

McCance, A.M., Moss, J.P., Fright, W.R., James, D.R., and Linney, A.D.: A three dimensional analysis of soft and hard tissue changes following bimaxillary orthognathic surgery in skeletal III patients, Br. J. Oral Maxillofac. Surg. **30**(5):305, 1992.

Nattestad, A., and Vedtofte, P.: Mandibular autorotation in orthognathic surgery: a new method of locating the center of mandibular rotation and determining its consequence in orthognathic surgery, J. Craniomaxillofac. Surg. 20(4):163, 1992.

Neff, C.: The size relationship between the maxillary and mandibular anterior segments of the dental arch, Angle Orthod. **27:**138, 1957.

Profitt, W.R., and White, R.P., Jr.: Who needs surgical-orthodontic treatment? Int. J. Adult Orthodont. Orthognath. Surg. **5**(2):81, 1990.

Profitt, W.R., Epker, B.N., and Hohl, T.A.: Treatment planning for dentofacial deformities. In Bell, W.H., Profitt, W.R., and White, R.P., editors: Surgical correction of dentofacial deformities. Philadelphia, 1981, W.B. Saunders Co.

Ricketts, R.M., et al.: Bioprogressive therapy, Book 1, Denver, 1979, Rocky Mountain Orthodontics.

Ricketts, R.M., et al.: Orthodontic diagnosis and planning, Denver, 1982, Rocky Mountain Orthodontics.

Turvey, T.A., et al.: Surgical-orthodontic treatment planning for simultaneous mobilization of the maxilla and mandible in the correction of dentofacial deformities. Oral Surg. **54:**491, 1982.

White, L.: The clinical use of occlusograms, J. Clin. Orthod. **16:**92, 1982.

that will occur with surgery are discussed, such as, "The lengthening of your lower jaw will bring your teeth together and increase your chin prominence." Moreover, despite previous patient input regarding desired facial esthetic changes, these desires must be illustrated to make certain the type of changes in facial appearance that will occur with the proposed surgery are indeed agreeable to the patient. This point is especially important when the patient has more subtle components of several deformities, such as vertical maxillary excess and mandibular retrusion.

Regarding intermaxillary fixation, the patient should never be guaranteed rigid fixation without intermaxillary fixation. The indications for rigid fixation versus skeletal suspension with intermaxillary fixation should be explained to the patient. The patient should be informed regarding where their particular case fits in the criteria for each and thus, the likelihood of rigid versus a combined approach. (The specific criteria for rigid versus intermaxillary fixation has been discussed in Chapter 2.)

Adjunctive surgical procedures should also be discussed at this time. These may include soft-tissue or skeletal augmentation cosmetic surgery and/or cortical cancellous bone harvests. Soft-tissue and skeletal augmentation cosmetic surgical procedures can enhance the final facial esthetic result or offset unfavorable facial esthetic changes that can accompany certain orthognathic procedures. The esthetic changes accompanying various orthognathic surgeries as described in Chapter 2 should be verbalized to the patient at this time. The soft-tissue and skeletal cosmetic procedures often used in conjunction with orthognathic surgery include malar augmentation, nasal/skeletal base augmentation, buccal lipectomy, and cervical facial lipectomy. Indications, techniques, and potential complications of these procedures are discussed as they are presented in this book.

If the planned orthognathic surgery will require a cortical cancellous or costochondral bone graft, these additional procedures should be outlined to the patient at this time also. The specific need for these additional procedures should be discussed in simple terms such as, "We are moving your upper jaw down and forward and it is best that we use some of your own bone to fill the void created by such movement." Similarly, the explanation of where and how the bone graft will be harvested should also be outlined in nonmedical terms. Indications, techniques, and potential complications of various methods of bone harvest are outlined in Volume III, Section VIII.

Approximately when will the patient be ready for the surgical phase of treatment?

On the basis of the definitive orthodontic-surgical treatment plan that has been developed, the patient is informed approximately when the surgery can be scheduled after the presurgical orthodontics has begun. It is emphasized that this is, at best, a time estimate, yet it does afford the patient some realistic expectations and permits them to plan accordingly. This may even have a bearing on when the patient decides to begin orthodontics. For example, a high school senior who plays basketball and baseball may not want to undergo surgery during these seasons. Accordingly, orthodontics can be initiated at an appropriate time to have it completed either sufficiently before or after these times. However, in this regard the patient is also informed that once the presurgical orthodontics are completed to the point at which surgery can actually be performed, the scheduling of the surgery is still elective and can be done when it is convenient and does not have to interfere with other important events in the patient's life.

What will the patient experience when hospitalized for surgery?

This includes a general discussion of the day-to-day routine the patient will experience while hospitalized for 1 to 2 days. This is done so that the patient and family know what to expect at each juncture and are not surprised by anything that occurs while in the hospital. This includes a discussion of the admitting evaluations, time of the proposed surgery, approximate length of surgery, general anesthesia, recovery room experience, and postoperative convalescence. Positive aspects of the experience are emphasized, such as, "The day after surgery you will be expected to be walking about the hospital and drinking fluids so that you may have your IV line removed." This positive approach helps to reassure the patient.

What will the patient experience after surgery?

This includes a factual estimate of probable length of hospitalization, amount of facial swelling, difficulties with speaking, special diet, time off from school or work, length of intermaxillary fixation if it will be necessary, physical limitations, and what will be experienced on release of intermaxillary fixation.

Realistic untoward sequelae or complications are also discussed. Factors such as numbness of the lips, potential for relapse, temporomandibular joint problems, and possibility of infection are important to include. These complications will vary with each specific surgery and rather than downplay them, it is best the potential risks are discussed openly. The patient will then be pleasantly surprised by normal sequelae.

What will be the costs involved?

Patients are informed that for the surgical phase of their treatment there will be three bills: the hospital's, the anesthesiologist's, and the surgeon's. Realistic estimates of the former two are given to the patient, and a surgical fee is quoted. Generally, the surgical fee is an inclusive one for in-hospital and all postoperative follow-up care for as long as the patient is seen postoperatively.

Desire to speak with previous patients

Certain patients may express this desire, or the surgeon may sense that it would be desirable. In either instance, it is advisable to arrange this without the surgeon being present.

ner in which his/her teeth come together, either with or without a splint in place. Furthermore, the patient is advised that he/she is to immediately return to the surgeon if there is any change in the bite, as occlusal elastics may be required to help control their bite.

JAW PHYSIOTHERAPY

The patient is advised that isometric and isotonic exercises, as described below, may be instituted 3 to 4 weeks postoperatively if limited opening is exhibited at that time.

Release of fixation

For patients in whom intermaxillary fixation was employed, the intermaxillary fixation is released by cutting the interdental and the intermediate skeletal stabilization wires. The occlusal splint, if used, remains secured to the arch to which it was wired intraoperatively. The patient is instructed to begin active jaw opening and protrusive exercises, but no chewing is permitted for 24 to 72 hours, at which time the patient is reevaluated. He/she is informed that during this time the teeth must continue to bite perfectly into the occlusal splint or the existing occlusion when no occlusal splint is used. *No elastics are used during this period because they will only mask relapse.*

When the patient is observed to bite perfectly into the splint or occlusion after the initial 24 to 72 hours, instructions are given to begin more vigorous isometric and isotonic exercises. This is to be done by the patient exercising 4 times daily as follows: first, the mouth is vigorously opened as widely as possible. Next, the patient is to bite into occlusion forcefully, and finally, to protrude the lower jaw as far as possible. While performing these exercises, the patient is given visual objectives regarding the desired interincisal opening and protrusive movements that are consistent with the measurements of their presurgical range of jaw movement. The following is a patient instruction sheet that the authors find helpful to give to all patients after release of intermaxillary fixation.

INSTRUCTIONS FOLLOWING UNWIRING OF THE JAWS

1. Jaw physiotherapy. On removal of the wires that hold your jaws together you are to do jaw exercises that are a combination of isometric and isotonic muscle exercises. These are intended to rapidly restore your jaw muscles to their presurgical function. In order to do this you are to exercise vigorously in front of a mirror for about 5 to 10 minutes at least three times a day. These exercises will not negatively affect your surgical result and are as easy as A, B, C.
    A. Forcefully open your mouth as widely as you can and keep it open for a few seconds.
    B. Place your teeth together and bite down firmly for a few seconds.
    C. Stick your lower jaw forward until your bottom teeth come in front of your upper teeth.

These exercises are to be repeated in sequence. When they are performed properly, usually all of the stiffness will be gone from your jaw within 7 to 10 days following the unwiring of your jaws. You can then discontinue the exercises. Normally one would be able to open wide enough at this point to place approximately three fingers between your upper and lower teeth.

2. *Diet.* During the first 1 to 2 weeks after removal of the wires that held your jaws together, you are *not to chew any foods.* Chewing during this period may displace or move the jaw segments and result in a severe problem, which may not be amenable to correction without additional surgery. However, you may eat foods that do not require chewing, such as mashed potatoes, pudding, jello, cottage cheese, etc.

3. *Observation of your bite.* During this period of jaw exercises and soft diet it is important that both you and your doctor periodically evaluate whether there is any change in your new bite. The manner in which your teeth come together, either with or without the plastic splint, was shown to you on removal of fixation. You must *self-monitor* your new bite several times a day for a few weeks after release of fixation in order to observe any changes.

   If there is any shift in this relationship, you should call your surgeon immediately so he/she can reevaluate your progress and make necessary adjustments. When this regimen of jaw exercises, proper diet, and observation of your bite is followed, it is extremely unusual to have any problems after your surgery. *When it is not followed,* significant problems can result that may not be correctable without additional surgery. If you have any questions about this at any time please do not hesitate to call our office.

About 1 week later, when the patient has resumed essentially a normal range of jaw movement and the teeth continue to bite perfectly into the splint or occlusion, the skeletal suspension wires, if used, are removed under light sedation or local anesthesia. Before removal, the wires are carefully cleaned where they enter the mucosa and are cut beneath the mucosa by forcing it down around the wire. Doing so prevents possible infection and avoids the need to use antibiotics. The patient is instructed to see the orthodontist within the next 48 hours to begin active postsurgical orthodontic finishing procedures. A return to normal masticatory function is gradually and progressively resumed over the subsequent 2 weeks. If at any time the patient does not occlude properly, after release of intermaxillary fixation the specific reason(s) is identified and appropriately managed (Chapter 5).

Lateral cephalometric radiograph

This is obtained to permit the definitive surgical cephalometric prediction tracing to be done and to document the presurgical soft-tissue, skeletal, and dental conditions. This radiograph may be the last progress film made by the orthodontist when no further significant orthodontic changes have occurred before surgery.

Panoramic or periapical radiographs

These are obtained to determine the position of the tooth roots, the surgical access for interdental osteotomies or ostectomies, and the periodontal conditions. The panoramic radiograph is also an excellent tool to aid in assessing the health of the maxillary sinuses, the symmetry of the nasal septum, the position of impacted teeth, the location and course of the inferior alveolar nerves, and the presence of intraosseous jaw pathology.

Properly articulated and mounted models

These are obtained to document further the presurgical occlusion. When indicated, these are duplicated and used to do the definitive model surgery and splint construction. The use of an anatomic articulator with a face-bow transfer is recommended in most cases involving segmental maxillary surgery, asymmetry, or simultaneous two-jaw procedures. Most other surgical procedures can be properly planned from models on a standard articulator and a carefully done surgical prediction tracing.

Immediate postsurgical records

Postsurgical radiographs and exams are made as soon as possible following surgery. Ideally they are made within 24 hours of surgery to identify any problems that need to be addressed while the patient is still hospitalized. They are also used to study and document the results of surgery. When discrepancies not within the surgeon's acceptable parameters of usual postoperative results exist in any of these records, the surgeon must deliberately address these discrepancies (complications) in a logical manner. The identification and management of such complications are discussed in Chapter 5.

The lateral cephalometric radiograph, panoramic radiograph, occlusal examination, and neurosensory examination are routinely made as soon as possible following surgery. These records are then systematically reviewed, and the results of that review are documented in the patient's chart. The specific manner in which each radiograph and clinical examination is done is outlined below.

Lateral cephalometric radiograph

The immediate postsurgical lateral cephalometric radiograph is compared with both the presurgical cephalometric tracing and the surgical prediction tracing. Assessment of the postsurgical result is done by superimposing the surgical prediction tracing atop the immediate postsurgical lateral cephalometric radiograph (Fig. 4-1). This superimposition is best done the same day these records are taken. The following are sequentially examined: (1) actual versus predicted skeletal results, and (2) condyle and mandibular proximal segment positions.

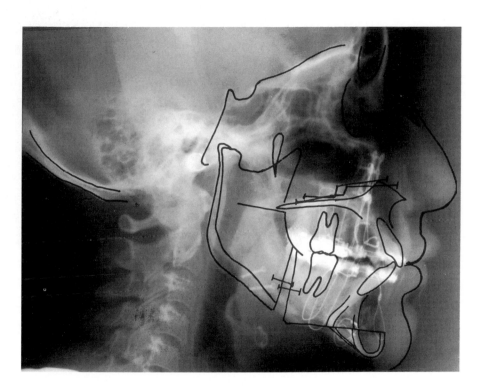

FIG. 4-1

1. Actual versus predicted skeletal results. Objectively comparing the actual versus predicted skeletal result is done by superimposing the prediction tracing atop the immediate postsurgical lateral cephalometric radiograph. Specific note is taken of the vertical and horizontal positions of the maxillary incisor, the occlusal plane, and pogonion. When the surgical result is outside the acceptable limits for the surgeon, the surgeon must logically examine the discrepancy and decide if reoperation is necessary.
2. Condyle and mandibular proximal segment positions. Condyle and mandibular proximal segment positions are reviewed using the aforementioned prediction/radiograph superimposition. Ideally, the proximal seg-

ments in the prediction tracing should closely approximate those in the postsurgical lateral cephalometric radiograph to assure the surgeon that the condyles and proximal segments are in acceptable positions. When the inferior border of the mandible (or proximal segment) on the radiograph lies below that on the tracing, the condyle has been pulled down out of the fossa (Fig. 4-2).

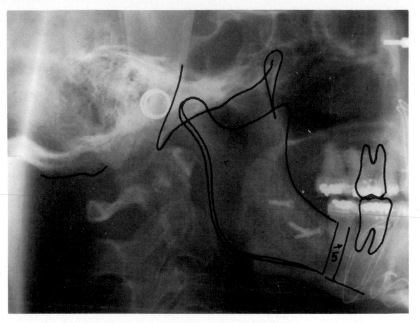

FIG. 4-2

When the posterior borders do not superimpose, there has been unplanned rotation of the mandible or proximal segment (Fig. 4-3). If either or both of these discrepancies exist between the predicted and actual result, the surgeon must decide if the achieved proximal segment position is clinically acceptable.

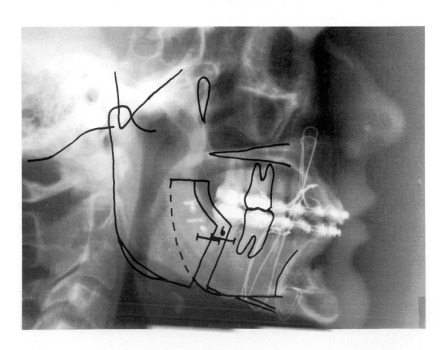

FIG. 4-3

Panoramic radiograph

The immediate postsurgical panoramic radiograph may be used to assess (1) the alveolar bone and teeth adjacent to osteotomies and ostectomies and (2) the status of wires, screws, and plates adjacent to sensory nerves and teeth.

1. Alveolar bone and teeth adjacent to osteotomies and ostectomies. The immediate postsurgical panoramic radiograph is used to assess the proximity of osteotomies and ostectomies to adjacent teeth. Ideally the lamina dura and apices of teeth adjacent to bony cuts should not be compromised. When osteotomies and/or ostectomies encroach on these structures, periodontal complications and/or tooth loss may result.

2. Status of wires, screws, and plates adjacent to sensory nerves and teeth. The status of intraosseous and skeletal suspension wires can be examined by reviewing the immediate postoperative panoramic radiograph. These wires should be tight (relatively straight) with close approximation to the bones around which they are looped. Space between the bone and wire or loops and/or kinks in the wire indicate that the wire is potentially ineffective and may need tightening.

Finally, the panoramic radiograph provides an excellent mechanism for evaluating the proximity of the ramus intraosseous screws to the inferior alveolar nerves. The information gained from a neurosensory exam and the panoramic radiograph can help a surgeon make an informed, deliberate decision regarding the need to remove one or more of these screws.

Clinical examination

An examination of the patient's occlusion and neurosensory status should be made soon after surgery. If rigid fixation is used without intermaxillary fixation, the patient should be able to bite repeatedly into the proper occlusion without significant shifting of the mandible; if the jaw is wired together, the teeth should be in tight approximation to one another without significant mobility.

When the patient is sufficiently alert and oriented following recovery from the general anesthetic, the neurosensory status of the lips and/or chin is evaluated by simple brush stroke discrimination. This may be accomplished by using a cotton-tipped applicator to brush gently the upper lip, lower lip, and/or chin depending on the potential for sensory nerve damage for the specific surgical procedure. Without exception, some decrease in sensation is expected. However, if directional brush stroke discrimination is absent—the patient is *unable* to discern the direction of a cotton-tipped applicator gently brushing the lips and/or chin—significant neurosensory damage is suspected.

Based on the above evaluation of the patient's postsurgical result, the surgeon can make an intelligent decision whether the patient has obtained an acceptable result or may require reoperation. Management of significant discrepancies between the expected result and that actually obtained is discussed in Chapter 5.

Release-of-fixation records

These records are made within a few minutes *after* release of intermaxillary fixation. They allow accurate assessment of the stability of the surgical result and document the occlusion achieved with surgery. Since most surgical relapse occurs during the period of intermaxillary fixation and immediately after release of fixation, these are perhaps the most important records with regard to evaluation of surgically related relapse. When significant problems exist, they must be corrected as discussed in the following chapter.

Lateral cephalometric radiograph

These are traced and compared with the immediate postsurgical cephalometric tracing as soon as possible. Any lack of skeletal stability and any compensatory dental changes are noted *and reported to the orthodontist* so that these factors can be dealt with appropriately during the postsurgical phase of orthodontics.

Photographs of the occlusion

Photographs are used to document the occlusal result achieved by the surgery. They are taken after removal of the occlusal splint and before the patient begins active postsurgical orthodontic treatment.

Postsurgical orthodontic progress records

Progress records may be taken by the orthodontist during the postsurgical phase of orthodontic treatment to monitor treatment progress. They may include one or more of the following.

Lateral cephalometric radiographs

These are taken as needed to check the dental movements that are actually occurring and to determine if the mechanics being employed are producing the desired or planned results. They are also used to evaluate the possible cause of postsurgical problems when compared with the immediate postsurgical and re-lease of fixation cephalometric radiographs to determine skeletal stability.

Panoramic or periapical radiographs

These are taken as needed to check root proximity in the locations where interdental osteotomies or ostectomies were done, to determine root parallelism during finishing, and to watch for any periodontal problems relative to the ortho-dontic mechanics being employed.

Study models

Study models are made to check treatment progress.

Completion-of-treatment records

Completion-of-treatment records are a duplication of the pretreatment records and serve to document the overall effect of the treatment. They are most often taken by the orthodontist at the time of appliance removal and the beginning of retention. These will include facial photographs, photographs of the occlusion, a lateral cephalometric radiograph, panoramic radiograph, and articulated dental models.

Finally, models that are improperly mounted on an articulator due to improper face bow technique or that are improperly related to one another due to the clinician's failure to recognize a significant discrepancy between centric relation and centric occlusion are a major liability in making proper and intelligent treatment planning decisions. Indeed, these inaccuracies produce the same esthetic and occlusal complications described for the improperly obtained cephalometric radiograph.

The techniques for doing surgical cephalometric prediction tracing and definitive model surgery are described in the chapters dealing with treatment of the various deformities. Herein, only the problems that may arise from the inaccurate transfer of the information gained by the prediction tracings and model surgery are addressed.

Transfer of surgical planning to the patient

The disparity between immediate presurgical planning and accurate intraoperative execution of that plan can be illustrated by the inaccurate transfer of reference lines made on the models prior to doing the model surgery to the patients' maxilla or mandible at the time of surgery.

For example, when performing superior repositioning of the maxilla, if the vertical reference lines placed on the maxillary model are oriented perpendicular to Frankfort horizontal and are transferred to the patient in any other orientation (i.e., *not* perpendicular to Frankfort horizontal), the actual surgical result obtained by the clinician who is relying on these vertical reference lines will not be the same as the result obtained on the model surgery. The effect of this loss of orientation is illustrated in Figs. 5-1 to 5-3, which depict a patient for whom a 6-mm

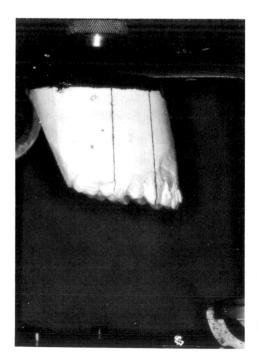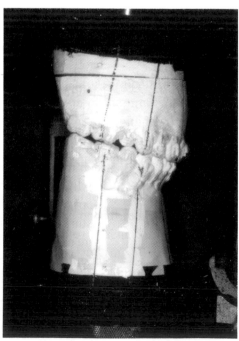

FIG. 5-1

superior repositioning of the maxilla is planned. The vertical reference lines made on the model for model surgery are perpendicular to Frankfort horizontal (Fig. 5-1). At surgery the vertical reference lines made on the patient's lateral maxillary wall are perpendicular to the maxillary occlusal plane (Fig. 5-2). When the sur-

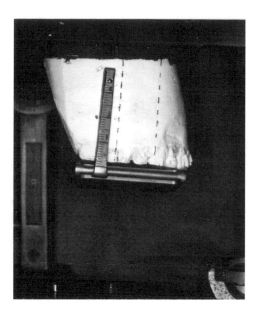

FIG. 5-2

geon subsequently uses the intraoperative vertical reference lines to duplicate the relationship that existed on the model surgery, the maxilla is placed well anterior to the desired position (Fig. 5-3). This error in the angulation of the reference lines would result in producing a Class II occlusion following surgery.

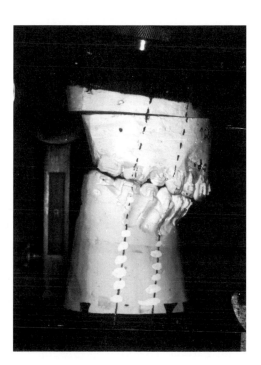

FIG. 5-3

INTEROPERATIVE COMPLICATIONS

The most common interoperative complications are: (1) unplanned fracturing (splitting) of the mandible, (2) damaging tooth roots adjacent to osteotomy sites resulting in ankylosis or periodontal defects, (3) unplanned injury (transection) of the mental or inferior alveolar nerve, (4) bleeding, and (5) difficulty in adequately stabilizing the repositioned osseous segments. These complications and their management are discussed in detail in the subsequent chapters that describe the various surgical procedures.

POSTSURGICAL COMPLICATIONS

Almost all the complications related to surgery occur during the first 2 months following surgery, that is, from immediately after surgery to shortly after completion of osseous healing. Thus, the need for critical evaluation of both the immediate postsurgical records and those at about 6 to 8 weeks (healing) is clear. Because different problems are generally noted to occur at different times following surgery, the following discussion is divided to describe the complications observed and corrected within the first week after surgery, during weeks 2 through 4, and during weeks 5 through 8.

The first week

The following radiographs and clinical exams are essential immediately following surgery.
A. Cephalometric radiograph
    1. Actual versus predicted result
    2. Condylar position
    3. Proximal segment position
B. Panoramic radiograph
    1. Alveolar bone and teeth adjacent to osteotomies or ostectomies
    2. Status of wires, screws, and plates relative to adjacent sensory nerves and teeth
C. Clinical examination
    1. Occlusion
    2. Neurosensory status

Cephalometric radiograph

ACTUAL VERSUS PREDICTED RESULT. To evaluate the actual versus predicted surgical result the cephalometric prediction tracing is superimposed on the immediate postoperative lateral cephalometric radiograph. Importantly, *if the cephalometric prediction tracing is to be a reliable referent, it must be accurately done.* Moreover, the actual postoperative clinical findings must confirm the cephalometric findings.

When a significant discrepancy exists between the cephalometric prediction tracing and the actual result achieved, a decision must be made regarding its relevance to the desired overall result. The discrepancy may be minor and of no significance (i.e., 4 mm of maxillary superior repositioning when 5 mm would have been ideal). However, if it is deemed significant, *the best and easiest time to rectify the problem is immediately.* For this reason, it is recommended that a cephalometric radiograph be obtained and these judgments made the day after surgery, while the patient is still in the hospital. For example, superior repositioning of the maxilla 5 mm in the incisor area was planned for a patient with vertical maxillary excess. However, the immediate postsurgical cephalometric radiograph reveals that the maxillary incisors actually moved 10 mm superiorly. This will result in a serious esthetic compromise, and reoperation with possible bone grafting must be discussed with the patient.

CONDYLAR POSITION. The postsurgical condyle position is evaluated in both the cephalometric and panoramic radiographs. It is difficult to distinguish left and right condyles in the cephalometric radiograph; therefore, while the cephalometric radiograph better illustrates the specific condylar position, the panoramic radiograph helps the surgeon identify the problematic side. The important thing is that the presurgical and immediate postsurgical radiographs demonstrate the same basic relation of the condyles to the fossas and eminences. The condylar position is best evaluated using the prediction tracing/immediate postsurgical lateral cephalometric radiograph superimposition. Any discrepancy in the position of the posterior and/or inferior borders of either the proximal segments of the mandible (mandibular or two-jaw surgery) or the entire mandible (isolated maxillary surgery) are noted and carefully studied. Ideally, the posterior and inferior borders of the mandible in the prediction tracing should superimpose precisely atop those in the postsurgical lateral cephalometric radiograph. When this is the case the surgeon can be certain that the condyles and proximal segments are in acceptable positions. However, if the postoperative lateral cephalometric radiograph shows the posterior border to be *anterior* to that in the prediction tracing and/or the inferior border to be *below* that in the prediction tracing, it is likely that a condyle has been distracted downward and forward out of the glenoid fossa. When this condition is unilateral, the immediate postoperative panoramic radiograph can be used to determine which side has the unfavorably positioned condyle. If a condyle is clearly displaced from the fossas (*diagnose*), the patient should be told (*inform*) and the condyle should be appropriately repositioned (*treat*). This might require only tightening of the skeletal suspension wires in a maxillary surgery case, or it may involve taking the patient back to the operating room and repositioning the condyle. New cephalometric and panoramic radiographs are then taken to determine the success of this treatment (*evaluate*).

PROXIMAL SEGMENT POSITION. Since the sagittal osteotomy is the most frequently done ramus osteotomy, this discussion pertains primarily to this procedure. Ideally, the position of the mandibular proximal segments will be unchanged in the preoperative and immediate postoperative radiographs. Again, this is easily evaluated by superimposing the prediction tracing atop the immediate postoperative cephalometric radiograph. To evaluate proximal segment position, the surgeon evaluates the superimposition of both the posterior and inferior borders of the mandibular proximal segments on the prediction tracing relative to those on the immediate postoperative cephalometric radiograph.

In mandibular advancement patients, if the proximal segment is rotated anteriorly more than 15 degrees, it will result in both an esthetic (loss of mandibular angle definition) and functional compromise (decreased masticatory efficiency occurs because the anterior rotation shortens and adversely reorients the direction of the major muscles of mastication, thereby producing decreased masticatory efficiency, poor chewing capacity, masticatory muscle fatigue, and even muscle pain in some patients). This anterior rotation is evidenced by the postsurgical mandibular posterior border being anterior and the inferior border being superior to the superimposed prediction tracing.

In the mandibular setback patient, if the proximal segment is rotated significantly posteriorly it will increase the propensity for relapse because the stretched muscles of mastication tend to return the proximal segment to its preoperative position, and in so doing, forces the distal mandible forward. This posterior rotation is evidenced by the postsurgical mandibular posterior border being posterior and the inferior border being inferior to the superimposed prediction tracing. When unfavorable proximal segment rotation exists (*diagnose*), the patient should be told of the problem (*inform*) and the proximal segment should be repositioned immediately (*treat*). The result of such repositioning is confirmed radiographically (*evaluate*).

Panoramic radiograph

ALVEOLAR BONE AND TEETH ADJACENT TO OSTEOTOMIES OR OSTECTOMIES. When interdental osteotomies or ostectomies are performed, the adjacent alveolar bone and teeth are evaluated in the postoperative radiographs for two problems: tooth root injury, including damage to the cementum or apex amputation, and possible bony defects in the interdental alveolar bone.

When tooth root injury exists, it can result in loss of a tooth, the need for endodontics, or ankylosis with subsequent inability to move the tooth orthodontically. The treatment decision in this instance is to inform the patient and the orthodontist of the injured tooth (teeth). The involved tooth (teeth) is then more critically evaluated both clinically and radiographically, on release of intermaxillary fixation.

If a defect exists in the crestal bone, it will usually result in either periodontal pathology (pocket) or poor bone healing in this area. The larger the bony defect, the more likely these complications are to occur. The problem is noted, the patient informed, and the defects more critically evaluated after release of fixation. Consultation with a periodontist is recommended in cases in which periodontal pathology is found to exist after release of fixation.

STATUS OF WIRES, SCREWS, AND PLATES RELATIVE TO ADJACENT SENSORY NERVES AND TEETH. When skeletal stabilization is used, the position and tightness of the wires are noted in the postoperative radiographs. They should be reasonably straight without unplanned twists or bends and *their vector should be such that they resist the known vectors of skeletal relapse for the specific deformity that was corrected.*

When bone plates and screws are used to effect stabilization of the maxilla and/or mandible the location of the screws relative to tooth roots and, in the mandible, the inferior alveolar nerve are carefully assessed in the postoperative panoramic radiograph. When the patient's neurosensory testing is unfavorable and bone screws in the mandible appear to encroach on the canal, serious consideration must be given to their immediate removal.

Clinical examination

OCCLUSION. The quality of the attained occlusion is carefully examined regardless of the type of fixation. When intermaxillary fixation is used, the patient is routinely asked at each postoperative visit to try to open the jaws forcefully. If movement occurs, the fixation wires are tightened.

In addition, when an occlusal splint is used, the position of the teeth in the splint is carefully checked. If the teeth are not properly interdigitated into the splint, appropriate wires are adjusted, tightened, or added to correct the problem. Since time has been taken to do model surgery and to make a splint, the teeth should be maintained properly in it during the period of fixation.

When rigid fixation is used it is critical immediately to evaluate the patient's ability to properly bite into good occlusion. This is best evaluated without elastics soon after surgery. When any malocclusion exists, the reason must be sought and immediately rectified.

NEUROSENSORY STATUS. As soon as the patient is alert and oriented following recovery from the general anesthetic, the sensory status of the tissue areas potentially affected by the surgery—lips, chin, etc.—are tested for directional discrimination and the results are recorded. Almost without exception there is a decrease in directional discrimination perception commensurate with a first- or second-degree nerve injury. When directional discrimination is absent (potential third- to fifth-degree injury) nociception testing must follow. Nociception testing involves the use of a sterile 26-gauge needle pricking the skin in the affected area. If the patient has no response to the pinprick, the surgeon must identify the probable cause, which may include a screw in or gross compression of the inferior alveolar nerve. If a screw is radiographically found to be placed in the inferior alveolar canal (*diagnose*), it is immediately documented, the patient informed (*inform*), the screw removed (*treat*), and the patient's neurosensory status monitored as discussed above (*evaluate*).

Weeks 2 through 4

When the immediate postoperative records are critically evaluated and any problems noted therein are appropriately corrected as previously discussed, there are few complications that occur during the period of intermaxillary fixation. Regardless of the method of fixation, skeletal or rigid, the patient is seen within the first 7 to 10 days after discharge from the hospital. At this examination the following features are noted:
1. Presence of proper occlusion
2. Teeth seated in the splint when one is used
3. Tightness of intermaxillary fixation when used
4. Status of incision lines

5. Oral hygiene
6. Level of sensory nerve dysfunction
7. Degree of facial edema
8. Level of general physical activity
9. Level of discomfort
10. Weight loss

Any alteration of these conditions beyond the expected must be noted. This may involve further investigation or may involve such actions as tightening the fixation wires, initiating patient irrigation of an open wound to prevent infection, or additional counseling of the patient regarding diet and weight loss. The important things here are that these factors are all noted and any abnormal findings are appropriately resolved. Patients who were placed in rigid fixation are monitored *without interarch elastics* during these early weekly visits, as wearing of interarch elastics serves to mask potential problems. If unfavorable occlusal changes occur, the reasons for them are diagnosed and appropriate treatment is instituted. Treatment may range from orthodontic compensation for the occlusal discrepancy to reoperation.

Weeks 5 through 8

There are two basic complications that occur during this period—occlusal relapse and failure to resume preoperative range of asymptomatic jaw function. When rigid fixation is used without intermaxilliary fixation, occlusal relapse may be observed earlier, as noted previously. Failure to resume the preoperative range of asymptomatic jaw function may occur in any patient regardless of the method of stabilization.

Occlusal relapse

When proper skeletal stabilization is used and the suspension wires are maintained tight during the period of intermaxillary fixation, relapse is rare unless the condyles were displaced at surgery. This normally is noted in the immediate postoperative radiographs and corrected at that time.

Regardless of the method of fixation, physical therapy is begun at about 3 to 5 weeks after surgery. At this time the patient is instructed in stretching the jaw (interincisal opening), clenching the teeth, and protruding the jaw and is seen again in 1 day. (The splint, if used, is left wired to the maxillary or mandibular teeth depending on the type of surgery performed.) The patient is instructed to *chew no foods* and told why this is important. *No elastics are used.* On reevaluation the following day the patient must be able to bite precisely into the splint or proper occlusion, indicating no skeletal relapse. If this is the case, the patient makes another appointment for 1 week later and is informed that if at any time before this appointment he/she is unable to bite properly into the splint, he/she is to call for an immediate appointment.

On reevaluation in 1 week, if the patient does not bite into the splint, the reason is ascertained (posterior occlusal interference versus relapse) and appropriate measures are taken. If relapse appears to be occurring at any time from 1 day to 1 week after release of fixation, complete new records are obtained and evaluated to determine the specific cause. Once the cause is known the appropriate measures to rectify the problem are instituted and progress is carefully monitored.

Failure to resume a full range of asymptomatic jaw function

Approximately 3 to 5 weeks after surgery, patients are instructed to initiate jaw exercises in front of a mirror for about 5 minutes at least three times a day. A measure of the preoperative interincisal opening is given to the patient, and the patient is informed that this opening is to be reachieved within 7 to 10 days after initiation of this jaw physiotherapy regimen. The patient is likewise instructed to perform protrusive exercises. Heat, massage, and nonsteroidal antiinflammatory drugs are recommended for stiff muscles. If the pretreatment interincisal opening is not achieved after 2 weeks of the active jaw physiotherapy regimen, passive physiotherapy is instituted.

Passive physiotherapy enlists the patient's fingers as an aid to opening. The same maneuvers as previously described are continued, except the patient now uses manual assistance to help reach the desired level of jaw function. As long as improvement is seen, it is best to allow the patient to continue. However, if the patient demonstrates an inability to achieve acceptable jaw function after instituting passive physiotherapy, the reason for failure must be diagnosed and addressed. Possible causes include lack of compliance, unusually prominent scars, or possible anterior displacement of the temporomandibular joint disk.

When the clinician determines that the restricted opening is likely the result of an anteriorly displaced temporomandibular joint disk, a pumping arthrocentesis is recommended as soon as the diagnosis is made. This is performed with the patient sedated and the affected joint anesthetized with 2 ml of 2% lidocaine without epinephrine. A 10-ml syringe filled with lactated Ringer's solution without epinephrine is then used to apply rhythmic hydraulic pressure to the upper joint space. This may be followed by deliberate manual brisement of the jaw. Passive physical therapy in and of itself does not result in a normal range of jaw movement. Following this, aggressive active and passive physiotherapy is continued for 1 or 2 additional weeks. If jaw opening remains limited an open arthroplasty may be indicated.

LONG-TERM COMPLICATIONS

Complications during the postsurgical orthodontic phase of treatment can be purely orthodontic or can be related directly to the surgery. The following discussion pertains to the problems directly related to surgery because a discussion of routine orthodontic complications is beyond the scope of this book. The majority of surgically related complications occur before this time in treatment and should have been noted and corrected previously. However, three specific areas of surgically related complications deserve further comment: (1) those related to surgical skeletal relapse, (2) those related to the interdental osteotomies or ostectomies, and (3) those related to the use of rigid fixation.

Complications related to surgical skeletal relapse

These complications are becoming much less frequent due to improved surgical techniques, use of skeletal stabilization, attention to the factors evaluated in the immediate postsurgical records, and observation of the patient during the period of intermaxillary fixation. Currently, surgical skeletal relapse either does not occur or is so minimal that appropriate postsurgical orthodontic treatment can easily and quickly correct any associated occlusal change.

However, a major complication can occur when dental fixation is used and there is skeletal relapse during the period of intermaxillary fixation. With the teeth tightly wired together, this skeletal relapse acts as an orthodontic force and 6 to 8 weeks of unplanned orthodontic tooth movement occurs. (This same phenomenon occurs when elastics are used during the period of healing in patients who have rigid fixation.) This usually involves significant extrusion of the anterior teeth or movements of all the teeth within one or both arches either anteriorly or posteriorly. After release of fixation, this "orthodontic" movement tends to relapse (reverse itself) to varying degrees as noted by the tendency for loss of the surgically attained occlusion. When this occurs, careful study of the immediate postsurgical records and release-of-fixation records allows the *degree of skeletal relapse* to be assessed. When it is minimal, elastic therapy (vertical, Class II, or Class III) will usually correct the problem. If orthodontic correction is attempted, *a reasonable time referent must be established to determine its feasibility*. If the orthodontic treatment has continually effected a positive change during the ensuing 2 to 3 months and the orthodontist believes the problems can be resolved with stable results, the orthodontic treatment is continued. If, on the other hand, there is either no measurable improvement or continued worsening of the occlusion despite appropriate orthodontic mechanics, it is advisable to reverse orthodontically the dental compensations that have been produced following the initial surgery and to reoperate.

The second major complication occurs when after surgery the condyles are out of their fossas by a significant amount. When dental intermaxillary fixation is used, relapse occurs as described in the preceding section. If skeletal fixation is used, relapse will usually become evident immediately on release of intermaxillary fixation as the condyles rapidly return to their fossa, acutely producing a Class II open-bite malocclusion. (A gradual return of the condyles to the fossa has occasionally been noted, particularly in patients who habitually postured their mandible forward before treatment.) When this occurs, despite appropriate orthodontic treatment, the occlusion progressively worsens. Reoperation is generally the only solution when this problem exists to a significant degree as determined by careful study of the records.

Complications related to interdental osteotomies

Two problems can occur following interdental osteotomies. First, one or more teeth adjacent to the surgical site may become ankylosed. Second, an interdental space present following the release of fixation may continue to reopen after it is closed orthodontically.

Ankylosed teeth are dealt with just as any other ankylosis. When the tooth is in an acceptable position, postsurgical orthodontic treatment may be completed and the ankylosed tooth restoratively modified as required to achieve the desired occlusal result. When the tooth prevents satisfactory completion of treatment, it may need to be extracted and replaced by a fixed prosthesis following the completion of treatment.

An interdental space that persists during the postsurgical orthodontic treatment is usually the result of a poorly planned or executed osteotomy, in which sufficient bone-to-bone contact in the alveolar area was not present following surgery and fibrous tissue fills the void during healing. The teeth adjacent to this space can be pulled together orthodontically, but they move apart rapidly when pressure is released. When esthetics is not a problem, the space can be left and the patient instructed to clean the area carefully so that a significant periodontal problem does not result. When the space creates an esthetic problem, the teeth can be approximated and splinted together or they can be brought into contact by crowning, placing facings, or bonding.

Complications related to rigid fixation
Neurosensory injury

Hardware used in the fixation of mandibular dentoosseous segments may injure the inferior alveolar nerve, thereby compromising the sensory perception from the lower lip and/or chin. Permanent sensory loss may occur if neurosensory injury caused by an intraosseous screw is ignored or not recognized early in the postoperative phase. When such a screw is present for a long time postoperatively (more than 6 weeks) it still should be removed and the neurosensory return monitored. If the degree of neurosensory return is unsatisfactory to the patient, he or she may elect to undergo a surgical exploration to investigate the injured site directly. Repair may involve a simple nerve decompression, or possibly a nerve graft. The specifics of such surgery are beyond the scope of this book, and the reader may refer to the bibliography at the end of this chapter for a more complete review of this subject.

Loose or exposed hardware

Plates and/or screws may become exposed a long time after surgery subsequent to an unrelated facial injury or dental infection. Additionally, hardware that has become even slightly mobile may result in an inflammatory response that causes swelling over the offending hardware or even partial exfoliation of the mobile fixation component. Hardware causing such a problem should be removed and such may often be done using only local anesthesia.

Temporomandibular joint condylar resorption

Condylar resorption is one form of late surgical relapse that is presumed to result from excessive loading of the joint structure. If improperly used for securing the proximal and distal mandibular segments, either positional or lag screws can result in excessive condylar torque and/or changes in intercondylar distance beyond the limits of normal remodeling. The excessive condylar loads thus produced can result in condylar resorption with subsequent development of a Class II occlusion with an anterior open bite over the first few years after treatment.

RECURRENT COMPLICATIONS

One final comment must be made before leaving the subject of complications. Having an occasional complication and dealing with it is part of the combined orthodontic-surgical correction of dentofacial deformities. However, in an effort to improve our treatment of these patients and avoid complications, the most important action to be taken is to *pay particular attention to any complication that becomes routine.* When the same problem is repeatedly noted, critical evaluation of the techniques that are being employed is mandatory. If an orthodontist continually has difficulty intruding lower incisors with a utility arch, the forces being used must be assessed to note if they are excessive or insufficient, and the form of the wire must be reviewed to determine if its anterior portion has the necessary labial root torque and its buccal portion is formed to avoid gingival impingement. If a surgeon notes that the condyles are routinely displaced from the fossas in the same direction following superior repositioning of the maxilla, he/she must evaluate, for example, whether the models are mounted properly on an anatomic articulator by the face-bow transfer, whether the cephalometric prediction tracings are being properly done, or whether the reference marks made on the models are properly transferred to the patient. When a defect is found in technique, the technique must be modified to correct that problem and the results of such a modification carefully and critically evaluated until the complication is no longer routine. Great care must be taken in making these changes in technique so that overcompensation and subsequent error in the opposite direction does not take place.

Specific records and meaningful use of them is critical to improve treatment results in the correction of dentofacial deformities. The intent here is not to give detailed descriptions of all possible complications and the methods to deal with each, for that would entail a book in itself. Rather, it is intended to convey a method that may be used in dealing with complications that all clinicians will experience from time to time. This method involves the use of records taken at the proper time to allow the clinician to *diagnose* the specific nature of the complications and to *inform* the patient of such. *Treatment* is then based on this diagnosis, and progress is carefully *evaluated* until the overall orthodontic surgical treatment is successfully completed.

REFERENCES

Aragon, S.B., Van Sickles, J.E, Dolwick, M.F., et al.: The effects of orthognathic surgery in mandibular range of motion, J. Oral Maxillofac. Surg. **43:**938, 1985.

Buckley, M.J, Tulloch, J.F.C., White, R.P., Jr., et al.: Complications of orthognathic surgery: a comparison between wire fixation and rigid internal fixation, Int. J. Adult Orthodont. Orthognath. Surg. **4:**69, 1989.

Epker, B.N., and LaBanc, J.P.: Orthognathic surgery: management of postoperative complications, Oral Maxillofac. Surg. Clin. North Am. **2**(4):901, 1990.

Ghali, G.E., and Epker, B.N.: Clinical neurosensory testing: practical applications, J. Oral Maxillofac. Surg. **47:**1074, 1989.

Gregg, J.M.: Post-traumatic trigeminal neuralgia: response to physiologic, surgical and pharmacologic therapies, Int. Dental J. **23:**43, 1978.

Lanigan, D.T., Hey, J.H., and West, R.A.: Hemorrhage following mandibular osteotomies: a report of 21 cases, J. Oral Maxillofac. Surg. **49**(7):713, 1991.

Lanigan, D.T., Hey, J.H., and West, R.A.: Major vascular complications of orthognathic surgery: false aneurysms and arteriovenous fistulas following orthognathic surgery, J. Oral Maxillofac. Surg. **49**(6):571, 1991.

Lanigan, D.T., Hey, J.H., and West, R.A.: Major vascular complications of orthognathic surgery: hemorrhage associated with Le Fort I osteotomies, J. Oral Maxillofac. Surg. **48**(6):561, 1990.

Nattestad, A., Vedtofte, P.: Pitfalls in orthognathic model surgery, Int. J. Oral Maxillofac. Surg. **23:**11, 1994.

Nishioka, G.J., Zysset, M.K., and Van Sickels, J.E.: Neurosensory disturbances with rigid fixation of the bilateral sagittal split osteotomy, J. Oral Maxillofac. Surg. **45:**20, 1987.

Nitzan, D.W., and Dolwick, M.F.: Temporomandibular joint fibrous ankylosis following orthognathic surgery: report of eight cases, Int. J. Adult Orthodont. Orthognath. Surg. **4:**7, 1989.

O'Ryan, F.: Complication of orthognathic surgery, Oral Maxillofac. Clin. North Am. **2**(3):593, 1990.

Phillips, R.M., and Bell, W.H.: Atrophy of mandibular condyles after sagittal ramus split osteotomy: report of case, J. Oral Surg. **36:**45, 1978.

Will, L.A., Joondeph, R., West, R.A., et al.: Condylar position following mandibular advancement: its relationship to relapse, J. Oral Maxillofac. Surg. **42:**578, 1984.

Wylie, G.A., and Epker, B.N.: Control of the condylar-proximal mandibular segments after sagittal split osteotomy to advance the mandible, Oral Surg. Oral Med. Oral Pathol. **62:**613, 1986.

Zaytoun, H.S., Phillips, C., and Terry, B.C.: Long term neurosensory deficits following transoral vertical ramus and sagittal split osteotomies for mandibular prognathism, J. Oral Maxillofac. Surg. **44:**193, 1986.

SECTION II CLASS II DENTOFACIAL DEFORMITIES

ESTHETIC CONSIDERATIONS WITHIN THE CLASS II PATIENT POPULATION

Section II, Class II Dentofacial Deformities, is composed of four chapters: Chapter 6, Class II Dentofacial Deformities Secondary to Mandibular Deficiency; Chapter 7, Class II Dentofacial Deformities Secondary to Vertical Maxillary Excess; Chapter 8, Class II Dentofacial Deformities Secondary to Vertical Maxillary Excess and Mandibular Deficiency; and Chapter 9, Class II Dentofacial Deformities with Open Bite. The three subgroups of the skeletal Class II deformity—mandibular deficiency, vertical maxillary excess, and their combination—are distinguished by virtue of their varied facial esthetic features and cephalometric findings, *not* by their occlusions. These esthetic and cephalometric features are used to determine the indicated corrective surgery. The treatment plan is not based to a major extent on the chin position, since this is easily corrected by an advancement genioplasty. *The decision to operate on the mandible, maxilla, or both jaws is based primarily on the vertical and anteroposterior position of the maxillary incisors.*

When the maxillary incisors are within the normal esthetic parameters outlined in Chapter 1, the patient has a Class II dentofacial deformity, and there is no open-bite malocclusion, the primary corrective surgery is generally bilateral sagittal split ramus osteotomies to advance the mandible, either with or without a genioplasty. Chapter 6 addresses this patient population.

When the maxillary incisor exposure is vertically excessive—greater than 3 to 4 mm in repose—the patient has increased length of the lower third face, and the patient has expressed esthetic concerns regarding these conditions, a LeFort I ostectomy is generally indicated to reposition the maxilla and the maxillary incisors into a normal vertical position. The anteroposterior position of the maxillary incisors is normalized at the same time as dictated by the esthetic relationships in the nasal, paranasal, and upper lip areas. After accomplishing this by cephalometric prediction tracing, if the mandible can be autorotated into an acceptable occlusal relation to the maxilla (± 2 or 3 mm), then the patient requires only maxillary surgery with or without a genioplasty, as discussed in Chapter 7. However, if the mandible must be advanced to occlude properly with the maxilla when the maxilla is placed into an esthetically normal vertical and anteroposterior position, simultaneous mandibular ramus surgery, with or without genioplasty, is indicated, as described in Chapter 8.

The presence of an open-bite malocclusion may require special treatment considerations; treatment for this condition is discussed in Chapter 9. An esthetic consideration unique to the Class II open-bite patient is that frequently the vertical relation of the upper incisors to the upper lip is within normal limits. When this is true *and the patient has a long lower third face*, the primary surgical procedure is designed to superiorly reposition the posterior maxilla more than the anterior, the vertical length of the lower third face is made normal by the autorotation of the mandible, and the chin position is normalized as necessary with a genioplasty and/or simultaneous mandibular advancement. When the patient *does not have a vertically long lower third face*, the correction of the open bite can, in select cases, be done by a mandibular advancement if special attention is given to specific technical aspects of the surgery.

OCCLUSAL CONSIDERATIONS FOR THE CLASS II PATIENT POPULATION

The arrangement of the teeth within the dental arches of the Class II patient is manifest in a number of variations. There may be no crowding, extreme crowding, or mild to moderate crowding. There may be normal overbite, deep overbite, or open bite. There may be a maxillary arch that is narrow, about right, or too wide relative to the mandibular arch. Each of these may require different orthodontic and surgical considerations.

Arch-width considerations

There are five generally accepted methods to correct arch-width problems: orthopedic maxillary expansion, orthodontic dental tipping, surgical mandibular narrowing, surgically assisted maxillary expansion, and surgical maxillary expansion. All of these have a place in the treatment of the Class II patient, but which is most appropriate depends on the magnitude of the problem, the age of the patient, and the orthognathic surgical procedure(s) indicated for the patient.

Surgical correction of a transverse problem is generally done when the magnitude of the problem is more than 4 mm and the primary surgical approach is to be in the maxilla. The maxilla is segmentalized into two, three, or four pieces at surgery and is expanded or constricted (rarely) as need be to fit the mandibular dentition (see Chapters 7, 8, and 9). The remaining four procedures are most frequently done in conjunction with correction of mandibular deficiency.

Orthopedic maxillary expansion is done when the transverse discrepancy is symmetric, greater than 4 mm, and the patient is *less* than 18 years of age. This is routine orthodontic practice and is not discussed in this book. After age 18, orthopedic maxillary expansion is best avoided as it frequently is not orthopedic, but involves extreme dental tipping, alveolar bending, and even the movement of teeth buccally through the buccal cortical plate. As such, relapse and/or severe periodontal problems are generally encountered. Rather, after age 18 when such expansion is desirable, surgically assisted maxillary expansion is done as described in the second approach discussed in Chapter 6.

If the transverse discrepancy is 4 to 6 mm at the molar and decreases in magnitude anteriorly, it can be corrected by surgically narrowing the mandible as it is being advanced (third approach discussed in Chapter 6). When the transverse discrepancy is accompanied by an anterior tooth mass discrepancy that requires extraction of a lower incisor, the entire mandible can be narrowed by removing a lower incisor and doing a midline ostectomy (also in the third approach discussed in Chapter 6).

When the transverse discrepancy is 4 mm or less, it can be corrected by routine orthodontic movement. It is assumed that this is indeed the case in the description of the three "usual" approaches in Chapter 6.

Overbite considerations

Some Class II patients have an anterior open bite. Only those rare open-bite patients with very specific and uncommon facial morphology are best corrected by mandibular advancement alone (third alternate approach discussed in Chapter 9). More commonly, for reasons of esthetics and stability, these patients are not treated by mandibular advancement, but rather by segmental maxillary superior repositioning (usual and first alternate approaches discussed in Chapter 9) or by simultaneous maxillary superior repositioning and mandibular advancement (second alternate approach discussed in Chapter 9).

Patients considered for correction of their Class II malocclusion by mandibular advancement usually have an overbite ranging from normal to extreme. When the deep bite is so extreme that leveling by usual orthodontic means is impossible, one or both arches can be treated segmentally and leveled surgically (fourth adjunctive approach or first alternate approach discussed in Chapter 6).

Patients with deep-bite Class II malocclusions *and short lower third face height* would benefit esthetically from leveling of their occlusal planes primarily by extrusion of the premolars and molars. Such is usually not possible by routine orthodontic treatment, as the muscular forces generated by these patients preclude the desired result. These patients can sometimes best be treated by placing a lingual bar of splint that engages only the incisors and terminal molars at surgery and using vertical elastics during fixation to produce the desired leveling by extrusion of the teeth in the buccal segments. This approach is discussed as part of the immediate presurgical planning (second usual approach discussed in Chapter 6).

More frequently the arches can be leveled orthodontically either by intrusion of incisors, or a combination of incisor intrusion, and premolar extrusion. Such is considered to be the case in the discussion of the "usual" approaches in Chapter 6.

Tooth mass/arch length considerations

The discrepancy between the tooth mass and arch length can vary in the Class II patient from none to extreme. Certainly when there is extreme crowding (<7 mm) extraction is the treatment of choice. Not doing so would require expansion of the dental arches beyond any reasonable expectation of stability and would generally require an increase in the existing dental compensation to the malocclusion—a treatment technique that is to be avoided from the standpoint of both stability and facial esthetics.

When no crowding exists it is difficult to rationalize extracting teeth unless the maxillary incisors are so prominent that not doing so would produce a double protrusion. When the usual dental compensations exist (protrusion of the lower incisors, retrusion of the upper incisors) and there is no periodontal reason to retract the lower anterior teeth, an esthetic chin projection can be produced more easily by surgical augmentation in concert with a smaller mandibular advancement than by retracting the lower anterior teeth and doing a larger advancement (second usual approach discussed in Chapter 6).

Thus, the question of extraction versus nonextraction exists only for the patient with dental compensations and mild to moderate crowding. Carefully done orthodontic-surgical prediction tracings (Chapter 2) are invaluable in planning treatment for these patients. Doing so will allow the clinician to explore different treatment options (extraction, interproximal recontouring, nonextraction) to decide which will most predictably produce the best result. It should be noted that the orthodontic concept of avoiding extractions because the patient has a deep bite is not applicable here because mandibular advancement surgery alters the forces of occlusion such that deep-bite relapse does not occur. While nonextraction treatment is not uncommon, extraction treatment is still most common due to crowding and the desire to reduce or eliminate the existing dental compensations (first usual approach discussed in Chapter 6).

Class II dentofacial deformities secondary to mandibular deficiency

The usual orthodontic-surgical approaches:

- *MANDIBULAR ADVANCEMENT*
- *MANDIBULAR ADVANCEMENT WITH ADVANCEMENT GENIOPLASTY*
- *THE CLASS II, DIVISION 2*

Introduction

The orthodontic surgical correction of the Class II dentofacial deformity secondary to mandibular deficiency is discussed in this chapter. For such patients the maxilla and maxillary incisors are within normal vertical and anteroposterior esthetic parameters. The patient has deficient chin projection, a Class II malocclusion, and no open bite (see Chapter 9). The usual surgical approach for correcting this deformity is bilateral sagittal split ramus osteotomies with or without an advancement genioplasty. The decision to include a genioplasty is based on the facial esthetics and patient's desires.

The adjunctive surgical procedures described in the second section of this chapter may be useful to produce the desired result when the malocclusion involves more than the usual anteroposterior discrepancy. These procedures include reduction genioplasty, orthodontic-surgical expansion of the maxilla, midsymphysis osteotomy (ostectomy) to narrow the mandible, and anterior mandibular subapical ostectomy to level an extreme curve of Spee.

The alternative surgical approaches described in the final section of this chapter are useful when certain unusual circumstances exist as described in the "contingency statement," which introduces the approach. These approaches include total subapical mandibular advancement and inferior repositioning of the maxilla with mandibular advancement.

First usual orthodontic-surgical approach: the patient with moderate overbite and moderate to severe crowding and/or dental compensations

MANDIBULAR ADVANCEMENT

Outline of treatment

Presurgical orthodontic treatment

1. Extract $\frac{5 \mid 5}{4 \mid 4}$
2. Place lower appliances, utility arch; begin lower canine retraction
3. Place upper appliances, align and level; begin upper molar advancement
4. Place Class III elastics as necessary
5. Finish lower canine retraction
6. Retract lower incisors
7. Coordinate arches
8. Records to determine the feasibility of surgery

Immediate presurgical planning

1. Surgical cephalometric prediction tracing
2. Model surgery
3. Occlusal splint construction as indicated

Orthognathic reconstructive surgery

1. Modified sagittal split ramus osteotomies

Postsurgical orthodontic treatment

1. Repair appliances as necessary
2. Check archwire coordination
3. Routine finishing procedures
4. Retain

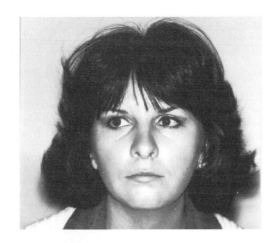

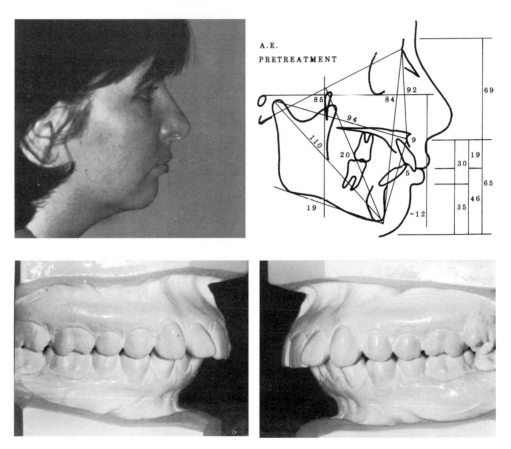

FIG. 6-1

Details of treatment

Presurgical orthodontic treatment

The first thing that is done for this patient is to mark on the chart, in a very conspicuous manner, that he/she is a surgical patient. This notifies the orthodontist, and more importantly the orthodontist's staff, that *this patient is not to receive routine treatment for their Class II malocclusion.* In addition, the visual treatment objectives are clearly illustrated on the chart, noting the desired presurgical dental movements. This information is taken from the orthodontic-surgical prediction tracing and allows the presurgical goals and anchorage requirements to be noted by simply glancing at the chart. Finally, a step-by-step plan to achieve these goals is written on the chart for reference (Fig. 6-2).

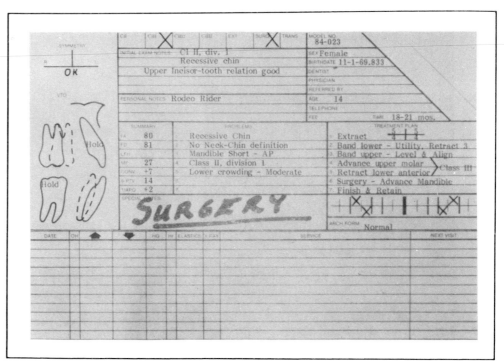

FIG. 6-2

The goal of presurgical orthodontic treatment is to place the teeth in their normal relation to the respective basal bones by removing the dental compensations to the existing skeletal deformity. In the Class II patient, this will usually involve intruding and retracting the lower incisors and advancing the upper molars (Fig. 6-3). This will increase the severity of the Class II occlusion. When the face is symmetric at the beginning of treatment, it is important that the magnitude of the Class II occlusion is equal on both sides and the dental midlines are coincident with the midline of the face to avoid the production of an asymmetric chin

PRETREATMENT POSITION ——————
DESIRED POSITION – – – – – –

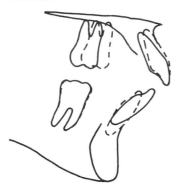

FIG. 6-3   NEEDED PRESURGICAL DENTAL MOVEMENT

when the mandible is advanced. Leveling, aligning, and arch coordination are done before surgery by standard approaches. Certainly not all patients will require extractions, but when moderate crowding exists with moderate dental compensations, no viable alternative exists. Treatment considerations when extractions are not necessary are discussed as the second usual approach, below. The following is the sequence of treatment when extractions are necessary.

The lower arch usually requires more time for presurgical preparation; thus, following appropriate separation, the appliances are placed on the lower teeth at the first banding appointment. Initial archwires consist of the following:

1. Stabilizing utility arch: a 16 × 16 archwire with labial root torque for the incisors, but without the molar tip backs used for incisor intrusion. (A standard utility arch with molar tip backs is used when incisor intrusion is desired.)

2. Buccal sectionals: 16 × 22 multistranded or other suitably flexible wire to level and align the posterior teeth from second molar through canine (Fig. 6-4). Elastic thread, power chain, etc. may be beneficial at this time in helping to resolve rotations or in beginning actual retraction of the canine teeth.

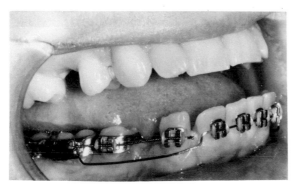
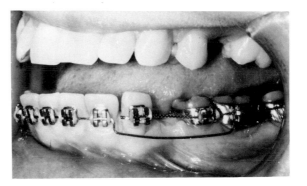

FIG. 6-4

The final presurgical phase is to coordinate the arch forms. This is done by placing continuous, coordinated archwires of increasing size until the desired arch form is achieved. Placing removable lingual arches with appropriate torque and width adjustments can also be helpful in producing arch coordination. When the clinician believes that coordination has been achieved, impressions are taken and feasibility model surgery is performed (Fig. 6-9).

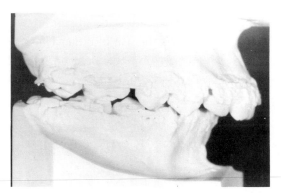 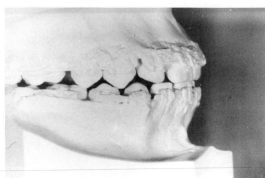

FIG. 6-9

When this model surgery reveals a problem, the archwires are adjusted and new impressions are made at subsequent visits until the orthodontist is pleased with the results achieved. It is not necessary for all teeth to fit one another perfectly, rather it is important to produce an occlusion at surgery that can be easily finished by routine orthodontic treatment. The primary goals are to achieve a Class I molar and canine relation without significant transverse or vertical problems. When these goals have been achieved, the patient is ready for surgery. The archwires are tied with ligature wires to prevent inadvertent disengagement of the wires, hooks are placed where desired (usually the canine teeth), and the patient is referred for surgery. When these goals have not been achieved, the following factors must be carefully studied and appropriate steps taken to remedy the problems.

1. *Tooth mass discrepancy*. Failure to note a preexisting tooth mass problem will preclude achieving a good Class I canine relationship. Either space is opened distal to the upper lateral incisors, or appropriate interproximal recontouring of the lower incisors is done to eliminate this problem.
2. *Lower incisor angulation*. Failure to upright the lower incisors adequately may produce a false tooth mass discrepancy by moving the contact points gingivally, thus increasing the effective mesiodistal width of the incisors and canines (Fig. 6-10).

**UPRIGHT
LOWER ANTERIORS**

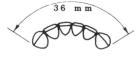

Contacts
Near Incisal Edge

**FLARED
LOWER ANTERIORS**

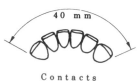

Contacts
More Gingivally

FIG. 6-10

3. *Leveling.* When the arches have not been sufficiently leveled, the excess overbite will either preclude achieving good canine and molar interdigitation, or it will create an open-bite in the premolar/first molar area. In the latter instance, if the final facial esthetic results will not be compromised by so doing, one may elect to proceed with surgery and use the "lingual bar" occlusal split with vertical elastics during fixation to rapidly effect leveling of the arches (see second usual approach, below).

4. *Transverse discrepancy.* When there is a transverse problem at this time and none was recognized before beginning treatment, one of two things has generally occurred. Either there was a transverse problem that was not recognized before beginning treatment, or the original arch width was not maintained. In the former instance, when the discrepancy is less than 6 mm, surgical narrowing of the mandible may be effective (see third adjunctive approach, below). If the discrepancy is greater than 6 mm, maxillary expansion must be considered (see second adjunctive approach, below). When either arch has been inadvertently expanded, a constricted removable lingual arch with lingual crown torque will simply and quickly resolve the problem.

The decision to proceed with surgery is made by obtaining new progress models and performing feasibility model surgery on them to determine its plausibility. When the model surgery permits surgical achievement of a Class I canine occlusion with acceptable overbite and overjet, and no posterior transverse problems, it is considered appropriate to proceed with surgery. The decision to proceed with surgery must be conjointly made by the surgeon and orthodontist, for the orthodontist must decide whether the surgically achievable occlusion can readily be finished after surgery or if it will present orthodontic problems that are best resolved before surgery. If it is elected to proceed with surgery, a new cephalometric radiograph is obtained and used as described in the following section.

Immediate presurgical planning

Definitive immediate presurgical planning is done after completing the necessary presurgical orthodontic treatment and after determining that the patient is ready for surgery by performing feasibility model surgery. This planning involves (1) making a surgical cephalometric prediction tracing, (2) performing definitive model surgery, and, when indicated, (3) constructing a surgical occlusal splint. Indispensable information that influences the precision and stability of surgery is gained from these steps.

The surgical cephalometric prediction tracing is made from a cephalometric radiograph obtained after the presurgical orthodontic treatment has been completed. Its purpose is to plan the details of the surgical movement, the method of fixation (rigid, semirigid, skeletal suspension), the intraosseous wire or screw positions, the necessity and magnitude of adjunctive procedures such as genioplasty, and soft-tissue cosmetic improvements.

The definitive model surgery is performed on models obtained at the time that the aforementioned cephalometric radiograph is made. It may be done on either a Class II, type I articulator (arbitrary hinge type) or a Class II, type III articulator (anatomic, adjustable type), depending on the specific type of surgery to be performed. This may be identical to the feasibility model surgery when the definitive model surgery need not be done on an anatomic articulator. Such is the case for most *symmetric* Class II dentofacial deformities secondary to mandibular deficiency.

SURGICAL CEPHALOMETRIC PREDICTION TRACING FOR MANDIBULAR ADVANCEMENT

Unlike the combined orthodontic-surgical prediction tracings discussed in detail in Chapter 2, the surgeon is bound by the position of the teeth that has been produced by the presurgical orthodontic treatment. As such, the surgical cephalometric prediction tracings are more simply and directly done. These prediction tracings provide much of the essential information required to perform the surgery properly. Furthermore, by superimposing the prediction tracing on the cephalometric radiograph obtained immediately following surgery the accuracy of the surgical changes can be studied. Significant discrepancies between the predicted and actual result may warrant additional surgical intervention before the patient leaves the hospital (Chapter 5).

The surgery is to be modified sagittal split osteotomies for mandibular advancement. As in all mandibular advancement patients a determination will be made regarding the need for and, if necessary, the magnitude of an advancement genioplasty.

The usual anatomic structures are traced from the presurgical cephalometric radiograph. Frankfort horizontal and subnasale perpendicular are constructed on this tracing as are the following surgical reference marks:

1. A line across the ramus parallel to and 3 to 5 mm above the mandibular occlusal plane (just above the lingula).
2. A line just distal to the mandibular second molar and perpendicular to the occlusal plane. (In large advancements this line may be between the first and second molars.)
3. A line crossing the above vertical line, parallel to and approximately 15 to 20 mm below the occlusal plane.
4. Two dots on the above horizontal line 10 mm apart, one on either side of the vertical line (no. 2 above).

5. A genioplasty line approximately 30 mm below the occlusal plane (below the mental foramina) and as parallel to the occlusal plane as possible. The angle this line makes with Frankfort horizontal will affect the vertical facial height as the genioplasty segment is advanced. If it is angled down anteriorly, the facial height will be increased; upward anteriorly, the facial height will be decreased. Moreover, the more this osteotomy is angled upward, the more uneven will be the inferior border of the mandible.

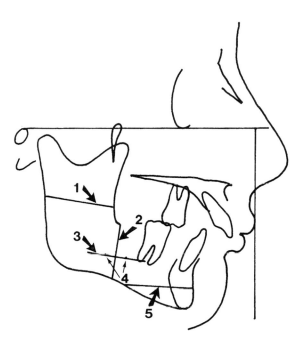

FIG. 6-11

Reference line no. 1 corresponds to the horizontal osteotomy of the sagittal split. Reference line no. 2 corresponds to the vertical osteotomy of the sagittal split. References 3 and 4 are constructed on the lateral aspect of the mandible at surgery. These reference marks are used as an aid in properly positioning the proximal segment and condyle intraoperatively by duplicating the changes determined from the prediction tracing. Reference line no. 5 corresponds to the horizontal osteotomy for a genioplasty when needed in conjunction with the mandibular advancement.

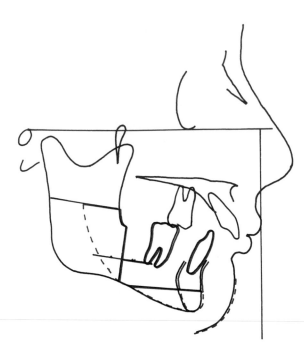

FIG. 6-12

The ***prediction*** (red line) is begun by tracing the mandible except for the bony and soft-tissue chin, and all the above reference marks except the dot on the proximal segment (no. 4) on a new piece of tracing acetate overlaid on the ***tracing*** (black line). The portion of the mandible below the genioplasty line and the soft-tissue chin are traced with a dashed line at this time. This approximates the actual anatomy (geometry) of the distal mandible that is repositioned at surgery. (*Note:* All superimpositions are shown slightly offset to better illustrate what is being traced.)

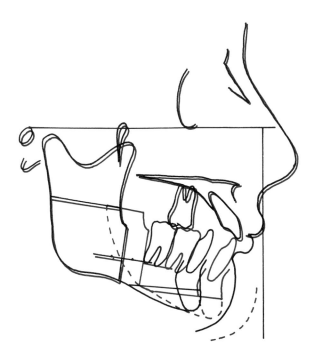

FIG. 6-13

The **prediction** is moved forward on the **tracing** to produce the ideal occlusal relation, and the stable structures, including the proximal mandible, are traced. The relation of the proximal and distal ramus segments are noted relative to their magnitude of change (increase distance between no. 4 references) and any vertical or rotational change (parallelism of two horizontal lines) so that the proper relation of the proximal and distal mandibular segments can be achieved at surgery. The geometry of the area where the proximal and distal segments overlap is studied to aid in decisions regarding the placement of the intraosseous screws. This is essential for good stability because proper placement of the screws affects control of the proximal segments and condyle positions.

SURGICAL OCCLUSAL SPLINT CONSTRUCTION

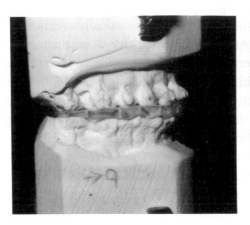 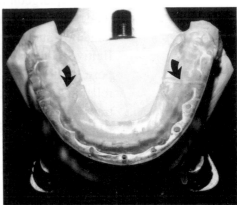

FIG. 6-17

If the occlusion is such that the models can unequivocally be positioned into an optimal occlusion, an occlusal splint need not be used. When this is not the case, an occlusal splint is constructed to ensure optimal positioning and stabilization of the mandibular distal segment. There is no overcorrection either antero-posteriorly or vertically.

The splint is not extended posteriorly beyond the mesial half of the terminal molars. Doing so often results in significant occlusal interferences both when rigid fixation is used without intermaxillary fixation and when the splint is left wired to the mandible during jaw physiotherapy after the release of intermaxillary fixation. The maxillary occlusal interdigitations are definite, but shallow, similarly to preclude occlusal interferences. When the surgical occlusal splint is to be secured to the mandibular dentition by circummandibular wires at the time of surgery, grooves are made in the splint between the premolars and molars (arrows) so that the circummandibular wires are located between the opposing maxillary teeth. This eliminates occlusal interferences where these wires pass over the occlusal aspect of the splint.

Orthognathic reconstructive surgery

MODIFIED SAGITTAL SPLIT RAMUS OSTEOTOMIES

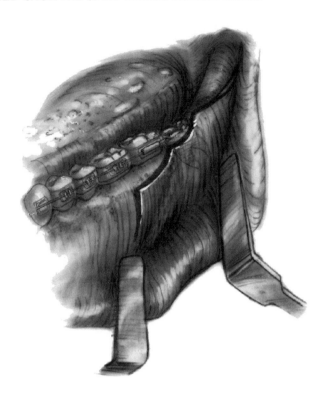

FIG. 6-18

To aid in hemostasis in the areas of the planned soft-tissue incisions and dissection, 5 to 10 ml of a local anesthetic with 1:100,000 epinephrine is injected. The lips are lubricated with a steroid ointment, and a bite block is inserted on the side opposite to that being operated on to open the mouth maximally. An incision is made over the lateral oblique ridge with a diathermy knife. The incision is made in a deliberate layered fashion; mucous, muscle, and periosteum, with each successive layer being retracted. This prevents excessive tissue cauterization, which predisposes to postoperative wound margin breakdown and excessive scarring. Extension of the incision too far superiorly will result in exposure of the buccal fat.

When impacted third molars exist, the surgeon should address the impaction with a definite surgical plan. Since the actual osteotomy is identical regardless of the presence or absence of a partially or completely impacted third molar, the difference lies in the design of the soft-tissue incision. When the third molar is fully impacted, no change is made in the previously described incision. However, in the presence of a partially erupted third molar, the incision must include the attached gingival cuff of the erupting tooth. If this is not done, a "button hole" which unnecessarily complicates an otherwise simple wound closure is left in the medial soft-tissue flap.

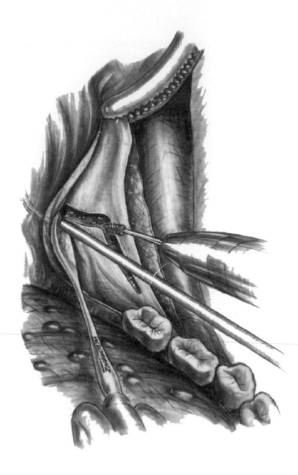

FIG. 6-19

The subperiosteal soft-tissue dissection is first carried superiorly, exposing the anterior border of the ramus of the mandible from the retromolar area almost to the tip of the coronoid process. A curved bone clamp is then used to grasp the coronoid process to retract the soft tissues and to hold the mandible anteriorly and laterally.

To achieve the medial subperiosteal dissection, first the tissues are carefully reflected subperiosteally from the internal oblique ridge, from its superiormost aspect inferiorly to the region of the second molar tooth. Once this is achieved the more posterior soft tissues are easily reflected subperiosteally, thereby exposing the lingula and often the entering inferior alveolar neurovascular bundle. The dissection proceeds posteriorly about 1 cm above and parallel to the *mandibular occlusion plane*. The sphenomandibular ligament can be stripped from the lingula area at this time. Doing so may be important in large advancements.

With the medial tissues retracted, the medial osteotomy is made parallel to the occlusal plane and is carried posteriorly just above and posterior to the lingula. The closer this osteotomy terminates to the mandibular foramen, the easier and more predictable the split will be, thus decreasing the chances of a pathologic split in this area. This osteotomy is made through the lingual cortex and medullary bone to a depth closely approximating the lateral cortex.

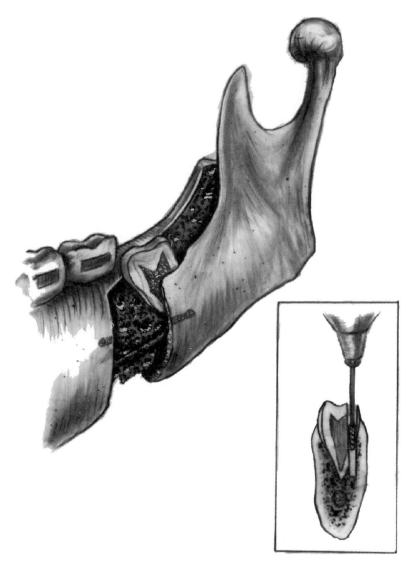

FIG. 6-20

The curved bone clamp is now moved inferiorly to engage the ramus just superior to the completed horizontal osteotomy. This allows greater inferior movement of the incision as the osteotomy proceeds down the anterior aspect of the ramus. The osteotomy is continued inferiorly through the anterolateral aspect of the ascending ramus cortex, well into the medullary bone, attempting to leave just the lateral cortex. This osteotomy usually ends lateral to the second molar tooth (Fig. 6-20). When an impacted third molar is present, the osteotomy is made in an identical fashion and whatever tooth structure encountered is treated as bone. This maximizes the amount of marrow remaining on the distal segment and promotes a "safe" split with the inferior alveolar nerve encased in the bone of the distal segment. When this osteotome is made such that the ascending ramus and retromolar trigone area are evenly divided mediolaterally, the split will more often occur such that the inferior alveolar neurovascular bundle is within the bone of the proximal segment. Such a split requires the tedious removal of the neurovascular bundle from the distal segment and increases the potential of producing a neurosensory defect.

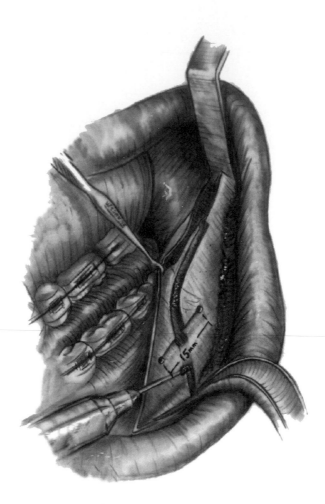

FIG. 6-21

After the anterior ramus osteotomy is completed, the bite block and bone clamp are removed, the jaw is closed, and the subperiosteal dissection is extended lateral to the molar teeth to the inferior border of the mandible. A channel retractor is inserted. A horizontal reference that reproduces the reference mark on the cephalometric prediction tracing is made in the lateral cortex using a 703 bur. This reference is made approximately 15 to 20 mm below and parallel to the mandibular occlusal plane. Unicortical holes are then made on this horizontal reference 10 mm apart (5 mm on either side of the planned vertical osteotomy). The use of this reference line in conjunction with the presurgical prediction tracing for the purpose of determining proximal segment and condylar position is discussed later in this chapter.

The lateral vertical osteotomy is completed to the inferior border of the mandible. This osteotomy is made at about a 45-degree angle to the outer cortex of the mandible. By so doing, it is easier to visualize the medullary bone, which helps to avoid making this osteotomy so deep as to inadvertently injure the inferior alveolar neurovascular bundle.

Next, the cortex of the inferior border of the mandible is completely osteotomized. If this osteotomy does not extend completely through the inferior border cortex, there is an increased risk of an unfavorable fracture. The arrow indicates the location of the desired fracture. The diagonal lines in Fig. 6-22 on the mandibular lateral cortex and inferior border indicate the bone cut with a 703 surgical bur. (Fig. 6-22)

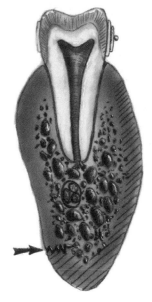

FIG. 6-22

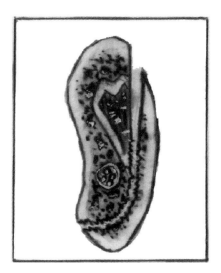

FIG. 6-23

The technique for completing a sagittal split ramus osteotomy associated with *any* partially erupted third molar is identical. All osteotomies are accomplished in a routine fashion except in the area of the erupting tooth, where the bur cuts through the tooth structure as though it did not exist. If bone is preferentially cut, as opposed to tooth structure, the bone will be significantly weakened and an unfavorable fracture may result when the actual split is attempted. In such instances, the buccal plate of the proximal segment often fractures directly adjacent to the impacted tooth. After the sagittal split is completed, the molar is removed by sectioning the tooth and/or selective removal of bone and elevation, with minimal leverage being applied.

One important deviation from the usual osteotomy plan may be necessary due to the location of the impacted tooth relative to the inferior alveolar nerve. If the tooth is entirely superior to the inferior alveolar neurovascular bundle, it is completely divided with the surgical bur through the osteotomy site. This allows the tooth to be sectioned easily after the sagittal split is accomplished.

On the other hand, if the impacted tooth's roots are inferior to, or closely associated with, the inferior alveolar neurovascular bundle, *only the portion of the tooth superior to the nerve is divided with the bur* (Fig. 6-23). Planning the location and amount of tooth division is best done by evaluating the preoperative panoramic radiograph.

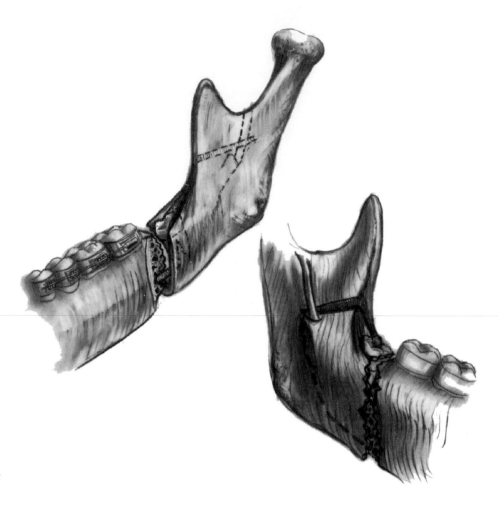

FIG. 6-24

    After the initial osteotomies are completed and the sagittal split is finalized, the impacted tooth is gently removed in fragments. Further sectioning of the impacted tooth may be required to avoid excessive levering during the extraction, but this is rarely necessary. If a tooth is not sectioned and excessive force is applied in an attempt to elevate it, an unfavorable lingual plate fracture may result as illustrated in Fig. 6-24.

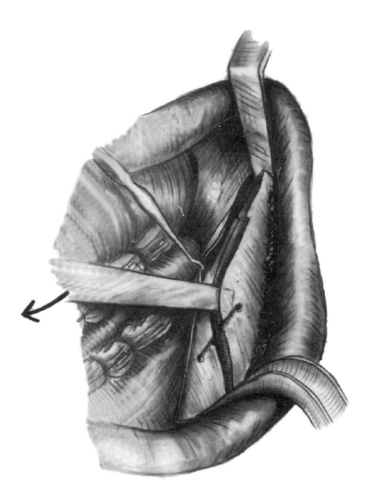

FIG. 6-25

Beginning at the superiormost aspect of the anterior ramus osteotomy, a thin straight calibrated osteotome is malleted into the osteotomy parallel to and just beneath the lateral cortex, to a depth of about 10 to 15 mm. This is done to ensure completeness of the cortical osteotomies and to initiate the actual plane of splitting such that the lateral cortex is separated from the medial cortex *and* attached medullary bone. This osteotome is not malleted so deeply that it might injure the inferior alveolar neurovascular bundle. For the same reason, it is not malleted into the vertical component of the osteotomy in the region overlying the inferior alveolar neurovascular bundle. In all instances it is important that the clinician determine the course of the nerve in the preoperative panoramic radiograph. In some individuals the nerve may be unusually high and the osteotome depth must be adjusted accordingly.

An osteotome is now malleted into the uppermost portion of the vertical osteotomy, in the region of the external oblique ridge, and is used to pry the proximal segment laterally by using the superior lateral aspect of the distal mandible in the region of the external oblique ridge as a fulcrum. *As splitting is initiated the inferior border is observed and must begin to open.* If it does not, the osteotomy through the inferior border is checked for completeness because, if it is incomplete, the probability of pathologic fracture of the buccal cortex is increased.

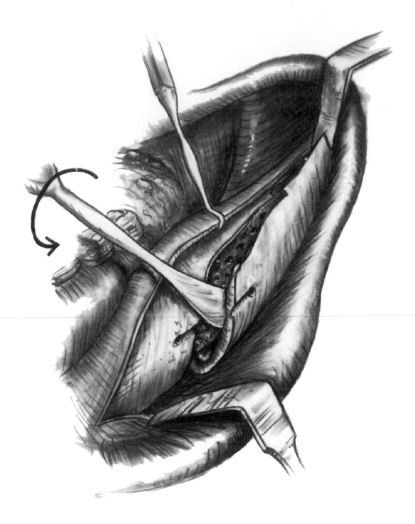

FIG. 6-26

Once movement of the inferior border is observed, opening of the superior osteotomy is checked. If this is not opening, the osteotomies are simultaneously checked in the superior and medial areas. *Incomplete osteotomies in either of these areas is the most common cause of difficulty in splitting and/or pathologic splitting of the mandible.* As the sagittal split separates and widens, the osteotome is replaced with a periosteal elevator, which is used to continue the split. The periosteal elevator uses the external oblique ridge as a fulcrum and may be rotated to increase the width of the split as well as to increase the surgeon's visibility of the progressing split.

As the opening of the split is being achieved, much like the opening of a new book, the inferior alveolar neurovascular bundle is identified within the medullary portion of the mandible. This is always done before attempting to complete the split. If it is favorably embedded within the medullary bone of the distal segment, the torquing of the proximal segment laterally is continued until the split is completed.

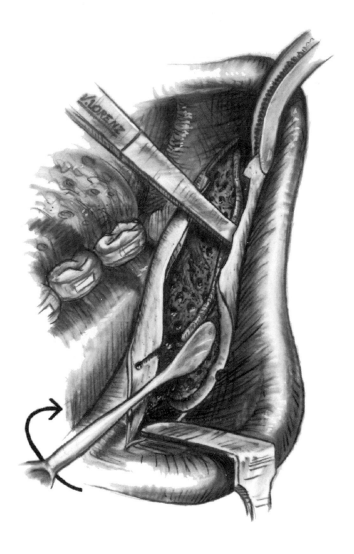

FIG. 6-27

If the inferior alveolar neurovascular bundle is adherent to the proximal segment and cannot be readily lifted free from the medullary bone of the proximal segment with a periosteal elevator as the split is being made, it is generally attached by remnants of the surrounding cortical bone that make up its canal. In such instances a small straight osteotome, directed at about a 45-degree angle to the lateral cortex, is carefully malleted to separate the neurovascular bundle from the lateral cortex. It is helpful for the surgeon to use surgical loops when accomplishing this maneuver.

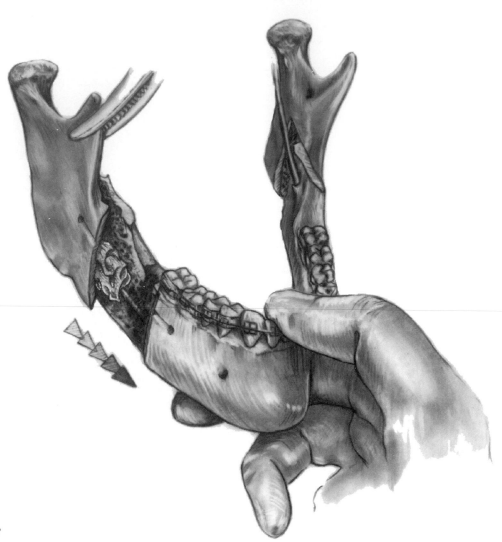

FIG. 6-28

After the splits are completed in both rami, the surrounding perimandibular soft tissues must be mobilized. Before beginning this mobilization a moist 2-by-2 in. gauze sponge is placed within the osteotomy site bilaterally to avoid traumatizing the inferior alveolar nerve with the sharp bone edges. Forceful movements of the *proximal* mandibular segments are avoided, since doing so can stretch or tear the temporomandibular joint ligaments. Further, such movements do not affect the desired mobilization of the perimandibular tissues necessary to permit passive advancement of the distal mandible. The desired mobilization of soft tissues is best accomplished by grasping the proximal segments with a bone clamp to maintain the proximal segment in its normal anatomic position while forcefully pulling the distal mandible forward into a Class III relation. This is a stretching action rather than a tearing one. *After adequate mobilization is achieved, the distal mandible is able to be positioned into the desired occlusal relation without the proximal segment being displaced by the tension from the perimandibular soft tissues.* This is important to reduce relapse, as discussed later in this section.

Fixation of the proximal and distal segments is generally accomplished using two or three intraosseous 2-mm titanium screws. Intraosseous screw placement is to achieve two essential objectives: (1) putting the condyle into its proper position within the glenoid fossa and (2) preventing rotation and shear slippage at the osteotomy site. These objectives are achieved by placing two or three bicortical screws. Specific indications for skeletal maxillomandibular fixation, semirigid fixation (two screws), and rigid skeletal fixation (three screws) without intermaxillary fixation are discussed in detail in Chapter 2. Only the techniques for securing the distal to the proximal segments will follow. Two basic techniques will be outlined: (1) skeletal maxillomandibular fixation with two positioning screws to maintain the proximal segment position and (2) rigid fixation without intermaxillary fixation with three screws used to secure proximal to distal segments.

The first technique may be used in all sagittal split ramus osteotomies regardless of the magnitude of advancement. This technique is currently used in all cases undergoing significant advancements (greater than 6 to 8 mm at pogonion, including any planned advancement genioplasty). The patient is first placed in skeletal maxillomandibular fixation. This is achieved by placing two 22-gauge piriform rim wires and two 22-gauge circummandibular wires in the premolar regions. The piriform rim wires are placed so that they form loops in the depth of the maxillary vestibule. The circummandibular wires are passed over the occlusal splint, when one is used, or interproximally when no splint is used. An intermediate 24-gauge wire is then passed between these two wires bilaterally and tightened to produce skeletal maxillomandibular fixation. Two supplemental interdental wires are sometimes added in the canine areas to prevent the maxillary teeth from becoming dislodged from the splint. This is important whenever the occlusal interdigitations of the maxillary teeth into the splint are not very deep and there is any tendency for the maxillary teeth to become displaced from the splint.

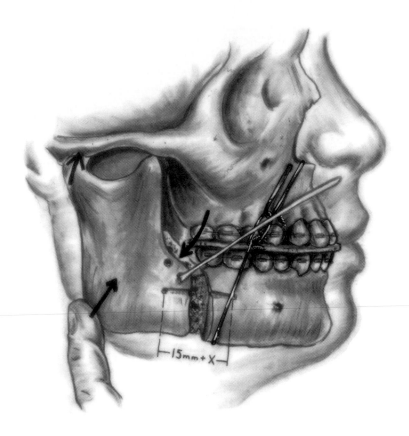

FIG. 6-29

After skeletal fixation is achieved, the proximal segments are positioned in the following manner. A hole is drilled in the superior-anterior corner of the proximal segment with a 703 bur (Fig. 6-29). This hole now serves as a purchase point for the placement of a wire director. Positioning of the proximal segment is accomplished using two hands, one holding the wire director to apply gentle pressure to the segment in an inferior-posterior direction while the second hand applies anterior-superior pressure at the mandibular angle facially. These simultaneously applied pressures result in a force vector in the condyle that is superior-anterior, thus properly seating the condyle. The horizontal reference line and holes on the lateral cortex of the mandible are measured to make certain that they correspond to the values determined from the cephalometric prediction tracing *before* screw placement.

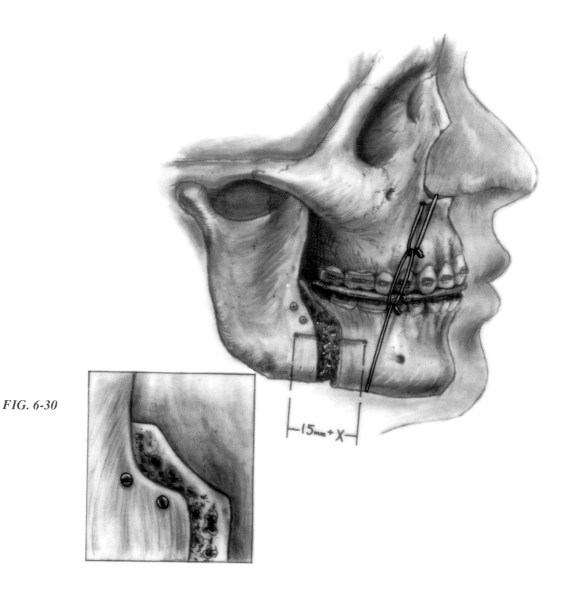

FIG. 6-30

Once the proper proximal segment position is obtained, *the first hole is drilled in the area of maximum passive bone contact* (Fig. 6-29). The first screw, generally 11 to 15 mm in length, is placed. The second hole is now drilled where the most optimal bone contact occurs, and the second screw is placed (Fig. 6-30). These screws are not tightened sufficiently to compress the segments together and cause potentially deleterious torquing of the condyles and/or nerve compression. When intermaxillary fixation is used, it is maintained for 3 weeks.

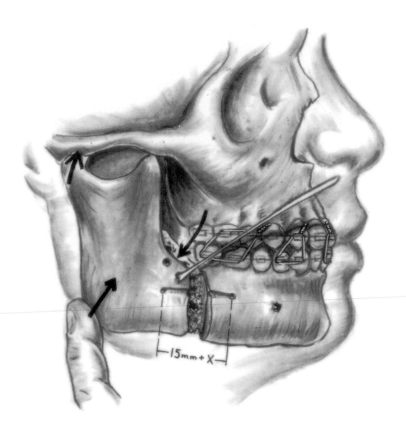

FIG. 6-31

When the indications for rigid fixation without maxillomandibular fixation have been met (as discussed in Chapter 2), the above technique is varied slightly. Intermaxillary *dental* fixation is placed in four areas—each canine and each first molar. In these instances the proximal segment positioning and screw placement is the same as previously described (Fig. 6-31).

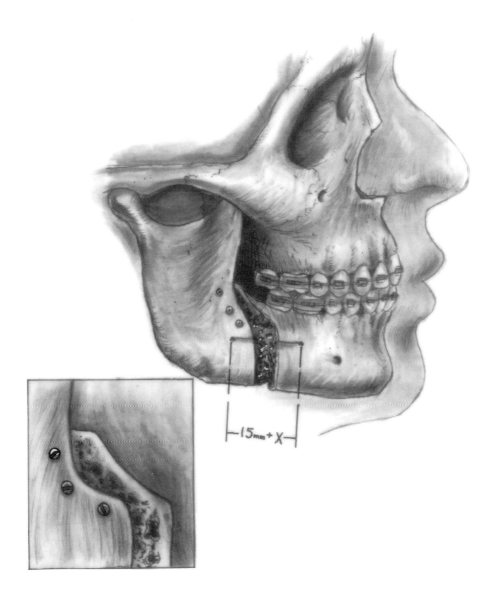

FIG. 6-32

    Three screws are placed to ensure adequate stability of the proximal and distal segments. The location of the third screw is either along the superior border or anteriorly below the neurovascular bundle.

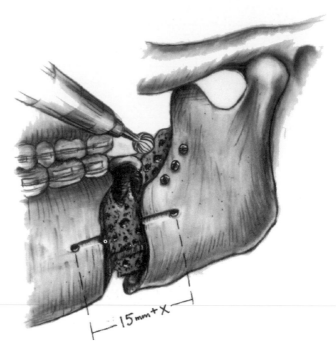

FIG. 6-33

In larger advancements (those greater than about 10 mm) the anterior ramus portion of the distal segment is partially removed after the intraosseous screws are placed to prevent it from encroaching on the maxillary tuberosity and/or obliterating the retromolar space.

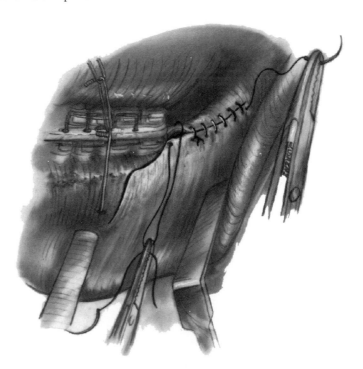

FIG. 6-34

The incisions are closed with running 3-0 chromic gut sutures. If the soft-tissue incision is made more medially than described, it is difficult or even impossible to locate the medial soft tissues and place sutures through them after the patient is placed into intermaxillary fixation. Therefore, in cases in which intermaxillary fixation is deemed necessary, two sutures are passed through the medial soft tissues in the region of the third molar after completion of all osteotomies, but *before* placing the patient into intermaxillary fixation. The needles are left attached and are retained laterally. The intermaxillary fixation is then achieved and the intraosseous screws are placed as described previously. The superior suture is passed through the lateral tissues and run superiorly, closing the superior limb of the incision. The lower limb of the incision is similarly closed with the inferior suture.

If skeletal maxillomandibular fixation has been used, the intermaxillary fixation is released about 3 weeks postoperatively by cutting the intermediate skeletal stabilization wires. Written instructions that address jaw physiotherapy, diet, and occlusal observation are given to all patients when their jaws are unwired (Chapter 4). The occlusal splint, if used, is maintained fixed to the mandible by the circummandibular wires. The patient is instructed to begin active jaw opening and protrusion, but no chewing is permitted for 24 to 72 hours, at which time the patient is reevaluated. He/she is informed that during this time the teeth must continue to bite perfectly into the occlusal splint or the existing occlusion when no occlusal splint is used. *No elastics are used because they will only mask relapse.* When the patient is observed to bite perfectly into the splint or occlusion, instructions are given to begin more vigorous isometric and isotonic exercises. This is to be done by the patient exercising four times daily as follows. First, the mouth is opened as widely as possible. Next, the patient is to bite into occlusion forcefully and then to protrude the lower jaw as far as possible. While performing these exercises, the patient is given visual objectives, consistent with the presurgical range of jaw movement, regarding the desired interincisal opening and protrusive movement. About 1 week later, when the patient has resumed essentially a normal and asymptomatic range of jaw movement and the occlusion is deemed stable, the piriform rim and circummandibular wires are removed under nitrous oxide/oxygen and local anesthesia. Before removal, the wires are carefully cleaned with peroxide where they enter the mucosa and are cut beneath the mucosa by forcing a wire cutter down around the wire. This prevents possible infection and avoids the need to use antibiotics. The patient is to see the orthodontist within the next 48 hours to begin active postsurgical orthodontic finishing procedures. A return to normal dietary consistency is gradually and progressively resumed over the subsequent 2 weeks. If the patient does not occlude properly at any time after release of intermaxillary fixation, the specific reason(s) is identified and appropriately managed (Chapter 5).

Postsurgical orthodontic treatment

The first orthodontic appointment is within 48 hours of the patient's release from the surgeon's active care. At this appointment both upper and lower archwires are removed, checked for damage, and adjusted or replaced as necessary. The fixed appliances are checked for damage (such as bent or broken brackets or squashed tubes), and loose or damaged appliances are replaced or recemented. The occlusion is checked, and the archwires are adjusted, applying any archwire mechanics or elastics that are appropriate to finish the occlusion as if the patient had never undergone a surgical procedure (Fig. 6-35). The patient is seen again in 2 to 3 days.

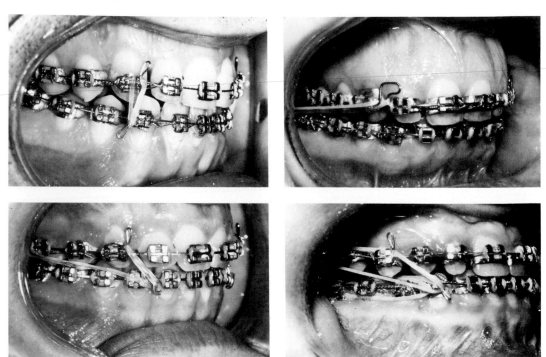

FIG. 6-35

Progress is assessed at the next appointment, paying particular attention to any acute occlusal changes that would indicate surgical instability. The appliances are adjusted if necessary, and the elastics are reviewed for their appropriateness. Usually nothing will be done at this appointment except to be sure that all that was done at the previous appointment was properly executed and that the patient is following instructions. The patient is seen again in 7 to 10 days.

The next appointment serves as a further check of progress. When no complications are noted, the patient is placed on routine 4-week recall for future adjustments. All succeeding appointments are routine in that appropriate archwire adjustments are made to perfect the occlusion, followed by appliance removal and retention in a usual manner.

In any instance when progress is not as expected, new records are obtained and compared to the records obtained at the release of fixation. The etiology of the problem can accordingly be determined and appropriate action taken to resolve the specific problem (see Chapter 5).

Factors affecting stability of treatment
Orthodontic factors

The following orthodontic factors are important in producing a stable result.

REMOVAL OF DENTAL COMPENSATIONS

This is done through properly chosen extractions, well-managed anchorage, Class III elastics, or a combination of the three. This does not preclude orthodontic relapse but creates a situation wherein any orthodontic relapse in the antero-posterior direction will tend to offset, rather than compound, any surgical skeletal relapse (Fig. 6-36).

PRESURGICAL ORTHO
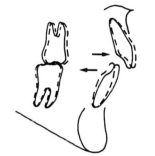

SURGERY
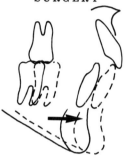

SURGICAL RELAPSE
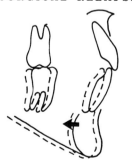

ORTHO RELAPSE
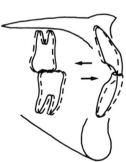

SURGICAL *MINUS* ORTHO RELAPSE
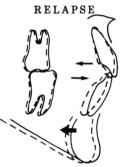

FIG. 6-36

CORRECTION OF TOOTH MASS DISCREPANCIES

When this is done, the surgeon will be able to produce a solid Class I posterior occlusion with normal overbite and overjet. Such an occlusion has less tendency for relapse because proper intercuspation of the teeth helps to stabilize the occlusion.

LEVELING OF BOTH ARCHES

This also is necessary to allow the surgeon to produce a good Class I occlusion with normal overbite and overjet and has the same stabilizing effect described above. Importantly, in combined orthodontic-surgical correction of the Class II dentofacial deformity, the method of this leveling—intrusion of anterior teeth versus extrusion of posterior teeth—is unimportant except in determining the vertical height of the lower third face. When maximal increase of lower face height is desired, the mandible can be advanced before complete orthodontic leveling using a special surgical splint to allow extrusion of the teeth in the buccal segments during fixation (see second usual approach, below). There is rarely if ever a tendency for a deep bite to develop postsurgically. This is perhaps because of the decrease in masticatory efficiency as a result of increasing the distance from the muscles of mastication to the dentition.

CORRECTION OF TRANSVERSE DISCREPANCIES

When there is a transverse discrepancy greater than 4 mm in a patient over 16 to 18 years of age, consideration must be given to correcting this with surgery. This may be variably achieved by simultaneous narrowing of the mandible, surgical widening of the maxilla, or orthodontic-surgical widening of the maxilla. Each of these methods is discussed later in this chapter. Determination of the magnitude of the transverse discrepancy must be made with the teeth approximating the Class I occlusion that is to be produced at surgery, and not from the existing Class II relation. One factor that can contribute to the production of an open bite postsurgically is relapse of the maxillary posterior teeth in a transverse direction, which tends to produce a cusp-to-cusp occlusion. This may cause the mandible to swing down and back and open the bite anteriorly (Fig. 6-37). This is especially true in light of the aforementioned decrease in masticatory efficiency.

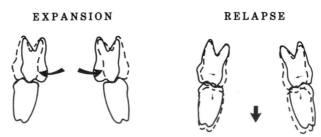

EXPANSION   **RELAPSE**

FIG. 6-37

PRODUCTION OF A DOUBLE PROTRUSION

When the mandibular advancement surgery involves clockwise rotation of the distal segment of the mandible, the teeth are advanced more than pogonion (Fig. 6-38). As such, it is easy to produce a bimaxillary protrusion that may ad-

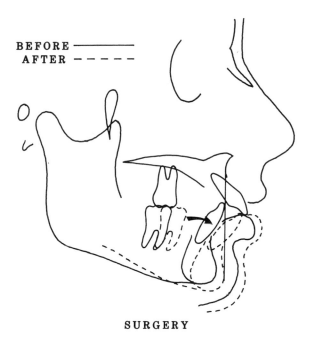

BEFORE ————
AFTER — — — —

FIG. 6-38   **SURGERY**

versely affect both the facial esthetics and the maintenance of incisor alignment following the removal of retention appliances. This can be avoided by retraction of the lower incisors or the addition of an advancement genioplasty.

Surgical factors

Surgical (skeletal) relapse subsequent to mandibular advancement surgery is, in large part, directly related to technique and occurs primarily during or immediately on release of intermaxillary fixation. The following factors are those that are most important to produce a stable result.

SOFT-TISSUE MOBILIZATION

After splitting of the rami has been achieved, the perimandibular soft tissues (that is, periosteum, ligaments, muscles, and submucosal tissues) tend to retain the proximal and distal segments in their original anatomic positions. If the distal segment of the mandible is not mobilized at this time as described in the preceding surgical technique section, the perimandibular soft-tissue tensions will contribute to skeletal relapse. As the distal mandible is advanced and stabilized, these soft-tissue tensions tend to displace the condyle anteriorly from the fossa and cause the proximal segment to rotate anteriorly and superiorly. The greater the magnitude of advancement, the greater will be this problem. In addition, and of equal importance, these soft-tissue tensions will also unfavorably load the distal segment. *This is perhaps the primary reason that it has been repeatedly noted that relapse of the distal segment occurs during the period of intermaxillary fixation, especially when fixation is achieved solely by interdental wiring.*

One additional comment is in order regarding mandibular advancement in the Class II patient with a significant overbite. The distal segment is often rotated clockwise significantly, and this results in a significant movement of the teeth with minimal advancement of pogonion. This rotational movement tends to reduce, but not eliminate, the potential for skeletal relapse, since pogonion is minimally advanced and there is minimal stretching of soft tissue. Further, the biomechanics of mastication are altered by this rotational advancement such that the patient actually possesses a reduced bite force after surgery. It is perhaps for this reason, at least in part, that little tendency for deep-bite relapse is noted when this deformity is corrected by combined orthodontic-surgical means.

DISTRACTION OF THE CONDYLE FROM THE FOSSA

This occurs when the soft tissues are not adequately mobilized or when the intraosseous screw placement is improper. *When condylar distraction occurs, relapse is inevitable.* The definitive surgical prediction tracing and the reference marks thereon serve as a guide to proximal segment position in each individual patient as nearly identical referents are transferred to the patient and used as a critical indicator of proximal segment position (see Fig. 6-21). The optimal fixation technique is done in such a way that the condyle/proximal segment is maintained in its presurgical position. When screw fixation without intermaxillary fixation is used, the proper condyle position is apparent immediately postoperatively as evidenced by the patient's being able to close into the planned occlusion *without elastics.* When any type of intermaxillary fixation is used, immediate postoperative radiographs must be used to confirm proper condyle position. If these records reveal measurable anteroinferior displacement, this will contribute to relapse if not corrected (see Chapter 5). A number of devices have been advocated to help control the condyle-proximal segment. These are all aids in this critical phase of the surgery.

METHOD OF FIXATION

Despite accomplishing adequate distal segment mobilization and proper condyle position, *relapse during bone healing occurs to variable degrees,* often to a significant degree. This is so with dental fixation and is related to the fact that when the teeth are used as the sole means of holding the advanced mandible forward, the periodontal ligaments are generally inadequate to withstand the loads applied to them. This becomes more problematic the farther the mandible is advanced, and is compounded when a simultaneous advancement genioplasty is performed. This relapse is manifest by skeletal relapse with accompanying anterior extrusion, posterior intrusion, and tipping of the teeth during the period of intermaxillary fixation. Unfortunately, when this occurs, these unplanned orthodontic movements are unstable and tend to reverse on release of the dental intermaxillary fixation. It is at this time that occlusal relapse is noted clinically. The orthodontist then attempts to counteract this relapse and is often unsuccessful. Moreover, this tends to compress forcefully the condyle distally and superiorly, which can have secondary effects as discussed later in this section. Accordingly, when the mandible is advanced more than 6 mm at pogonion, it is best maintained with skeletal fixation wires that are placed such that their vector of force counteracts the well-documented downward and backward pattern of skeletal relapse (see Fig. 6-30). These wires must be of sufficient strength to resist stretching and are tightened as indicated during the period of intermaxillary fixation.

In cases of skeletal advancements greater than 6 to 8 mm, especially with simultaneous advancement genioplasty and three-screw fixation without maxillomandibular fixation, relapse occurs during healing (first 6 to 8 weeks) due to rotation and slippage at the osteotomy site. These large advancements produce chronic compressive condylar loading. In many instances these patients experience secondary (first year) relapse due to condylar modeling resorption—osteolysis. Accordingly, it is recommended that these cases be stabilized for 3 weeks postoperatively with skeletal maxillomandibular fixation.

ADDITIONAL FACTORS

The amount of skeletal advancement, duration of intermaxillary fixation, and suprahyoid muscle pull are additional factors that can influence the stability of results but to a lesser degree. Accordingly, for individuals in whom the amount of skeletal advancement is great (10 to 12 mm at pogonion) the length of skeletal maxillomandibular fixation is increased to 4 to 6 weeks, and consideration is given for suprahyoid myotomies (see Chapters 8 and 9). The latter can perhaps be best assessed by the ease or difficulty with which the *patient can protrude* the mandible into a Class III occlusion before surgery. If the patient is unable to do this, or can only do it with considerable effort, suprahyoid myotomies are to be considered. In addition, clinical assessment of tension in the suprahyoid area by palpation during maximum protrusion is a useful clinical guide. When the cephalometric prediction tracing reveals that more than 30% lengthening (stretch) of the suprahyoid muscles will occur with the planned advancement, suprahyoid myotomies will aid in reducing the soft-tissue tensions that can contribute to relapse.

Age-related factors

The relationship of the age of the patient with Class II dentofacial deformity and the stability of combined orthodontic-surgical treatment—specifically, at what age can the mandible be successfully advanced surgically—has been debated, often emotionally, with many authorities stating that surgery must be delayed until facial growth is completed. After about age 6 years, there is proportionate growth of the maxilla and mandible as evidenced by the fact that an individual with non-syndrome-related Class II deformity, without vertical maxillary excess or open bite, neither improves nor worsens with growth. The patient who is retrognathic at age 6 years will remain retrognathic, and the degree of the

Class II occlusion will remain essentially unchanged, unless therapy is undertaken to change it.

To address the relationship of age, growth, and stability logically, two essential questions must be answered. First, what effect will mandibular advancement surgery have on the subsequent growth of the patient? And second, what effect will the subsequent growth have on the occlusal and esthetic result attained by the surgery?

EFFECT OF MANDIBULAR ADVANCEMENT ON SUBSEQUENT FACIAL GROWTH

Proximal segment control as discussed in the surgical technique section earlier in this chapter becomes even more critical when operating on the growing individual. When mandibular growth (relocation) following mandibular advancement surgery is more vertical than expected, this correlates well with the fact that either the proximal segment was rotated in a counterclockwise direction at surgery or skeletal relapse occurred. This observation has been confirmed in animal studies that have evaluated the effects of proximal segment rotation on subsequent facial growth. These studies support the contention that more horizontal growth (relocation) occurs when the proximal segment is rotated clockwise and more vertical relocation occurs when this segment is rotated counterclockwise. Thus, some control of the vector of facial relocation—horizontal versus vertical— following mandibular advancement surgery is possible and is related to the details of surgical technique. A probable biomechanical explanation for these findings has been proposed and is discussed in detail in the literature cited at the end of this chapter.

Several additional factors must be considered that can and do result in either some modification of the subsequent growth vector or lack of maintenance of the achieved occlusion. The factors include: (1) alteration of the biomechanics of mastication as they relate to maxillary growth, (2) alteration of the biomechanics of the condylar cartilage as they pertain to subsequent growth, and (3) possible damage to condylar cartilage ("growth center").

ALTERATION OF THE BIOMECHANICS OF MASTICATION AS THEY RELATE TO MAXILLARY GROWTH. There is a direct relation between the magnitude of vertical maxillary growth and the magnitude of masticatory loading—the greater the masticatory loading, the less vertical maxillary growth. Since the efficiency of the masticatory mechanism (Class III lever) is decreased as the lower teeth are advanced (increased distance of the teeth from the muscles of mastication) with mandibular advancement there will theoretically occur a decreased magnitude of masticatory loading (masticatory efficiency), which in principle can result in increased vertical maxillary growth. Although this has not been noted to affect the actual stability of the surgical result, it is a factor that tends to result in an increased vertical growth pattern after surgical advancement of the mandible during growth.

ALTERATION OF THE BIOMECHANICS OF THE CONDYLAR CARTILAGE AS THEY PERTAIN TO SUBSEQUENT GROWTH. Both compressive and tensile loading directly influence the rate and direction of cartilaginous growth. With the significant alterations in condylar cartilage loading that occur with mandibular advancement surgery, it follows that alterations in the magnitude and direction of subsequent condylar cartilage growth can occur. If the resultant loading is either excessively increased or decreased, unfavorable growth can result that will also tend to result in a more vertical than horizontal facial growth pattern. Excessively increased loading, as discussed next, is most likely to occur.

POSSIBLE DAMAGE TO CONDYLAR CARTILAGE. This factor cannot be separated from the previous factor. However, when the intermaxillary stabilization is not adequate and skeletal relapse occurs during the period of fixation, the condyles are chronically and forcefully compressed posterosuperiorly into the glenoid fossas during the entire period of fixation. Thus, compressive injury to the condylar cartilages can occur and result in decreased subsequent mandibular growth. This would result in a tendency for the occlusion to become a Class II open bite.

EFFECT OF SUBSEQUENT GROWTH ON THE OCCLUSAL AND ESTHETIC RESULT ATTAINED AT SURGERY

When the surgery is meticulously done to prevent surgical relapse, the post-surgical growth that occurs, regardless of its actual vector, has little if any effect on the occlusion that was achieved at surgery. The occlusal result attained at surgery is maintained.

The presurgical orthodontic treatment is usually completed by about age 12 to 14 years. By this age between 85% and 95% of the facial growth is completed. Thus, even if growth following surgery is not completely normal, very little change in facial appearance will occur. For example, the average female exhibits only about 3 mm Condylion-Gnathion of growth between age 14 and 18 years. Indeed, the mandible can be advanced at even a younger age, but this is only advocated for the child who is experiencing psychologic difficulties resulting from his/her facial appearance or for syndrome-related dentofacial deformities.

Results of treatment

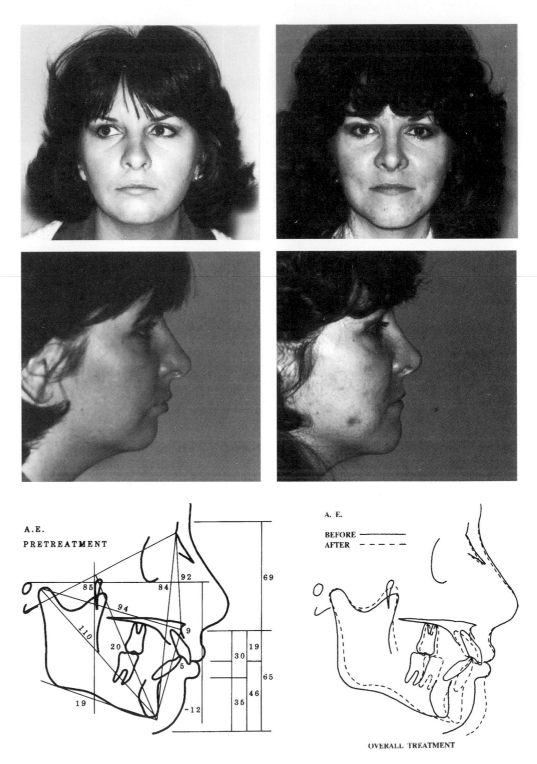

FIG. 6-39

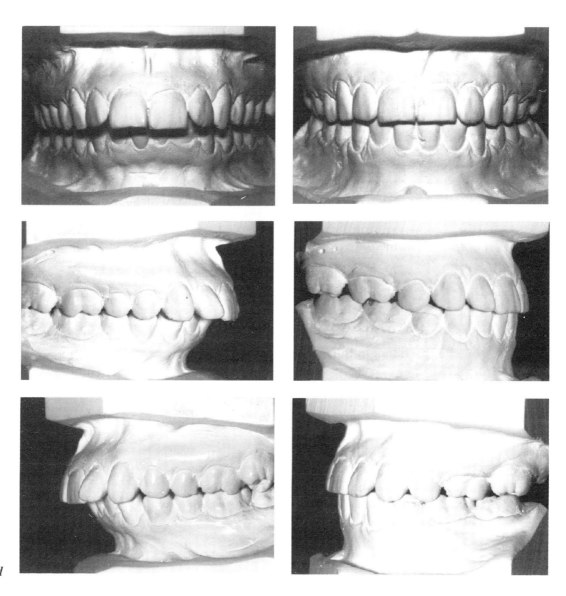

FIG. 6-39, cont'd

in both arches, arch coordination is achieved. Tip-back bends may be used to finish leveling, and wearing of Class III elastics is continued until the desired anteroposterior tooth positions are achieved. Progress models are now made to evaluate the occlusion that can be produced at surgery. If this feasibility surgery results in a satisfactory occlusion, the archwires are tied with ligature wires, elastic hooks are placed where appropriate (usually the canines), and the patient is referred for surgery.

With this method of treatment, the biggest problem encountered is a tendency for the lower incisors to become too protrusive. Thus, almost without exception, the patient needs to wear Class III elastics. Excessive flaring of the lower incisors is to be avoided because it diminishes the amount of advancement possible, increases the potential for relapse, and often produces a relative tooth mass discrepancy (Chapter 2). When excessive flaring cannot be avoided by use of Class III elastics and/or interproximal recontouring, it is necessary to extract teeth and to use the mechanics sequence described in the first section of this chapter. Importantly, extractions need not be avoided for fear of deep-bite relapse, because when the mandible is advanced surgically, deep-bite relapse tends not to occur.

LEVELING TO THE FUNCTIONAL OCCLUSAL PLANE

BEFORE ————————

AFTER — — — — —

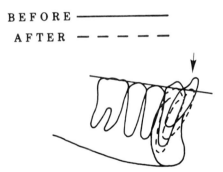

FIG. 6-42

Most patients would optimally benefit from having their mandible advanced along the functional occlusal plane. So doing produces maximal chin projection, thus reducing the size of genioplasty required and produces little, if any, increase in lower face height. Their deep bite is primarily due to an increased curve of Spee in the lower arch while the upper curve of Spee is within normal limits. This is in contrast to the Class II, division 2 deformity in which the upper curve is also usually reversed, increasing the deep bite even more (see third usual approach). Thus, the lower arch will generally take more preparation and is begun first unless the upper anterior teeth must be moved to provide room for placement of the lower anterior brackets.

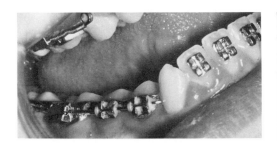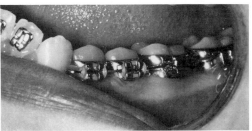

FIG. 6-43

Appliances are placed on the lower posterior teeth (second molar through first premolar), and these segments are leveled to define the functional occlusal plane (Fig. 6-43).

Appliances are then placed on the lower incisors, and a 16 × 16 utility arch is placed to begin incisor intrusion (Fig. 6-44).

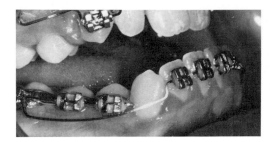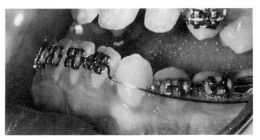

FIG. 6-44

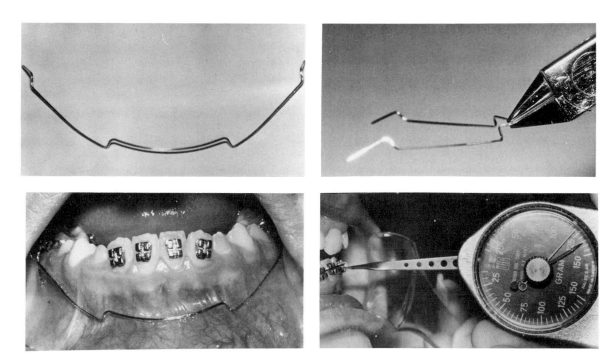

FIG. 6-45

This utility arch must have (1) labial root torque across the incisor section to keep the incisor roots away from the lingual cortical plate during intrusion and (2) tip-back bends at the molars sufficient to produce 80 to 100 g of intrusive force across the incisor section (Fig. 6-45).

Once lower incisor intrusion is begun, the appliances are placed on the upper arch and routine leveling and aligning are started. Archwires in the upper arch are increased in size until ideal archwires are placed. (For patients who require upper incisor intrusion, the upper arch can be treated exactly as described for the lower arch.)

When the lower incisors are level with the posterior segments, a continuous 16 × 16 or 16 × 22 archwire is placed. This wire steps down at the canine teeth, but otherwise is ideal in shape. Appliances are placed on the lower canines (it may be impossible to place a bracket because of interference from the maxillary teeth, and a button or cleat may be used). Elastic thread is used to intrude the canines to the desired level (Fig. 6-46). Intrusive forces of 35 to 50 g per tooth are adequate for canine intrusion; *excessive forces preclude intrusive movements.*

FIG. 6-46

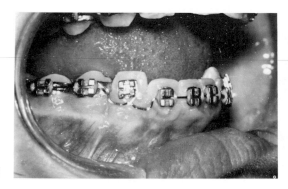 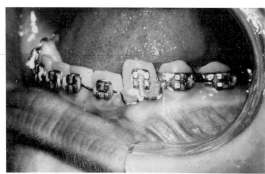

Once the canines are at the desired level, an ideal 16 × 22 lower archwire is placed and the upper and lower arches are coordinated. Class III elastics are now worn until the desired anteroposterior relationship is achieved. Judicious interproximal recontouring may also help in this respect. Elastics are avoided until this phase of treatment is reached because they may elevate the functional plane by decreasing the anterior intrusion if used before this time. Study models are now made to check arch coordination and leveling by doing feasibility surgery, and a cephalometric radiograph is taken to check the vertical and anteroposterior dental relationships. Once the presurgical treatment goals have been met, the archwires are tied with ligature wires, hooks are placed where appropriate (usually the canines), and the patient is referred for surgery.

The above method is not perfect, and the lower occlusal plane will probably not exactly match the pretreatment functional occlusal plane but will be very close to it. In cases in which this vertical difference is *critical,* surgical leveling of the curve of Spee by a lower anterior subapical procedure must be considered, as described later in this chapter (see forth adjunctive approach).

Immediate presurgical planning
SURGICAL CEPHALOMETRIC PREDICTION TRACING FOR MANDIBULAR ADVANCEMENT WITH ADVANCEMENT GENIOPLASTY

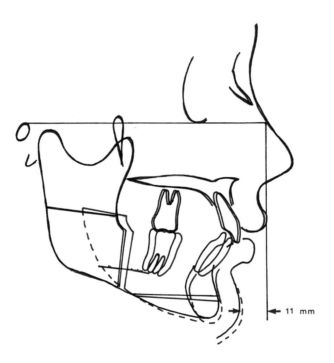

11 mm

FIG. 6-47

The surgical prediction is begun exactly as described previously in this chapter on pages 202 to 206. The cephalometric radiograph is traced, Frankfort horizontal, subnasale perpendicular, and several surgical reference marks are placed thereon. This drawing is referred to as the ***tracing*** (black lines). The ***prediction*** (red lines) is begun by tracing the distal mandible on a new piece of acetate paper and advancing it into the optimal occlusal relationship. The "fixed" structures are traced and the chin projection is checked for adequacy relative to subnasale perpendicular.

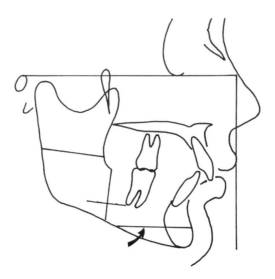

FIG. 6-48

When the chin projection is not adequate as in Fig. 6-47, a genioplasty is added to the ***prediction*** using the genioplasty line previously constructed on the ***tracing*** and transferred to the ***prediction*** to indicate the desired level and angulation of the horizontal osteotomy.

To review, this genioplasty reference line for the genioplasty (See arrow in Fig. 6-48) is drawn beneath the mental foramina, at least 30 mm below the lower occlusal plane, and as parallel to the occlusal plane as possible. The angle this line makes with Frankfort horizontal effects the vertical facial height as the genioplasty segment is advanced. If it is angled down anteriorly, the facial height will be increased; upward anteriorly, the facial height will be decreased. Moreover, the more this osteotomy is angled upward, the more uneven will be the inferior border of the mandible. This reference line is reproduced on the mandible at surgery by using two vertical measurements easily identified on a cephalometric radiograph: (1) the distance from the lower incisor edge to the osteotomy and, (2) the distance from the first premolar orthodontic bracket to the osteotomy.

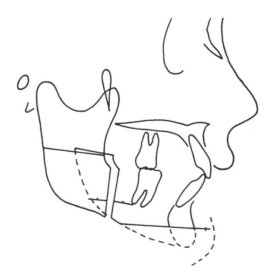

FIG. 6-49

The genioplasty is added to the ***prediction*** by extending the genioplasty line anteriorly on the ***prediction*** approximately 1.4 times the amount of soft-tissue augmentation desired.* A reference mark is also placed on this line anteriorly the amount of soft-tissue augmentation desired.

*N.B. The figure of 1.4 used herein is based on a ratio of soft tissue to hard tissue movement of 0.7:1 (1 ÷ 0.7 = 1.4). Current data suggests that the amount of soft tissue augmentation for a given amount of bone movement is dependent upon the amount of bone movement. The soft tissue moves almost 1:1 for bony movements less than 5 mm and decreases in movement reaching a ratio of 0.5:1 for bone movements over 15 mm. This ratio is also affected by the amount of mandibular advancement accompanying the genioplasty; the larger the advancement, the smaller the ratio of soft tissue movement produced by a genioplasty. Each clinician is encouraged to develop his or her own parameters by carefully observing the results obtained.

As a general rule, it is unesthetic to advance the bony chin more than a few millimeters anterior to the lower incisor teeth as may occur if one relies solely on subnasale perpendicular norms to plan treatment of an advancement genioplasty. No single parameter ideally defines the anteroposterior chin relation. Thus, the NB:Po and A-Po relations are also studied to determine the ideal position of the chin relative to these hard-tissue landmarks. Ideally, the incisal edge of the lower incisor lies equally as far ahead of the NB line as does the bony pogonion. Thus, if the lower incisor is 6 mm ahead of the NB line, so too should be pogonion. Also, the incisal edge of the lower incisor ideally lies 1 ± 2 mm ahead of the A-Po line. Accordingly, a line drawn from Point A through a point 1 mm behind the lower incisor tip and extended inferiorly would define the anterior location of pogonion. By adding the information from these two relations to that obtained from the subnasale perpendicular evaluation, the chin can be optimally repositioned. Usually the desired amount of augmentation as determined by these three methods is nearly the same. However, a discrepancy may exist when the soft tissue covering the chin is extremely thin or (rarely) when it is excessively thick. When consider-

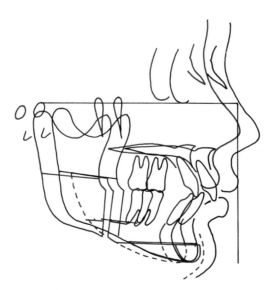

FIG. 6-50

able variance exists between these parameters, the bony chin is *not* advanced anterior to a line drawn from nasion through the tip of the lower incisors.

The proposed genioplasty is added to the **prediction** by sliding the **prediction** backward on the **tracing** keeping the genioplasty lines superimposed until the desired amount of bony augmentation is produced (the end of the anteriorly extended genioplasty line). The bony augmentation is traced.

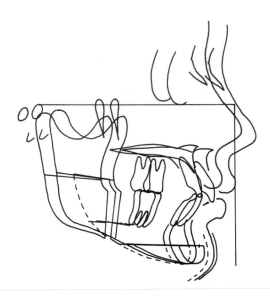

FIG. 6-51

The corresponding soft-tissue change is illustrated by sliding the ***prediction*** anteriorly along the genioplasty line to the reference mark previously placed in accordance with the expected ratio of soft-tissue to hard-tissue change and tracing the soft-tissue chin.

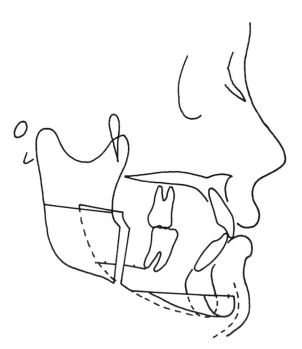

FIG. 6-52

The ***prediction*** is finished by completing the soft tissues of the lower lip as described in Chapter 2. This tracing provides the essential information properly to reposition and stabilize both the sagittal osteotomy sites and the genioplasty at surgery.

MODEL SURGERY

Most commonly the model surgery will be as previously described in the first usual approach. Occasionally, however, the dental arches will not be completely level either because it was not possible or because it was not desirable to do so during the presurgical orthodontic treatment. In such instances one may proceed with surgery if a Class I relationship can be achieved with no transverse discrepancy. The teeth will contact anteriorly and posteriorly with an open-bite relationship buccally in the premolar/first molar area. Importantly, *the most posterior molars must be in occlusal contact to preclude damage to the condyle following surgery*. Figure 6-53 illustrates this. The photos on the left depict the preoperative state of the patient's occlusion (Class II deep bite). The photos on the right depict the final model surgery. All the remaining occlusal discrepancies will be corrected orthodonically post-oper-

FIG. 6-53   atively.

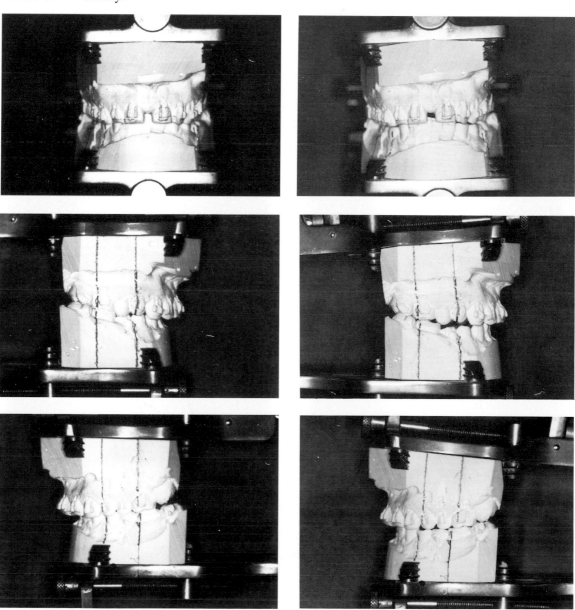

OCCLUSAL SPLINT CONSTRUCTION

Usually the occlusal splint is constructed as described in the first usual approach, above. However, when the occlusal planes are as described in the preceding paragraph, a "lingual bar" occlusal splint can be used to allow extrusion of the teeth in the buccal segments during the period of fixation. Such an occlusal splint is constructed as follows.

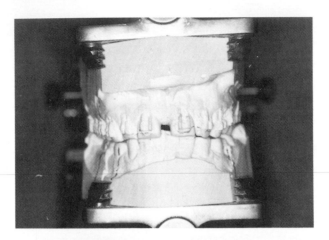

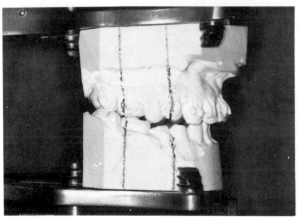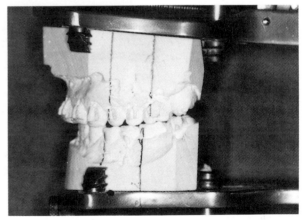

FIG. 6-54   Occlusal models are mounted on an articulator in Class I occlusion acceptable to the orthodontist completing the case. In deep-bite patients, this will create an open bite in the area of the premolars and perhaps the first molar.

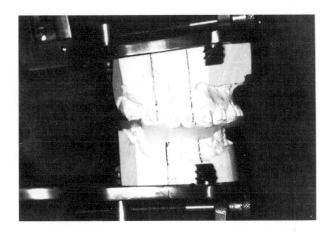

FIG. 6-55

Soft white utility wax is placed in the area of the open bite to prevent the flow of soft acrylic onto the occlusal surfaces of the teeth that are not in direct contact.

Orthodontic acrylic is now placed such that the terminal molars and anterior teeth are occlusally encased into the splint. An acrylic lingual bar connects these occlusal contact areas. The splint is finally trimmed and holes are drilled.

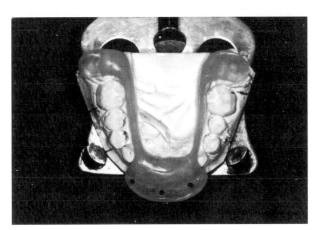 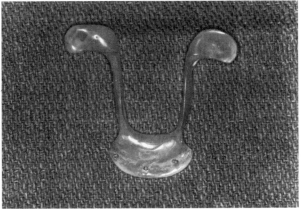

FIG. 6-56

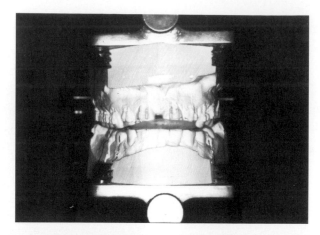

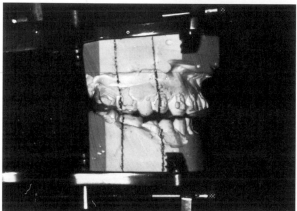

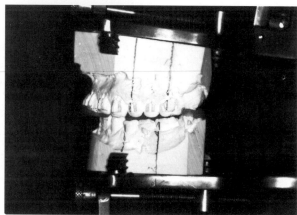

FIG. 6-56, cont'd

At surgery the orthodontic wire is cut at the interproximal area anterior to where the excessive curve of Spee begins. (Optionally, the orthodontist may place segmental wires or no wires prior to the surgery.) Interarch elastics are placed that will result in the eruption of these teeth to effect the closure of the open bite postoperatively. The exact location of orthodontic arch wire cutting and interarch elastics is case-dependent and is customized to fit the occlusal needs of each particular case (see "Postsurgical Orthodontic Treatment").

Orthognathic reconstructive surgery

MODIFIED SAGITTAL RAMUS OSTEOTOMIES WITH ADVANCEMENT GENIOPLASTY

When advancement genioplasty is to be performed along with the bilateral sagittal split ramus osteotomies the genioplasty is completed first, then the sagittal split ramus osteotomies. The primary reason is that this sequence minimizes the danger of displacement of the proximal segments due to surgical manipulation.

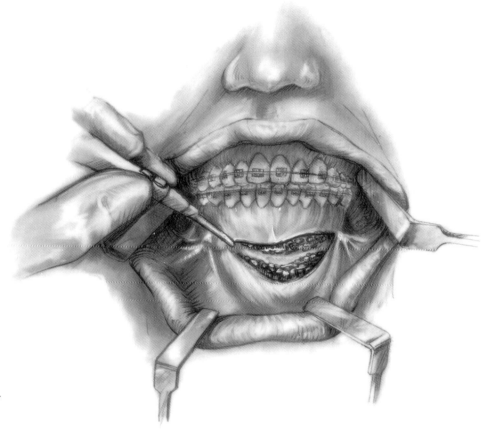

FIG. 6-57

About 5 minutes before making the incision, 5 to 10 ml of local anesthetic with 1:100,000 epinephrine is injected into the vestibule of the mandible in the location of the proposed genioplasty soft-tissue incision. The lips are lubricated as necessary during the procedure with steroid ointment. On retraction of the lower lip, the larger mucosal branches of the mental nerves can often be visualized through the mucosa. The incision is made in a layered fashion to the bone with a diathermy knife, being careful to avoid direct injury to the mental nerves. This incision passes tangentially through the submucosal tissues, the mentalis muscles, and finally the periosteum.

The subperiosteal dissection is first completed anteriorly to expose the inferior border of the mandible, and a symphysis retractor is inserted. The dissection is next extended posteriorly along the inferior borders of the mandible. Exposure of the mental nerves as they exit from the mandible is easily achieved with this approach, thus minimizing the chance of injury to them. Once exposed, the mental nerves are not deliberately dissected free from the surrounding soft tissues. This limited nerve dissection decreases mental nerve paresthesia of both the lower lip and chin.

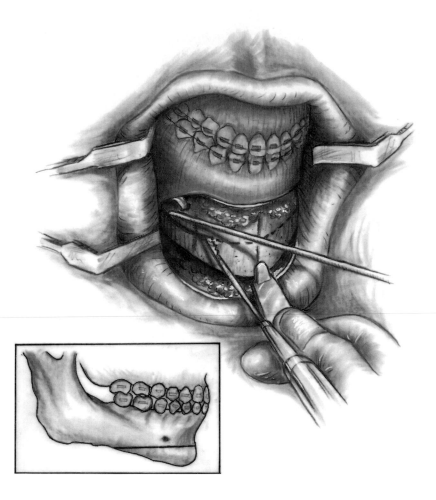

FIG. 6-58

The mandibular midline is marked, as well as the indicated vertical referents in the symphysis and premolar region as determined in the cephalometric prediction tracing. The planned horizontal osteotomy is made with a reciprocating saw. While doing so, it is prudent to protect the mental nerve with a suction tip to prevent nerve injury if the blade inadvertently bounces out of the osteotomy. This osteotomy is made 4 to 5 mm below the mental foramina and extends posteriorly to end in the molar area. This posterior extension of the horizontal osteotomy results in greater bone contact in large advancements, a good lateral ledge of bone, and avoids the unesthetic inferior border notch that is produced by shorter and/or steeper osteotomies.

Prior to performing the osteotomy it is helpful to mark its intended location on the outer cortex. The horizontal osteotomy is begun at its most posterior extent and the inferior border is completely cut through at this point. The blade is then laid on the surface of the symphysis bone with its tip still in the most posterior extent of the bony cut. This technique helps stabilize the reciprocating saw during saw movements. After grooving the outer cortex of the symphysis, the blade is repositioned to cut the bone at about a 45-degree angle to its surface, with the surgeon remaining cognizant of the thickness of the symphysis. All too often the replicating saw blade is hubbed to the outer cortex of bone and the lingual musculature is carelessly macerated by the overextended saw blade. The cut now extends to the midline of the symphysis. The same procedure is repeated on the opposite side in a symmetric fashion.

After the horizontal osteotomy is completed the inferior portion is mobilized by grasping it with a bone-holding forceps and pulling it anteriorly. When intraosseous skeletal suspension is to be used, additional lingual attachments of the anterior bellies of the digastric muscles may need to be removed from the most posterior aspect of the mobilized segment to make it possible to place the wires around the inferior border. However, it is important to maintain maximal attachment of the suprahyoid musculature to the mobilized segment to maintain its vascular pedicle. When the symphysis is stripped of its blood supply (that is, advanced as a free graft), it will resorb approximately 50%.

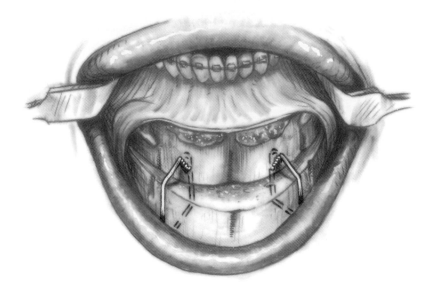

FIG. 6-59

Holes are placed bilaterally completely through the superior bone segment just posterior to the mental foramina. Then, while the mobilized segment is held in its planned position with a bone clamp, notches are made in the inferior border 2 to 3 mm posterior to the aforementioned holes so that the wires will hold the inferior segment forward when they are tightened. Two 22- or 24-gauge wires are passed through the holes, beneath the inferior border of the mobilized segment, and are tightened while maintaining the mobilized segment in its proper position.

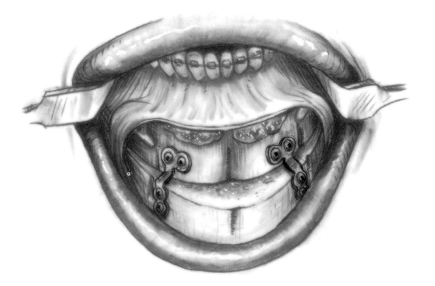

FIG. 6-60

Alternatively, bone plates can be used, but they produce no known advantage. The predetermined amount of advancement is checked by measuring with calipers, and right-to-left symmetry is maintained by aligning the midline mark and ensuring that the lateral "shelves" of the genioplasty segment are symmetrically positioned bilaterally. The surgical site is packed and the remaining surgical procedures are completed. If a cervical facial lipectomy is planned, it is accomplished just prior to closure at the completion of the orthognathic surgical procedures. The details of cervical-facial lipectomy are discussed in usual approach three, below.

When large chin advancements are performed or the patient has a pointed chin and/or parasymphysis depressions preoperatively (see Fig. 6-66), it is helpful to place a hydroxylapatite microfibrillar collagen mixture on the bony shelf created by the sliding osteotomy, especially laterally. The hydroxylapatite/microfibrillar putty mixture and soft-tissue closure described in the following paragraphs are accomplished *at the very end of the skeletal orthognathic surgery*. It is discussed here only to avoid disrupting the "flow" of the advancement genioplasty surgery.

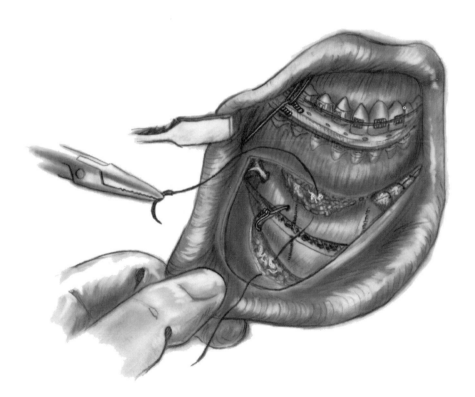

FIG. 6-61

Just prior to closure, the chin is rechecked for advancement and symmetry as the chin segment may have inadvertently been moved during other bony or soft-tissue manipulations. The initial soft-tissue closure is achieved by carefully reapproximating the mentalis muscles. Suturing of the mentalis muscles and associated periosteum is important to prevent ptosis of the lower lip with the resultant unsightly exposure of the lower anterior teeth. The mucosa is closed with running 3-0 chromic gut sutures and a tape dressing is applied to afford additional soft-tissue support and reduce edema. This dressing is left in place for 2 to 3 days.

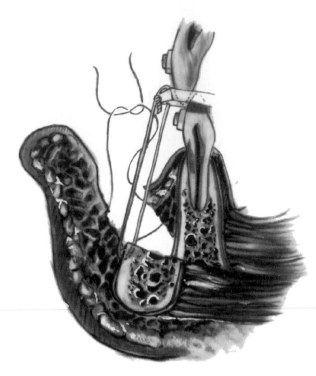

FIG. 6-62

When the lateral wires do not afford excellent stabilization of the advanced portion of the mandibular symphysis, such as in a major advancement, additional wire stabilization may be needed to prevent any downward and backward tipping of the segment secondary to the suprahyoid muscle pull. This is achieved by passing a wire from the center of the anteriormost aspect of the advanced segment to the occlusal splint. (If no splint is used, the orthodontic wire or brackets may be used.) This wire is removed when the piriform rim and circummandibular wires are removed.

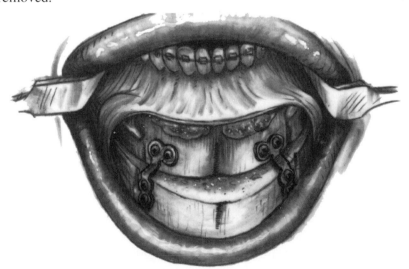

FIG. 6-63

A second option to stabilizing the genioplasty segment of the mandible is the usage of two L plates. All other surgical aspects of the advancement genioplasty are identical, except that stabilization of the segments is accomplished as illustrated in Fig. 6-63.

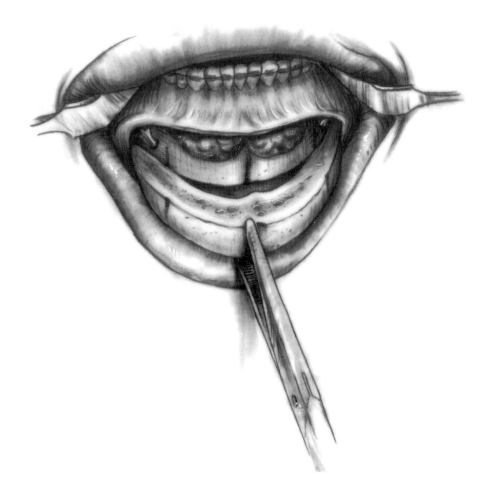

FIG. 6-64

Finally, with regard to advancement genioplasty, the maximum advancement genioplasty is discussed. This procedure is used when the amount of planned advancement of bony pogonion exceeds the thickness of the symphysis and allows unstable superior telescoping of the chin segment. The maximum advancement genioplasty technique uses two 2.0-mm diameter screws, placed bilaterally approximately 5 mm anterior to the mental nerve and superior to the horizontal osteotomy. The chin segment is then advanced such that the entire mobilized segment telescopes above the stable segment of the mandibular symphysis.

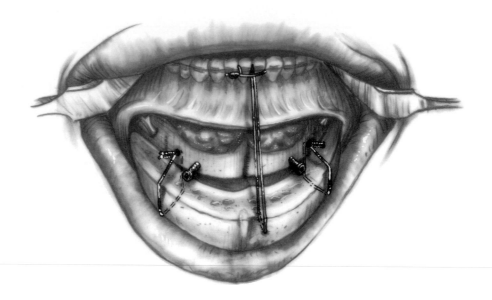

FIG. 6-65

The two screws placed as described above prevent further superior telescoping and act as positive stops, as well as a mechanism to secure the chin segment. To secure the genioplasty segment against the two screws, 24-gauge stainless steel wires are then placed as previously described. An additional wire in the midline of the chin segment may be used to stabilize the chin further if necessary and may be placed as illustrated in Fig. 6-65.

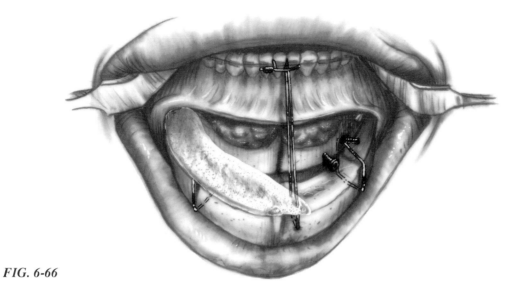

FIG. 6-66

As described previously for larger chin advancements, a putty mixture of hydroxylapatite and microfibrillar collagen* may be used to refine the contour around the large bony shelf created by the maximum advancement genioplasty. The sagittal split ramus osteotomies for mandible advancement are now done as described previously (first usual approach, above).

---

*Helitene, LifeSciences Company, Plainsboro, N.J. 08536.

Postsurgical orthodontic treatment

The postsurgical orthodontic treatment is completed as described above in the first usual approach. The exception to this is the patient who has had a "lingual bar" splint placed at surgery to allow leveling of the dental arches by extrusion of the teeth in the buccal segments. While the specific needs may vary with each individual patient, the following principles apply.

1. The most effective elastic traction is produced by 3.5-oz elastic, one-eighth of an inch less in length than the number of teeth to which it is attached in eighths (i.e., if five teeth are to be incorporated, then a 1/2-in. elastic is used—5 teeth/8 − 1/8 = 1/2 in.).
2. The elastic is woven anteriorly from lower to upper teeth using either brackets and/or hooks to secure them (Fig. 6-67).

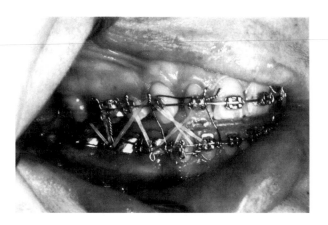

FIG. 6-67

3. The elastic should be changed by the patient or the doctor at least twice a day after surgical soreness has dissipated.
4. When differential extrusive movement is desired, the hierarchy of movement from most movement to least movement is:

Most movement	No wire
	Small flexible wire
	Large stiff wire
Least movement	Splint stabilization

Thus, differential extrusion of upper and lower teeth is possible to varying degrees using the following mechanical principles:

1. If equal movement is desired then either no archwire is placed or the same size archwire is placed in both arches.
2. If more movement of the teeth in one arch is desired either no archwire is placed in the arch to be moved farthest or a larger archwire is placed in the arch to be moved the least.
3. If no movement is desired in one arch, this is achieved by incorporating into the splint small wires that extend from the lingual bar and rest on the occlusal surface of the tooth (teeth) to be stabilized. Elastic traction is then placed as described above.

Factors affecting stability of treatment
Orthodontic factors

The factors affecting stability are the same as those described in detail in the first usual approach, above. They include removal of dental compensations, correction of tooth mass discrepancies, leveling of both arches, correction of any transverse discrepancy, and avoiding production of a double protrusion.

Surgical factors

The soft-tissue and skeletal mechanisms that contribute to surgical relapse were previously discussed in this chapter. One point is noteworthy, however, regarding the amount of advancement of pogonion. When the clinician considers the type of fixation that will be used for a particular case or the factors effecting skeletal relapse, it is *the total skeletal advancement of the mandible at pogonion* that must be considered. Therefore, if a treatment plan consists of a 4-mm sagittal split advancement and a 6-mm advancement genioplasty, *the total skeletal advancement is 10 mm (4 mm + 6 mm)*. It is this 10-mm advancement of pogonion that the surgeon should keep in mind when choosing a method of fixation or contemplating reasons for skeletal relapse.

Age-related factors

The age-related factors affecting the stability of this procedure are the same as those discussed in detail in the first usual approach, above.

Results of treatment

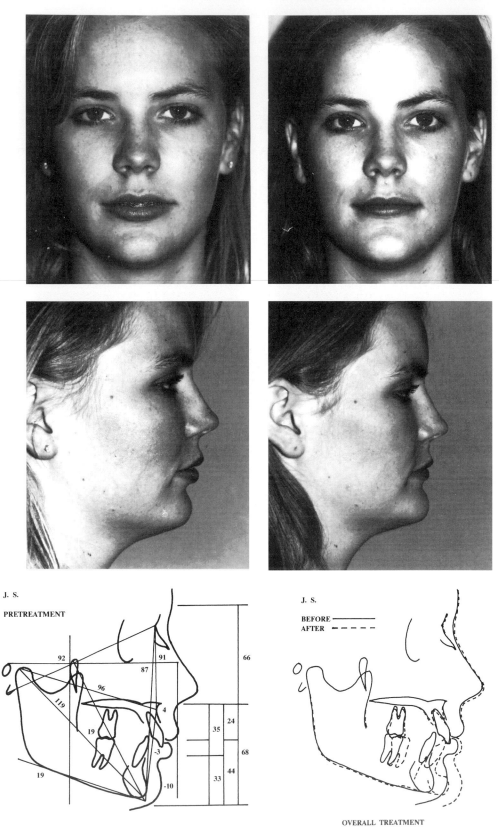

FIG. 6-68

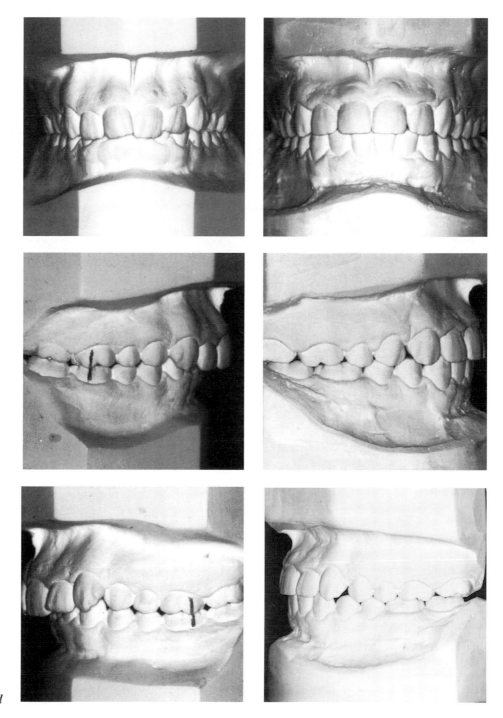

FIG. 6-68, cont'd

Third usual orthodontic-surgical approach: the patient with
a typical Class II, division 2 malocclusion

MANDIBULAR ADVANCEMENT

Outline of treatment

Presurgical orthodontic treatment

1. Place upper appliances; torque and intrude upper central incisors
2. Place lower appliances; align and level upper and lower arches
3. Coordinate arches while using Class III elastics as necessary
4. Impression for feasibility model surgery

Immediate presurgical planning

1. Surgical cephalometric prediction tracing
2. Model surgery
3. Occlusal splint construction as indicated

Orthognathic reconstructive surgery

1. Modified sagittal split ramus osteotomies

Postsurgical orthodontic treatment

1. Repair appliances as necessary
2. Check archwire coordination
3. Routine finishing procedures
4. Retain

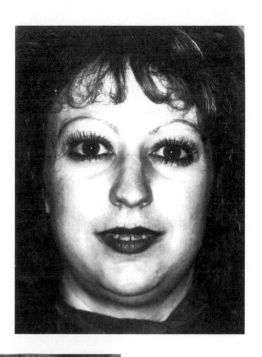

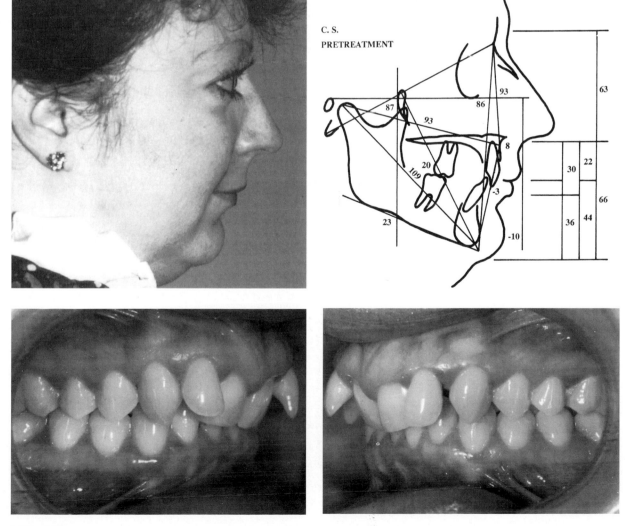

FIG. 6-69

Details of treatment

Presurgical orthodontic treatment

The goal of the presurgical orthodontic treatment for the patient with a Class II, division 2, deformity is to produce a Class II, division 1, malocclusion so that the mandible can be advanced. This requires intruding, advancing, and torquing the upper central (and sometimes lateral) incisors. When this is done, there will be little if any effect on the upper lip drape (esthetics) because before treatment there is a void between the upper lip and the upper central incisors as the upper lip support is produced by the lateral incisors and/or the lower lip. The upper arch may or may not require expansion to accommodate the advanced mandible. Generally, the transverse discrepancy is minimal and can be stably treated by orthodontic tooth movement. However, when the discrepancy is more than 6 mm in a patient over age 18 years, combined orthodontic and surgical expansion is required (see second adjunctive approach, above). In addition, the lower arch must be aligned and leveled.

In treatment planning for combined orthodontic-surgical correction of the Class II, division 2, dentofacial deformity, the preferred method of leveling the arches is important because this will have an effect on the changes produced at surgery in both the horizontal and vertical dimensions of the lower third face. For example, if the pogonion is prominent and the lower third face is short, it is desirable that the presurgical arch-leveling minimally intrude anterior teeth and instead extrude premolars (that is, leveling to the molar-incisor occlusal plane). When this is done, the subsequent surgery to advance the mandible will maximally increase lower face height and minimally increase the chin projection (see "Integration of Cephalometric Prediction Tracings," Chapter 2).

The first action taken is to note on the patient's chart that he/she is a surgical patient. This serves to alert both the clinician and his/her staff that this patient will not receive routine orthodontic treatment for the malocclusion. Treatment begins by placing appliances only on the upper molars and central incisors. A 16 × 16 utility arch with advancing springs is placed to begin intrusion as well as advancing and torquing the incisors (Fig. 6-70).

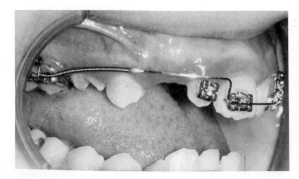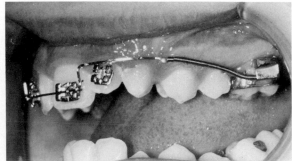

FIG. 6-70

The lower appliances are placed once the upper incisors have been advanced sufficiently to lower appliance placement on the lower incisors without occlusal interference. The lower arch is aligned and leveled. When an increase in the lower face height is desired as part of the treatment, this leveling can be done with continuous wires, gradually increasing in size and employing tip-back bends and vertical elastics in the premolar area, if desired, until the teeth are in the appropriate position. This method of leveling usually will produce more extrusion of the buccal segments than incisor intrusion; thus, the lower face height will be increased when the mandible is advanced.

Conversely, when an increase in the lower face height is not desired, leveling is done in the following manner:

1. Sectional archwires are placed from the second molar through the first premolar to level these teeth and thus establish the functional occlusal plane.
2. A 16×16 utility arch is placed with intrusive force for the incisors.
3. Once the incisors are level with the buccal segments, a continuous stabilizing archwire is placed and stepped around the canines, and elastic thread is used to intrude the canines to the level desired.
4. An ideal, continuous archwire is placed.

This technique is discussed and illustrated in detail in the preceding section of this chapter. It can be used in either arch or both arches as needed to achieve the desired leveling for the specific patient being treated.

The rest of the upper appliances are placed once the central incisors are advanced and level with the upper lateral incisors. The remaining leveling and aligning in the upper arch is routine: beginning with small, flexible wires, working to a rectangular ideal archwire coordinated with the lower ideal archwire. In most instances, a wire larger than 16×22 is rarely used, but the Class II, division 2, deformity may be an exception. When additional torque is desired for the upper central incisors, a 17×25 or even an 18×25 may be helpful.

Once both upper and lower arches are in coordinated archwires, a progress cephalometric radiograph is made to check the anteroposterior position of the teeth. Appropriate elastics, usually Class III, are used if necessary to produce the desired presurgical overjet. Once it appears that the presurgical orthodontic goals have been accomplished, models are made and feasibility model surgery is done. The primary goals are to achieve a Class I molar and canine relation without significant transverse or vertical problems. It is not necessary for all teeth to fit one another perfectly. Rather the goal is that the occlusion produced at surgery can be easily finished by routine orthodontic treatment. When these goals have been achieved, the patient is ready for surgery. The archwires are tied with ligature wires to prevent inadvertent disengagement of the wires, elastic hooks are placed where appropriate (usually the canines), and the patient is referred for surgery. If these goals have not been met, the factors described above chapter must be carefully studied and appropriate steps taken to correct the problems.

Immediate presurgical planning

Once the dental arches have been corrected sufficiently to allow the planned surgery to be done, the immediate presurgical planning is done as described in the preceding sections of this chapter.

Orthognathic reconstructive surgery

The major surgical procedure is a mandibular advancement most usually done by the modified sagittal split ramus osteotomy. This may be done in concert with an advancement genioplasty when it is determined to be necessary by the surgical prediction tracing. Because the total improvement in facial appearance is a major goal in combined orthodontic-surgical treatment, several adjunctive procedures are now commonly used in conjunction with orthognathic reconstructive surgery. One such procedure—the cervicofacial lipectomy—is applicable as an adjunct in the correction of a wide variety of facial deformities, but is presented here because the patient presented in this section is an excellent example of the improvement afforded by its use.

ADJUNCTIVE COSMETIC PROCEDURE—TRANSORAL CERVICAL FACIAL LIPECTOMY

Orthognathic surgical procedures may improve or worsen the cervicomental or neck-chin esthetics (Table 6-1). In instances in which improvement such as mandibular advancement and/or advancement genioplasty is expected, the surgeon must critically determine if the change in the neck-chin angle can be additionally improved by the simultaneous removal of excessive cervical-facial fat. Conversely, if the planned orthognathic procedure will predictably worsen the cervicomental esthetics, as is the case with correction of mandibular prognathism, a simultaneous cervical facial lipectomy may be used to negate these untoward effects. In either instance, the existence of cervical-facial lipomatosis without redundant skin is a relative indication for simultaneous cervical-facial lipectomy. The transoral technique is preferred to the transfacial technique when a mandibular anterior vestibular incision is used with the planned orthognathic surgery. Such incisions are necessary to accomplish a genioplasty and/or a mandibular subapical procedure, and therefore, are easily used to gain access to the cervical-facial fat.

TABLE 6-1. *EFFECT OF ORTHOGNATHIC PROCEDURES ON NECK-CHIN ESTHETICS*

Improved	*Worsened*
Mandibular advancement	Mandibular setback
Advancement genioplasty	Reduction genioplasty
Superior maxillary repositioning	Inferior maxillary repositioning
Any combination of the above	Any combination of the above

When no orthognathic procedure is performed in the mandibular symphysis region, or tissue redundancy exists in the cervical facial area, a cervical facial lipectomy is best accomplished transfacially. This approach is described in Chapter 10. In the following section, only the transoral cervical-facial lipectomy is described.

The cervical-facial lipectomy is performed after completion of all planned orthognathic surgical procedures so that the pressure dressing can be applied immediately after its completion to minimize hematoma and excessive edema. When cervical-facial liposuction is planned, the area to be treated for fat reduction is marked with an indelible pen while the patient is sitting upright and before they are taken to the surgical suite. The inferior border of the mandible and the anterior borders of the sternocleidomastoid muscles are marked. Inferiorly, the location of the thyroid cartilage is used to draw a horizontal line connecting the two lines defining the anterior borders of the sternocleidomastoid muscles. In addition, areas that manifest an excess of subcutaneous fat are highlighted with the marking pen. These most frequently exist in the submental and occasionally in the jowl areas.

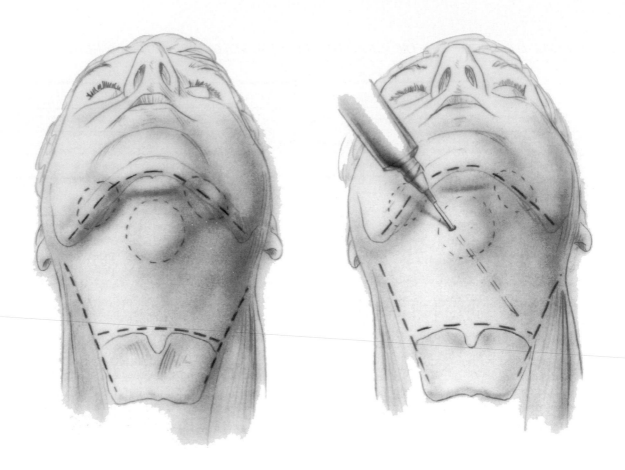

FIG. 6-71   *FIG. 6-72*

The neck is instilled with approximately 20 ml of 1% lidocaine with 1:200,000 epinephrine using an 18-gauge 5-in. spinal needle. This infiltration is carried out in the subcutaneous-supraplatysmal muscle tissue plane throughout the entire area outlined previously. After infiltration, approximately 10 minutes is allowed to elapse prior to beginning the surgical procedure. During this time the infiltration will generally cause noticeable blanching of the area.

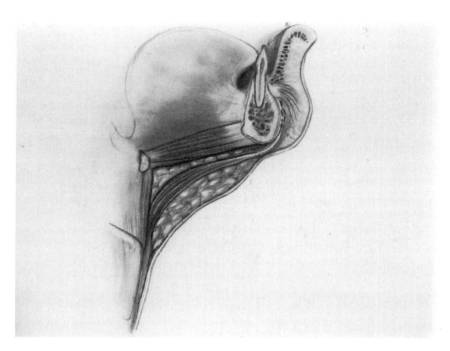

FIG. 6-73

Figure 6-73 illustrates the anatomic relationships in the chin and cervical area. The fat to be removed is located superficial to the platysma muscle and is approached through the traditional vestibular incision. The subperiosteal dissection is carried out, elevating the periosteum, overlying muscles, and mucosa, down to and including the inferior border of the mandible.

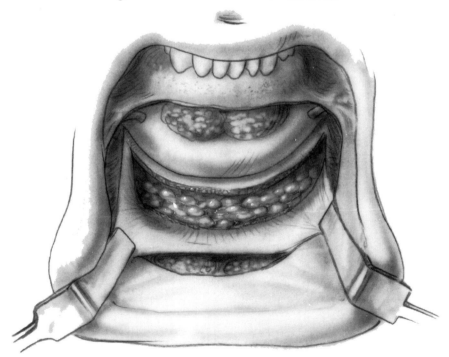

FIG. 6-74

The periosteum and underlying platysma muscle are incised at the level of the inferior mandibular border. This affords easy entry into the submental-cervical region deep to the skin and superficial to the platysma muscle. The entry incision into this space is best located distal to the prominent submental skin crease, when one exists, to avoid accentuation of this region postoperatively.

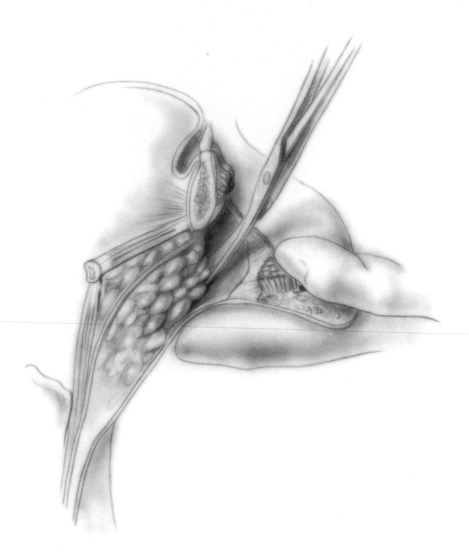

FIG. 6-75

Dissecting scissors with cutting edges on the outer and inner sides of each blade are used to create a subcutaneous pocket, while leaving a small amount of fat attached to the dermis. This dissection is then extended to the boundaries of the presurgical markings. The fat is suctioned with 8- to 10-mm suction cannulas at between 0.5 and 1.0 atmosphere of suction pressure. This is initially done with the opening directed deeply toward the platysma, using a raking and sweeping motion. Visual inspection and the "pinch test" is used to ensure optimal fat removal and determine the need to remove any subplatysmal fat.

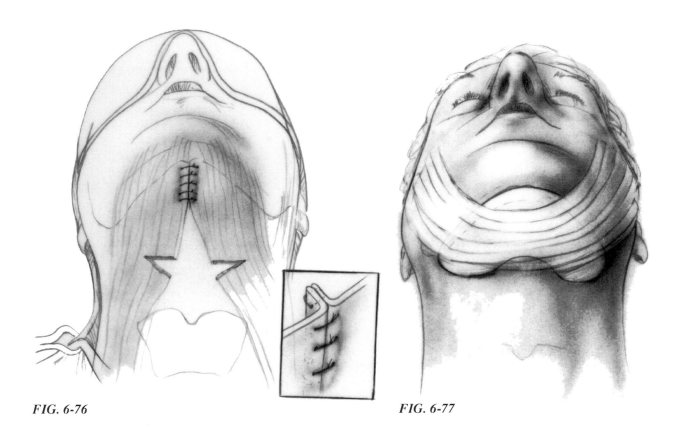

FIG. 6-76   **FIG. 6-77**

Once all the fat has been removed from the platysma, a dehiscence is often seen in the midline of the muscle. When significant subplatysmal fat is present, this fat is removed through the dehiscence. When dehiscence of the platysma has been performed, it is plicated using an absorbable suture. Closure of the incision is now completed in layers with care to reapproximate the mentalis muscle accurately to circumvent lower lip ptosis.

A pressure dressing, made from an arm board cut and fashioned to fit within the confines of the mandibular inferior border and half-inch paper tape, is placed and left for 3 to 5 days. This provides a firm stint during the initial healing phase. Such a rigid board ensures good subcutaneous adaptation and reduces the risk of hematoma formation. No drains are used.

Postsurgical orthodontic treatment

The postsurgical orthodontic treatment for the Class II, division 2, malocclusion is as described previously in this chapter and is not repeated here.

Factors affecting stability

The factors affecting stability are the same as previously discussed in this chapter and are not repeated here.

Results of treatment

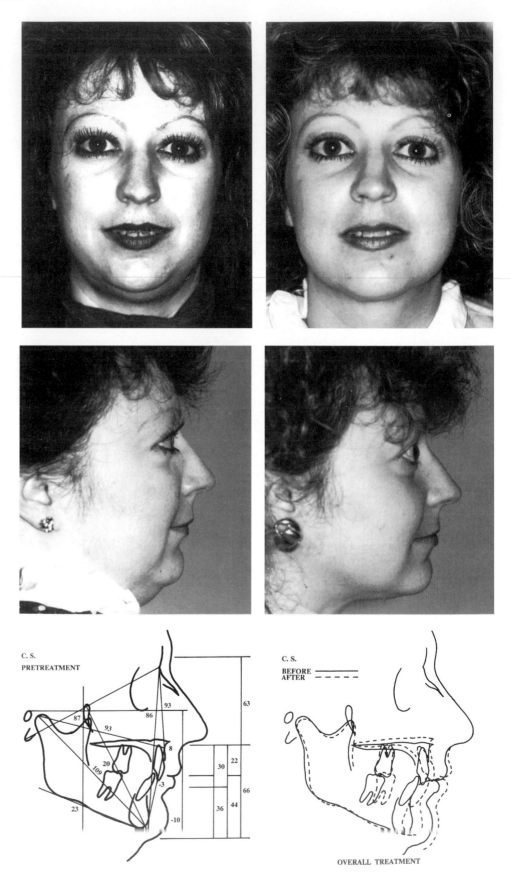

C. S.
PRETREATMENT

93
87   86
93
8
63
20
109
-3
30   22
23
36   44   66
-10

C. S.

BEFORE ————
AFTER - - - - -

FIG. 6-78

OVERALL TREATMENT

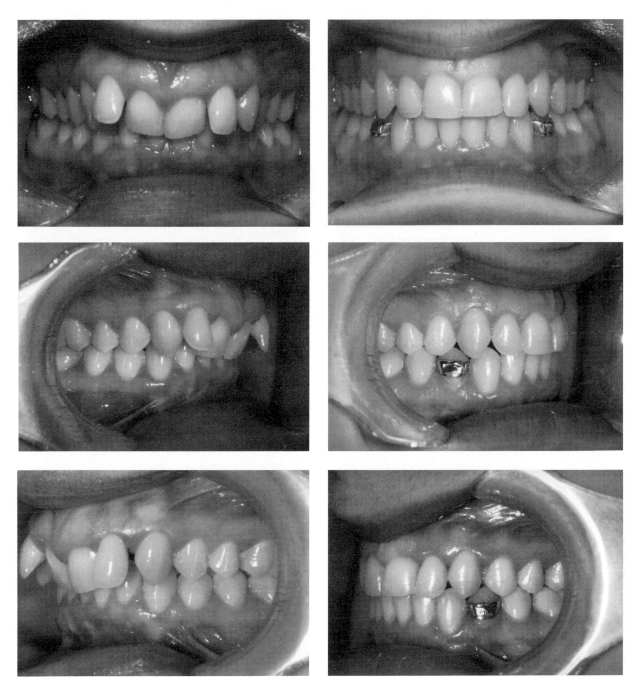

FIG. 6-78, cont'd

Adjunctive orthodontic-surgical procedures:
- *MANDIBULAR ADVANCEMENT WITH REDUCTION GENIOPLASTY*
- *ORTHODONTIC-SURGICAL MAXILLARY EXPANSION FOLLOWED BY MANDIBULAR ADVANCEMENT*
- *MANDIBULAR ADVANCEMENT WITH NARROWING BY MANDIBULAR MIDLINE OSTEOTOMY*
- *MANDIBULAR ADVANCEMENT WITH ANTERIOR MANDIBULAR SUBAPICAL OSTECTOMY*

MANDIBULAR ADVANCEMENT WITH REDUCTION GENIOPLASTY

Contingency statement

In certain patients with Class II dentofacial deformities there exists adequate (normal) projection of the chin while the mandibular dentoalveolus is retruded. When this condition exists, advancement of the mandible will result in excessive protrusion of the chin. In such instances either sagittal mandibular advancement with simultaneous reduction genioplasty or total subapical mandibular advancement should be considered. The former procedure is technically easier. However, the most important factor in making this decision is the actual magnitude of the discrepancy between the lower incisor and pogonion positions. When the anteroposterior discrepancy is less than 5 mm, good esthetics can generally be achieved with routine mandibular advancement and a properly performed anteroposterior reduction genioplasty. As this difference approaches 8 to 10 mm, poor esthetic results are achieved with reduction genioplasty because when major posterior movements are done by this approach, the labiomental fold is eliminated, the chin is made to look very square, and the submental area exhibits a permanent increased fullness. Thus, when a large discrepancy exists between the lower incisor and pogonion position, the total subapical mandibular advancement becomes the treatment of choice (see first alternate approach, above). Mandibular advancement with reduction genioplasty is discussed in this section.

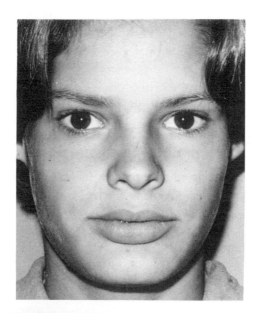

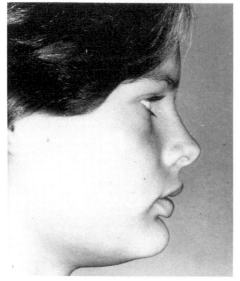

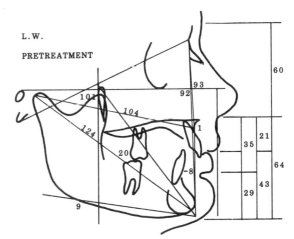

L.W.

PRETREATMENT

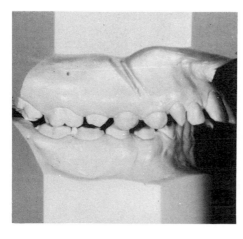

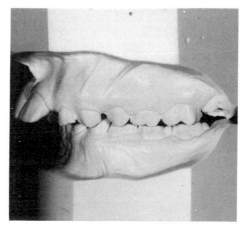

FIG. 6-79

Details of treatment

Presurgical orthodontic treatment

The patient who is considered for mandibular advancement with reduction genioplasty generally has mandibular dentoalveolar retrusion. As such, orthodontically placing the lower incisors in the proper relation to the anteroposterior line, while correcting the malocclusion, would require advancing the lower incisors beyond their supporting alveolar bone. The surgical posterior repositioning of pogonion makes it possible for the lower incisors to be placed in their optimal position without excessive advancement.

A prediction tracing must be done to determine the specific orthodontic mechanics to be used and the need for extractions. When a reduction genioplasty is to be included, the first step in making the prediction tracing is to reduce pogonion by an amount that will produce optimal mandibular anatomy and then complete the tracing as described in Chapter 2. The presurgical orthodontic treatment is done as described previously in this chapter. Most frequently such treatment will be nonextraction, but there will be instances when extractions are necessary. Regardless, the presurgical goals are to level, align, and coordinate the arches to permit the lower arch to be advanced into a Class I occlusion with good overbite and overjet and without transverse problems. Furthermore, when the face is symmetric, it is important that the maxillary dental midline is coincident with the midline of the face and the magnitude of the Class II occlusion is the same on each side to avoid an asymmetric mandibular advancement and the potential production of an asymmetric chin. The specific presurgical orthodontic mechanics necessary to treat this patient were presented above, and the appropriate discussion should be reviewed for more detailed information.

Orthognathic reconstructive surgery

When sagittal mandibular advancement and reduction genioplasty are done simultaneously, the sequencing of the surgical procedures is first to perform the reduction genioplasty to completion. Completing the genioplasty before the sagittal splits reduces the potential for disrupting the screws used to secure the proximal and distal segments. Additionally, this sequence avoids cutting the circum-mandibular wires (if used) since they are passed after the reduction genioplasty is completed.

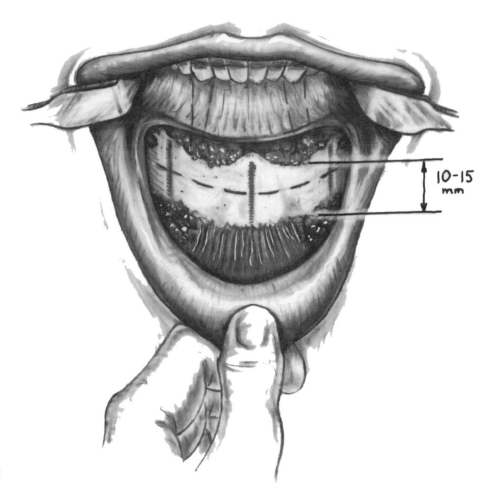

10-15 mm

FIG. 6-80

About 10 minutes after the region has been injected with a local anesthetic with 1:100,000 epinephrine, an incision is made in the depth of the labial vestibule with a diathermy knife from about the distal of the canine on one side to the same location on the opposite side. The subperiosteal dissection is very limited, and *the symphysis is not degloved,* since degloving produces unpredictable soft-tissue results. The subperiosteal dissection is done to expose approximately 10 mm of bone anteriorly in the area just beneath the tooth root apices. This subperiosteal dissection is then carried posteriorly to expose the mental neurovascular bundles bilaterally and finally the inferior border of the mandible distal to them in the region beneath the molar teeth.

Three references are scored into the mandibular symphysis with a bur to maintain symmetry when the chin is repositioned. These references include midline and bilateral bone scores just anterior to the mental foramen. Also, two holes are drilled into each of these lines—one 5 mm above and one 5 mm below the planned location of the horizontal osteotomy. These will permit accurate caliper determination of any indicated vertical change. This is discussed in more detail below.

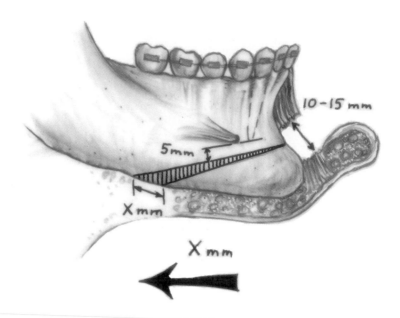

FIG. 6-81

Calipers are used to measure the level of the horizontal osteotomy so that it passes at least 5 mm beneath the canine apices and the mental foramen bilaterally and external posteriorly to the inferior border. Next the *two proposed osteotomy lines* are scribed into the bone as noted. The distance *X* is equivalent to that to which the chin segment will be retropositioned. This manner of performing the osteotomies and ostectomy avoids protrusion of the posterior corner of the mobilized segment, which will create an irregular inferior mandibular border.

The horizontal osteotomy is completed with a reciprocating saw while protecting the mental neurovascular bundle with the suction tip. The saw is held in one hand and a finger of the opposite hand is held facially to detect the tip of the saw as it cuts through the posterior and lingual aspects of the inferior border of the mandible. So doing avoids unnecessary extension of the saw blade into the soft tissues with the potential for laceration of the facial vein and/or artery.

When performing this procedure the most inferior osteotomy is completed first, so that the more superior osteotomy can then be more readily achieved on the "stable" component of the mandible. The linear distance between the two most proximal extents of the inferior and superior osteotomies will be equivalent to the linear amount that the chin will be set back. *X* in Figs. 6-81 through 6-85 represent the amount of genioplasty set back.

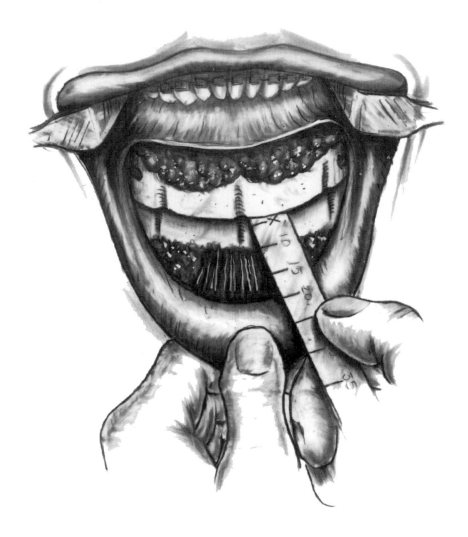

FIG. 6-82

After completion of both horizontal osteotomies, which creates a triangular ostectomy from each side of the mandible, the inferior segment is repositioned posteriorly the amount determined from the cephalometric prediction tracing and checked by measurement. The lateral referent lines are used to determine both the magnitude of retropositioning and symmetry of the repositioned chin segment. At this time marks are made with a bur where the holes are to be drilled to wire the segments together.

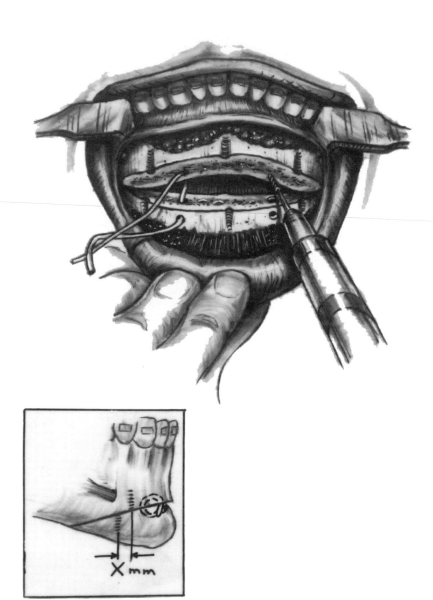

FIG. 6-83

Appropriately positioned holes are placed through the lingual cortex of the superior bone bilaterally and the labial cortex of the inferior (mobilized) segment. These will retract the chin segment when they are tightened. The exact locations of these holes is important. The desired anteroposterior change may not occur when the wires are tightened if these holes are placed arbitrarily.

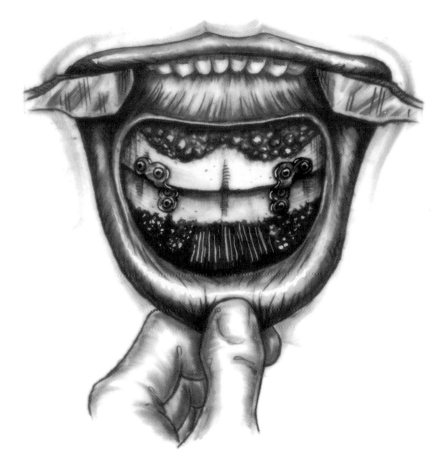

FIG. 6-84

The use of small L-shaped bone plates is an alternate method of stabilization, but when doing so, care must be exercised that the superior bone holes and screws do not injure the tooth roots.

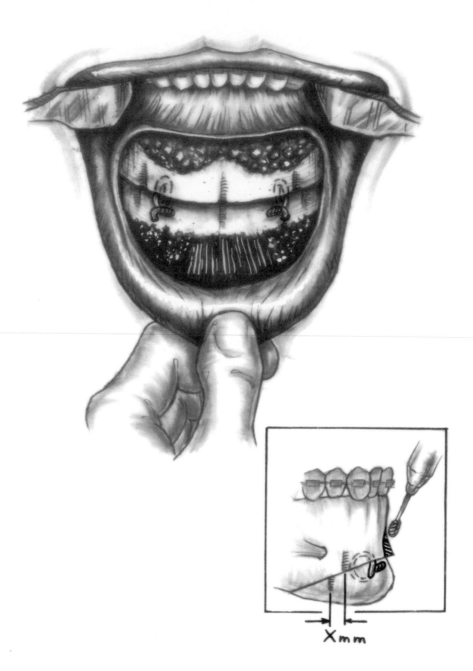

FIG. 6-85

    A small sharp ridge of bone is usually present where the superior osteotomy was made. This may be smoothed using a round bur (Fig. 6-85). Care must be taken not to shave the facial surfaces of adjacent root apices. If this procedure is necessary, it is completed prior to the placement of bone plates since this recontouring will affect the final shape of these plates.

The genioplasty site is packed to reduce residual bleeding and the sagittal splits are now performed to completion. The surgical details of the sagittal splits have been discussed previously in this chapter, and the reader may review that portion of the text if so desired. Following the mucosal closure of the sagittal splits, the genioplasty incision is closed in a deliberate layered fashion.

The mentalis muscles and associated periosteum are first reapproximated with 3-0 chromic gut suture, and then the mucosa is closed with a running horizontal mattress suture. A multilayered tape pressure dressing is applied and left in place for 2 to 5 days. This dressing extends posteriorly the extent of the genioplasty to maintain the healing soft tissues tightly against bone and to minimize the sequelae of increased soft-tissue fullness in these regions. After removal of the pressure dressing, a nighttime elastic neck dressing is helpful and heat is applied to the area to accelerate reduction of the edema and/or ecchymosis. After 10 to 14 days the patient is to begin lower lip exercises to reduce the inevitable tightness in this area more rapidly. The patient is maintained on a no-chew diet for 10 to 14 days after surgery to preclude disrupting the vestibular incision.

About 6 weeks following surgery the area is considered sufficiently healed so that the patient can return to unlimited physical activities.

Postsurgical orthodontic treatment

The addition at a reduction genioplasty to the mandibular advancement procedure has no effect on the postsurgical orthodontic care. Patient appointments and mechanics are used just as described for the "usual" patients earlier in this chapter. The reader is encouraged to review this as desired.

Factors affecting stability of treatment
Orthodontic factors

The addition of a reduction genioplasty to the mandibular advancement procedure has little if any effect on the orthodontic stability, except as it relates to allowing the lower incisor to anteroposterior relationship to be normalized without excessive flaring of the lower incisors. In this respect any increase in stability is attributed to the fact that less orthodontic movement is necessary to produce the desired esthetic and occlusal results.

All other factors relating to orthodontic stability in mandibular advancement procedures are applicable here except concerns for producing a double protrusion. These factors include the following:
1. Making the occlusion more Class II before surgery
2. Properly managing tooth mass discrepancies before surgery
3. Adequately leveling upper and lower arches before surgery
4. Properly managing any transverse discrepancy before surgery
5. Being aware that deep-bite relapse is not common

These factors are discussed in detail earlier in this chapter and may be reviewed for more information.

Surgical factors

Surgical factors related to the stability of the surgically advanced mandible have been discussed in detail earlier in this chapter and are not repeated here.

The skeletal stability of the reduction genioplasty is generally excellent if it is done as a well-pedicled, vascularized bone segment. If, instead, it is done as a free bone segment, unpredictable resorption will occur. Similarly, the primary factor in obtaining the optimal soft-tissue esthetic result is related to removing minimal soft tissue from the inferior (mobilized) segment. When the inferior chin segment is not degloved, the skeletal movement of the symphysis carries the soft tissue with it in nearly a 1:1 ratio and optimizes the predicted esthetic result. This requires considerable care at surgery and makes the operation much more tedious than advancement genioplasty wherein the chin is degloved. Finally, a tightly applied pressure dressing is helpful to optimize the desired soft-tissue result.

Age-related factors

Factors related to age and mandibular advancement have been previously discussed in the usual treatment section of this chapter. The addition of a reduction genioplasty will have no effect on subsequent growth, and any growth after surgery will not reestablish the prominent pogonion once it is surgically reduced.

Results of treatment

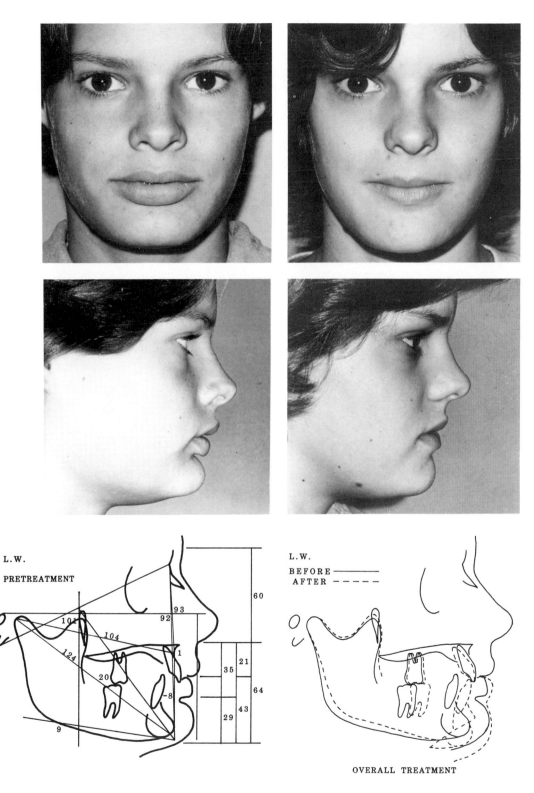

FIG. 6-86

ORTHODONTIC-SURGICAL MAXILLARY EXPANSION FOLLOWED BY MANDIBULAR ADVANCEMENT

Contingency statement

When mandibular advancement surgery is planned for an adult patient (over 18 years of age) and a transverse discrepancy of 6 mm or more exists due to maxillary constriction, combined orthodontic-surgical expansion of the maxilla is recommended as a part of the treatment plan. The need for this is determined by observation after placing the models into the desired anteroposterior position (that is, mandible advanced) or measuring the transverse relations between the maxillary and mandibular teeth (cusp to appropriate fossa) in the molar, premolar, and canine areas. When the diagnosis of a transverse discrepancy is made, a distinction must be made between a transverse discrepancy that exists as the result of dental tipping and a true transverse maxillary skeletal discrepancy. This is done by evaluating the buccolingual inclination of the posterior teeth. When the discrepancy is the result of lingual tipping of the maxillary teeth or buccal tipping of the mandibular teeth, routine orthodontic uprighting of the teeth is usually sufficient to correct the problem.

Orthodontic-surgical expansion of the maxilla is recommended when the transverse discrepancy is truly skeletal—transverse maxillary deficiency. This is generally done as the first phase of treatment, unless compensatory lingual tipping or extreme malalignment of the mandibular teeth exists. When these conditions exist, it is advisable initially to upright and align the lower teeth, placing them into their proper positions relative to the basal bone, so that the proper amount of maxillary expansion can be accurately achieved.

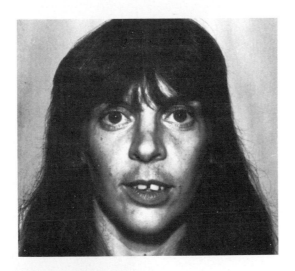

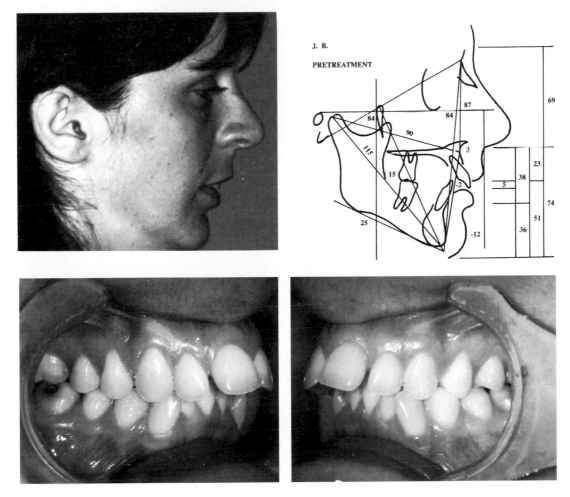

FIG. 6-87

Details of treatment
Presurgical orthodontic treatment

The first thing that is done for this patient is to mark prominently on the chart that combined orthodontics and surgery are to be used so that the entire staff knows that routine Class II procedures will not apply to this patient.

At the first appointment separators are placed mesial and distal to the teeth that will support the expansion appliance (usually first molars and first premolars). One week later, bands are fit on these teeth and an impression is made. The bands are carefully removed and placed into the impression, and the impression is poured, producing a working model on which to construct the expansion appliance. Separators are again placed. The following week the appliance is cemented but not activated (Fig. 6-88). The patient is now ready for the surgical procedure.

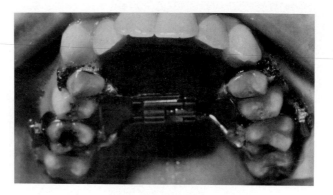

FIG. 6-88

Three things are important regarding the expansion appliance used. First, the appliance is ideally a fixed appliance. Second, the appliance must be capable of the desired amount of expansion without need for refabrication. Third, the appliance is preferably tooth-borne both to allow surgical access and to avoid possible palatal soft-tissue necrosis. This latter consideration is important, since *after surgical mobilization the major blood supply to the dentoosseous segments being moved comes from the palatal mucosa.*

Orthognathic reconstructive surgery

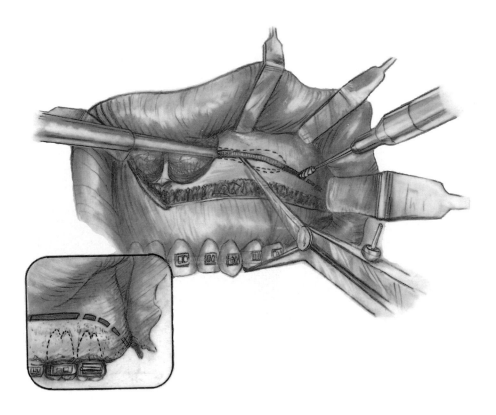

FIG. 6-89

With the patient under general anesthesia or intravenous sedation, a local anesthetic with 1:100,000 epinephrine is injected into the depth of the maxillary vestibule from tuberosity to tuberosity about 5 to 10 minutes before making the initial incision. An incision is made in the depth of the vestibule with a diathermy knife from the region of the first molar on one side to the midline. The soft tissues are reflected subperiosteally, first superiorly from the lateral aspect of the maxilla. Next, the dissection is done to expose the anterior floor of the nose and piriform aperture area. Finally, the subperiosteal dissection is carried posteriorly to the pterygoid-maxillary junction.

The level of the lateral maxillary osteotomy is determined with calipers, making it at least 5 mm above the tooth-root apices. This is approximately 30 to 35 mm above the cusp tip of the maxillary canine in the piriform area and 25 mm above the cusp tips of the maxillary molars.

As the osteotomy is being done anteriorly, a periosteal elevator is maintained beneath the nasal mucoperiosteum to protect it. Once the lateral maxillary wall osteotomy is distal to the terminal molar tooth it is tapered inferiorly to avoid, or at least minimize, the need for pterygoid-maxillary separation by a traditional osteotomy with a pterygoid osteotome. The inferiorly tapered lateral wall osteotomy is readily done with a small curved osteotome.

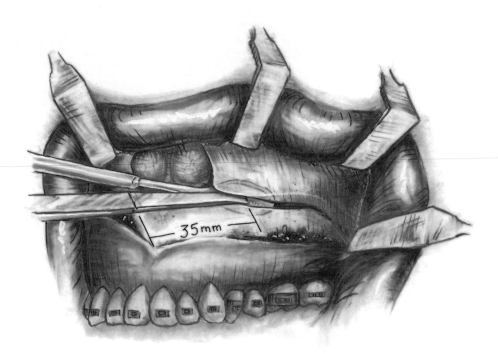

FIG. 6-90

On completion of the lateral maxillary wall osteotomy, a periosteal elevator is passed subperiosteally well distally into the lateral wall of the nose. This is used to protect the nasal mucoperiosteum while a small curved osteotome is malleted posteriorly to complete the lateral nasal wall osteotomy. This osteotomy is stopped short of the greater palatine bone (about 35 mm posterior to the piriform rim). The same soft-tissue incision is now made on the opposite side, and the identical dissection and osteotomies are completed.

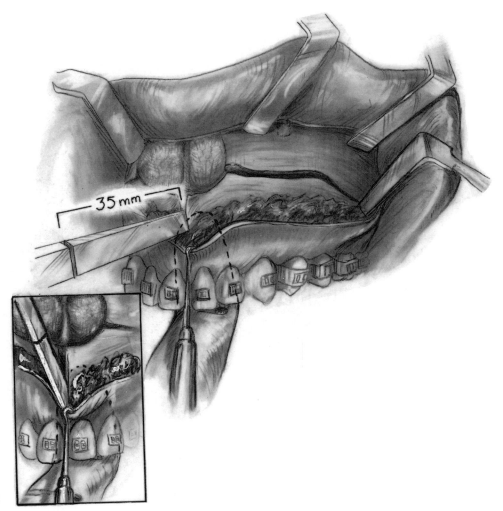

FIG. 6-91

The midline of the anterior maxillary alveolus is separated with a small straight osteotome. When this osteotome is malleted, a finger is placed palatally to feel it as it passes through the palatal aspect of the bone and, thereby, to avoid incising the palatal mucosa. The midpalatal osteotomy is similarly accomplished by malleting this osteotome posteriorly, parallel to the palatal plane, to ensure separation of the entire midpalatal suture. This also results in separation of the nasal septum and avoids the need for additional nasal-septal osteotomies by use of a nasal septal osteotome.

All essential osteotomies have now been completed, and mobilization of the maxilla is next achieved. This is done by manually applying a downward force on the maxilla. However, unlike the usual LeFort I down-fracture, *the maxilla is mobilized only 10 to 15 mm inferiorly*. This is done to ensure completeness of all osteotomies and fractures, especially posteriorly, yet it does not make the maxilla unnecessarily mobile.

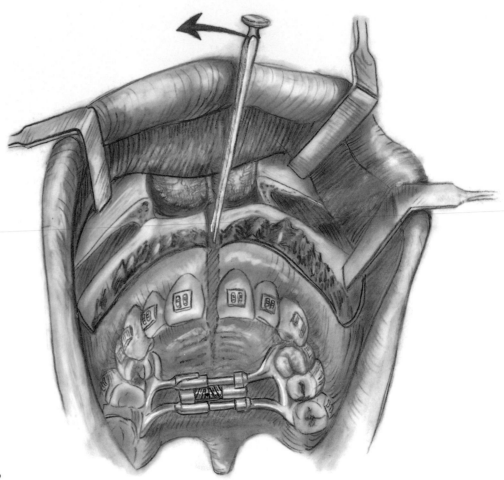

FIG. 6-92

Finally, the midpalatal osteotomy is similarly mobilized by inserting an osteotome into it and torquing it right to left until an obvious 2-to-4-mm opening occurs anteriorly. More separation is not possible because of the presence of the orthodontic expansion appliance.

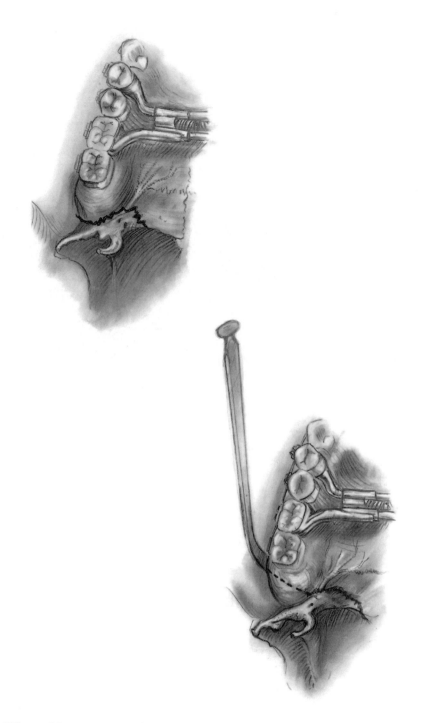

FIG. 6-93

When this sequence of osteotomies and subsequent mobilization is done, fractures will generally occur posteriorly between the maxilla, pterygoid plates, and palatine bones. However, if it becomes apparent that this area is not mobilized adequately, a small curved osteotome is inserted in the tuberosity region and malleted medioposteriorly. As this is being done, a finger is placed palatally to detect the osteotome passing through this region. Before removal of this osteotome, it is torqued anteriorly and posteriorly to ensure completeness of the osteotomy and fractures in this area. This is generally not necessary in younger patients, but may be in older individuals.

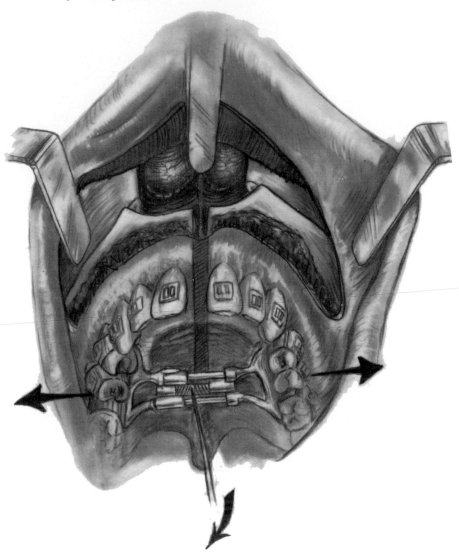

FIG. 6-94

The expansion device is now activated so that the maxilla is actually expanded 3 to 5 mm before closure of the soft-tissue incisions. More than 5 mm of expansion is contraindicated to avoid tearing the gingival tissue between the central incisors, which may result in permanent loss of the papilla. As the activation is done, a midline diastema opens between the incisors, and the lateral maxillary walls will be noted to expand. It is essential at this time to note that the expansion is occurring bilaterally and symmetrically. If only unilateral expansion is noted, the mobilization is incomplete and the osteotomies must be checked and completed on the stable side, otherwise unilateral, asymmetric expansion will result. If asymmetric expansion occurs, it is also advisable to make certain the nasal septum is separated by use of a nasal septal osteotome.

The soft tissues are closed, and the remainder of the predetermined expansion is completed over the next week or two. This must be carefully checked and measured, as overexpansion is contraindicated. No fixation is employed, and the patient is forewarned that *mastication is prohibited for the next 4 to 6 weeks* until bony union is achieved. Further, the patient is informed that this procedure will result in a large midline diastema that will require subsequent orthodontic closure, as discussed in the postsurgical orthodontic section.

Postsurgical orthodontic treatment

Following surgery, the patient is informed about appliance activation (two one-quarter turns per day), and this process is closely observed. The patient is seen 2 to 5 days following surgery to check his/her understanding of the activation procedure and to measure the progress closely. The patient is then seen at appropriate intervals (usually every few days) until the desired expansion has been achieved. At this time the appliance is stabilized so that it cannot unscrew and decrease the amount of expansion achieved. This can be done by passing a dead soft 0.014 wire through the hole used to activate the appliance and tying it to the anterior bar of the appliance (Fig. 6-95).

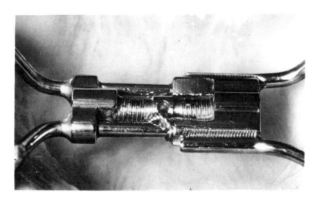

FIG. 6-95

When combined orthodontic-surgical expansion is done, two aspects are entirely different than when routine orthopedic expansion is done. First, there is no need to overexpand unless the upper posterior teeth are to be tipped lingually as part of the remaining orthodontic treatment. Indeed, expansion done in this manner and appropriately stabilized is so stable that overexpansion can be corrected only by subsequent lingual tipping of the upper teeth. Second, the midline diastema produced frequently will not close by itself as occurs in orthopedic expansion. It is important that active orthodontic closure of this diastema is not begun until there is radiographic evidence that bone has formed between the incisors. This usually occurs 8 to 10 weeks following surgery.

After the maxillary expansion appliance has been stabilized, the orthodontic treatment of the lower arch is begun. Most frequently, patients who require maxillary expansion will be treated without extraction; however, in some instances extractions may be necessary. In either instance, the treatment sequence described earlier in this chapter may be followed. Importantly, intermaxillary elastics are not used for 6 to 8 weeks following combined orthodontic-surgical maxillary expansion unless it is desired to move the entire maxilla. When this is desirable, the movement will be quite rapid and care must be taken that the maxilla is not pulled downward by the vertical component of such mechanics, thus producing an undesirable effect.

Approximately 8 weeks following surgery, the remaining upper appliances are placed, and leveling and aligning is begun with an appropriately flexible wire. It is advantageous to leave the expansion appliance in place until the upper diastema is closed to ensure maintenance of the appropriate arch width. However, when speech considerations make this inappropriate (rarely), the expansion appliance can be removed and arch width maintained by a removable lingual arch-wire. No active closure of the diastema is begun until bone is radiographically evident between the incisors (Fig. 6-96). Once bone is seen, the space is closed with an elastic thread or chain.

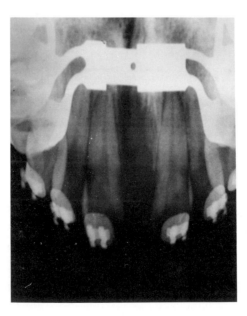 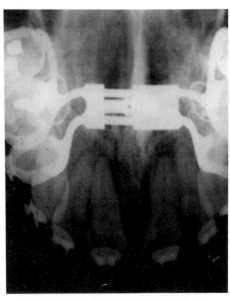

FIG. 6-96

Once the maxillary diastema is closed, the expansion appliance is removed. If maxillary extractions are necessary, they are done at this time and appropriate mechanics are instituted to close the extraction spaces while maintaining anchorage requirements. After the spaces are closed or when extractions are not necessary, the remaining orthodontic treatment is directed toward leveling, aligning, and coordinating arch forms for the mandibular advancement. As in all cases, progress is monitored by cephalometric radiographs and study models to determine when the patient is ready for the second surgical procedure—mandibular advancement.

Factors affecting stability of treatment
Orthodontic factors

APPLIANCE CONSTRUCTION AND CEMENTATION

The expansion appliance must be well made with tightly fitting bands and well-done solder joints. It must be well cemented so that there is minimal chance that the appliance will break or come loose during the manipulation of the maxilla at the time of or following surgery. Finally, it is ideally tooth-borne to minimize the possibility of soft-tissue impingement, which may compromise the blood supply to the palatal tissues and thus create the various sequelae of avascular necrosis.

APPLIANCE ACTIVATION

It is important that the appliance be activated 3 to 4 mm at surgery to check that equal mobilization of both sides of the maxilla is occurring and that skeletal movement is produced. Following surgery, the patient activates the appliance at a much slower rate—two one-quarter turns per day—to avoid excessive stretching or tearing of the palatal and alveolar mucoperiosteum. If this occurs in the region between the maxillary central incisors, a resultant periodontal or gingival defect will result. The latter is often manifest clinically as loss of the interdental papilla.

APPLIANCE STABILIZATION

The expansion appliance must be stabilized for a minimum of 8 weeks after completion of expansion for good bony union to take place. This is done by placing a ligature wire through the activation hole and tying it to ensure that the expansion appliance cannot unwind. It is preferable to maintain the appliance in place until the midline diastema is closed by the active postsurgical orthodontics.

MAINTENANCE OF ARCH WIDTH

The archwires placed following expansion must be carefully made to conform to the desired arch width. Either the expansion appliance or a lingual arch can be used to ensure that maxillary arch width is maintained. Experience has shown that it is quite easy to produce undesired construction in the canine and first premolar area while closing the midline diastema. Maintaining this width with the expansion appliance or a lingual arch is a simple, safe, and efficient method to avoid this possible problem.

Furthermore, there must be a conscious effort on the part of the orthodontist to maintain the original lower arch width even when the maxilla is to be expanded. This does not mean that the few teeth that are obviously in linguoversion cannot be incorporated into the arch form, but that general width of the lower arch is maintained and generalized expansion of all teeth is avoided. When the mandibular arch is excessively expanded, the maxillary arch will likewise be expanded beyond any physiologic limit and both arches will tend to collapse following treatment.

Surgical factors

COMPLETENESS OF THE OSTEOTOMIES

The stability of results with this integrated orthodontic-surgical approach for expansion of the maxilla is excellent as long as the osteotomies are complete. Doing so ensures subsequent skeletal, as opposed to dental, expansion. The obvious areas of potential incompleteness are in the regions of the pterygoid-palatine-maxillary sutures and nasal septum. These regions may need to be additionally osteotomized by use of a curved pterygoid maxillary osteotome or nasal septal osteotome if doubt exists as to the completeness of the osteotomies or fracturing in these areas when observing the actual opening of the midline diastema and movement of the lateral maxillary walls during the expansion done before soft-tissue closure.

Indeed, it is important to appreciate that the stability of this procedure is such that overexpansion is contraindicated. If overexpansion occurs, it will require subsequent orthodontic treatment to narrow the dental arch by lingual tipping.

RETENTION OF THE EXPANDED MAXILLA

Once the predetermined magnitude of expansion of the maxilla is achieved, bone defects will exist in the midpalatal and lateral maxillary wall areas. It will require about 8 weeks for reasonable bony union to occur. Accordingly, during this time the palatal expansion must be maintained. After radiographic evidence of bone filling of the midpalatal defect is evident, the expansion appliance can be removed without concern of relapse.

Age-related factors

Since the transverse growth of the maxilla is virtually complete by age 12 to 14 years and it is not generally advocated to perform combined orthodontic-surgical expansion of the maxilla in individuals less than 16 to 18 years of age, this surgery will have no effect on subsequent maxillary growth. There are, however, select individuals who, although less than 16 to 18 years of age, would benefit from combined orthodontic-surgical expansion.

For some patients between 12 and 18 years, in whom traditional orthopedic maxillary expansion does not occur within 5 to 7 days, as evidenced by a radiographically demonstrable midline defect in the maxilla, the appearance of the appropriately sized anterior midline diastema, and the absence of unusual tipping of the posterior teeth, combined orthodontic-surgical expansion is indicated. In such individuals, the surgical intervention will again have no adverse effect on transverse maxillary growth, since it is essentially complete. Moreover, surgical intervention seems to lessen the magnitude of subsequent vertical maxillary growth, which is generally a benefit for patients who have a high mandibular plane angle and exhibit a predominantly vertical growth pattern.

Results of treatment

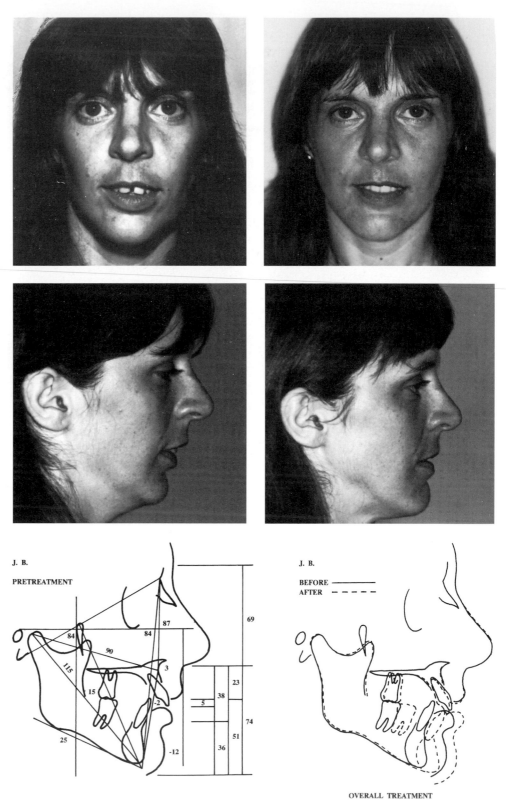

FIG. 6-97

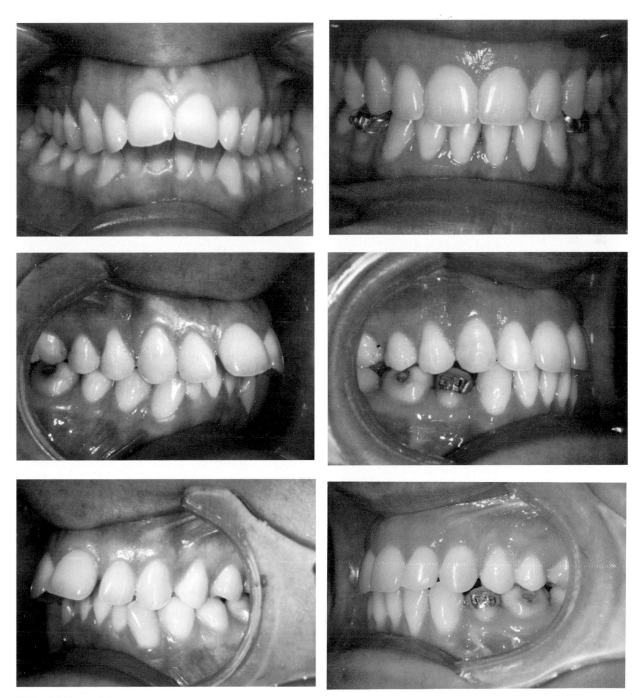

FIG. 6-97, cont'd

MANDIBULAR ADVANCEMENT WITH NARROWING BY MANDIBULAR MIDLINE OSTEOTOMY

Contingency statement

In select cases the maxillary arch form and skeletal position is acceptable, but a small (5 mm or less) transverse discrepancy results when *the models are placed into a Class I relationship*. Additionally, this discrepancy is greater in the molar region than in the canine area. In these instances a mandibular advancement with midline osteotomy to narrow the mandible may be indicated. Because of the geometry involved, the anterior midline osteotomy is most effective in narrowing the intermolar width, while producing less change in intercanine width.

A variation may exist wherein the entire lower arch is slightly wide and the lower intercanine width is excessive. If this condition is accompanied by a tooth mass discrepancy in which extraction of a lower incisor is the treatment of choice, it is often possible to do an anterior ostectomy with extraction of a lower incisor and surgical reapproximation of the remaining incisors to correct the tooth mass problem simultaneously with the mandibular advancement and narrowing.

Whether or not the anterior midline osteotomy or ostectomy with extraction of an incisor will adequately correct an existing transverse discrepancy must be determined by carefully done feasibility model surgery. Importantly, this procedure, when indicated, eliminates the need for a LeFort I osteotomy to normalize the maxillary and mandibular transverse widths. Most frequently there is need to narrow the lower arch; expansion is rarely indicated.

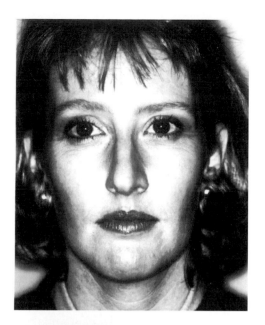

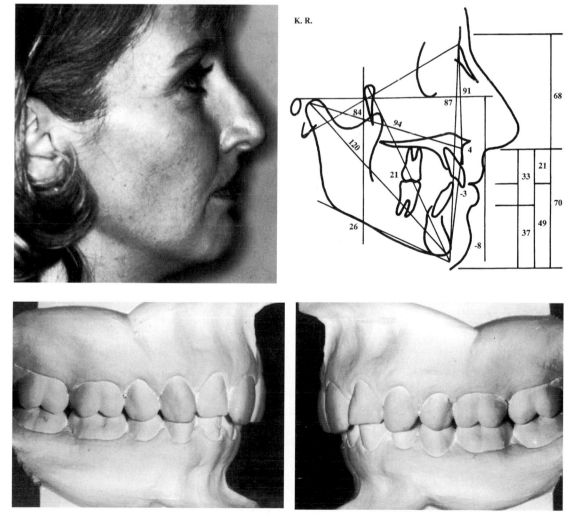

FIG. 6-98

Details of treatment

Presurgical orthodontic treatment

This procedure may be done as an elective method to correct a small transverse discrepancy that exists before treatment, or as a result of the discovery of such a discrepancy in the immediate presurgical records. It is generally the preferred method of correcting a pretreatment transverse discrepancy that is too large to be stably corrected by routine orthodontic treatment (greater than 4 mm) but not so large as to require maxillary expansion (less than 6 mm).

When a midsymphysis osteotomy to narrow the intermolar width is planned, careful consideration must be given regarding the magnitude of the pretreatment transverse discrepancy and what effects (increase versus decrease) the presurgical orthodontic treatment will have on it. This is so since the amount of intermolar constriction that can be predictably achieved with stable results at surgery is limited to about 6 mm. Consequently, when the pretreatment transverse discrepancy is less than 6 mm and this technique is to be used to correct the problem, it is recommended that a passive removable lingual arch be placed in both arches at the beginning of treatment to eliminate the possibility of inadvertent expansion in either arch during leveling and aligning. The remainder of the presurgical treatment is as described earlier in this chapter. The removable lingual arch is removed from the lower arch immediately before surgery.

When a lower midline ostectomy with extraction of a lower incisor is planned, the conditions set out in the contingency statement at the beginning of this section must be specifically met. This procedure is not indicated when there is significant crowding in the lower incisor area and the tooth mass warrants removal of a lower incisor, because when the lower anterior crowding is significant, the intercanine width is not excessive or is minimally so. In this situation it is preferable to extract a lower incisor and orthodontically eliminate the crowding and align the anterior teeth while closing the space.

Most commonly, the presurgical orthodontic treatment for a lower midline ostectomy with extraction of a lower incisor will consist of placing upper and lower appliances, followed by leveling and aligning the teeth by the simplest method appropriate. It is quite acceptable to use coordinated upper and lower arches before surgery, since the removal of a lower incisor during the midline body ostectomy will not significantly affect the arch shape but will serve primarily to narrow the intercanine distance and to a lesser extent the intermolar distance. Once the patient is ready for surgery, the lower archwire is segmentalized, the archwires are secured with ligature wires, and the orthodontic attachment is removed from the incisor to be extracted.

A transverse discrepancy is sometimes discovered as part of the immediate presurgical planning. It may have been overlooked in the original planning, inadvertently produced during the presurgical orthodontic treatment, or not fully corrected during the presurgical treatment. Regardless of the cause, if the transverse discrepancy is within the limits of good surgical technique as determined by feasibility model surgery, it can be corrected as part of the mandibular advancement surgery.

Orthognathic reconstructive surgery

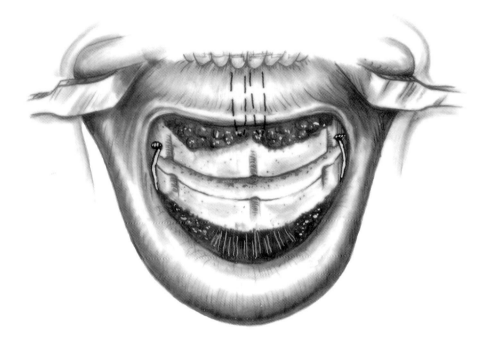

FIG. 6-99

When the mandibular midline osteotomy is performed in conjunction with bilateral sagittal split ramus osteotomies with advancement of the mandible *and* advancement genioplasty, the surgical sequence is as follows. If an advancement genioplasty is to be performed, it is accomplished to completion as previously described at the onset of the orthognathic procedures. The genial segment is best secured with interosseous wires, rather than plates, to permit the physical manipulation of the mandible after completion of the sagittal split osteotomies and midsymphysis osteotomy/ostectomy.

The bilateral sagittal ramus osteotomies are done to completion but the proximal segments are not fixed. The sagittal split sites are packed and attention is directed to the midsymphysis ostectomy.

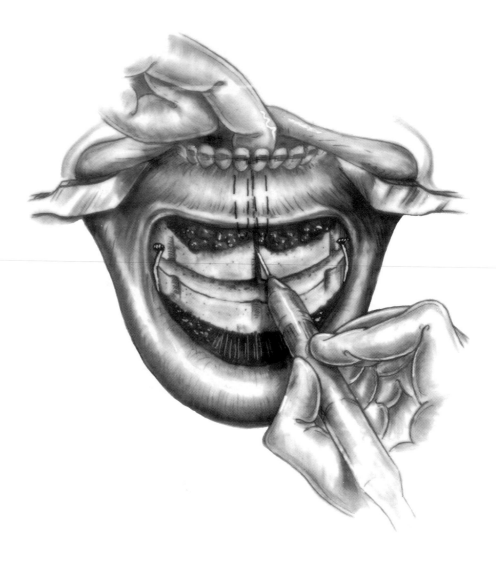

FIG. 6-100

A periosteal elevator is used to perform a limited subperiosteal dissection to expose the area between the lower central incisors. A 701 cross-cut fissure bur or fine reciprocating saw is used to initiate the mandibular midline ostectomy through the buccal cortex between the lower anterior teeth and extending inferiorly to the location of the genioplasty osteotomy. It is important that the cut extend only through the buccal cortex in the area of the lower central incisor tooth roots. However, inferior to these same roots apices, both the buccal and lingual cortex may be cut to the level of the horizontal osteotomy.

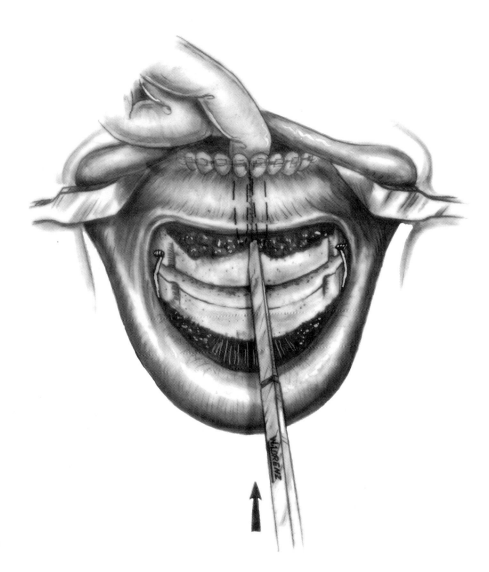

FIG. 6-101

The osteotomy between the lower central incisor tooth roots is completed with a fine thin osteotome. The osteotome is malleted between the lower central incisor tooth roots until its leading edge can be palpated with the surgeon's index finger on the lingual surface of these same teeth.

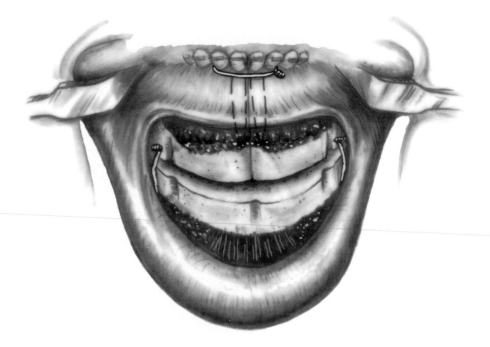

FIG. 6-102

After the osteotome has been malleted through the lingual cortex from the midroot region inferiorly to connect with the through-and-through bur cut, the residual split up through the crest of the dental alveolus between the lower central incisors is accomplished with a periosteal elevator, which is used in a lever-type fashion. Generally, some lingual cortical bone will have to be removed to permit the intermolar narrowing without widening (opening) the buccal osteotomy or producing a space between the adjacent teeth. This is easily accomplished after the separation of the symphysis is completed. A 24-gauge bridle wire is then passed between the mandibular lateral incisors bilaterally. This wire is then twisted to secure gross movements of the two mandibular dental osseous segments but not completely secured. The same basic operative approach is used when a tooth is to be removed and an ostectomy performed to narrow the mandible while correcting an anterior tooth mass discrepancy.

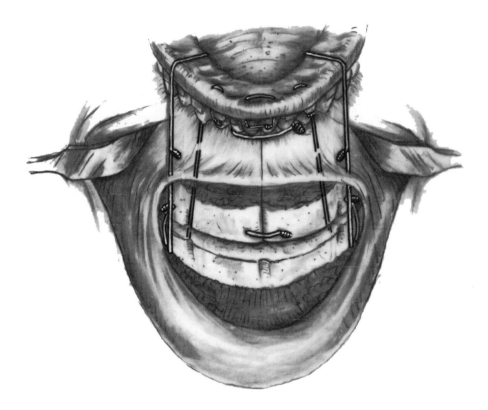

FIG. 6-103

If skeletal maxillomandibular fixation is to be used, and an occlusal splint is required, the occlusal splint is wired to the mandibular teeth using dental fixation. Stainless steel circummandibular wires (22 gauge) are now passed over the splint and tightened in the area between the mandibular second bicuspid and first molar. If a splint is not required, the circummandibular wire is placed beneath the orthodontic arch wire between the mandibular second bicuspid and first molar and secured. The bridle wire between the mandibular lateral incisors may now be fully tightened.

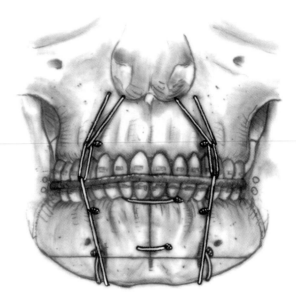

FIG. 6-104

The mandibular dentoosseous units are now skeletally stabilized using a 24-gauge stainless steel wire intermediate between a 22-gauge piriform rim wire and the 22-gauge circummandibular wires bilaterally. This skeletal maxillomandibular fixation technique was previously described in detail in this chapter. The proximal segments of the sagittal splits are now positioned and secured with two or three interosseous bone screws as previously outlined.

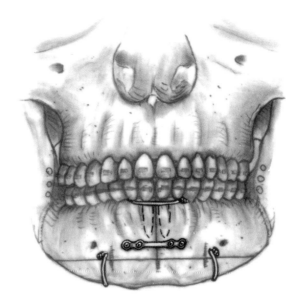

FIG. 6-105

If rigid fixation is to be used, the mandibular dentoosseous units are secured to the maxilla using 26-gauge stainless steel interdental wires. The midline ostectomy is now plated with a 4- to 6-hole miniplate, placed no less than 5 mm below adjacent root apices.

The proximal segments of the sagittal split ramus osteotomies are now rigidly secured using three interosseous screws as outlined previously in this chapter. Interdental fixation is released and the occlusion is passively checked for accuracy. All operative sites are now irrigated and closed with 3-0 chromic suture.

When the midline osteotomy is performed to *narrow* the mandibular arch width, the reduced distance between the most posterior aspects of the distal segment is generally favorable with respect to condylar proximal segment position and adaptation of the proximal segments to the distal segments. Accordingly, there need not be undue concern regarding abnormal effects of narrowing on condylar torque.

Results of treatment

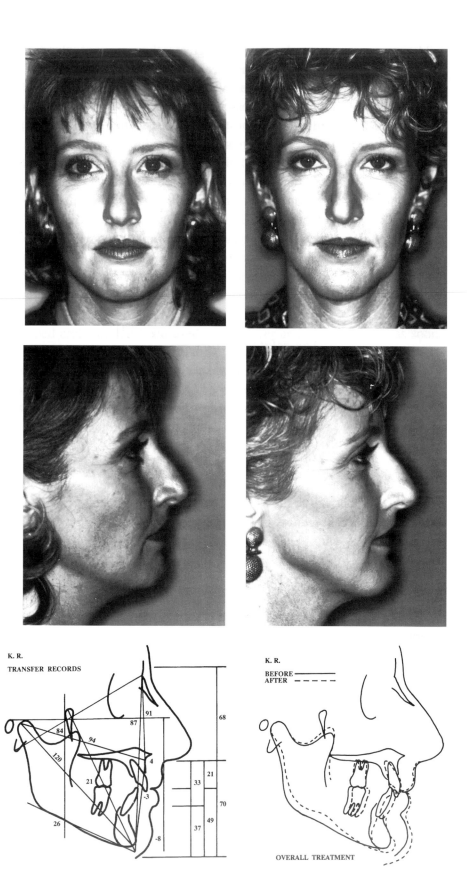

K. R.
TRANSFER RECORDS

K. R.
BEFORE ————
AFTER ———— ————

OVERALL TREATMENT

FIG. 6-106

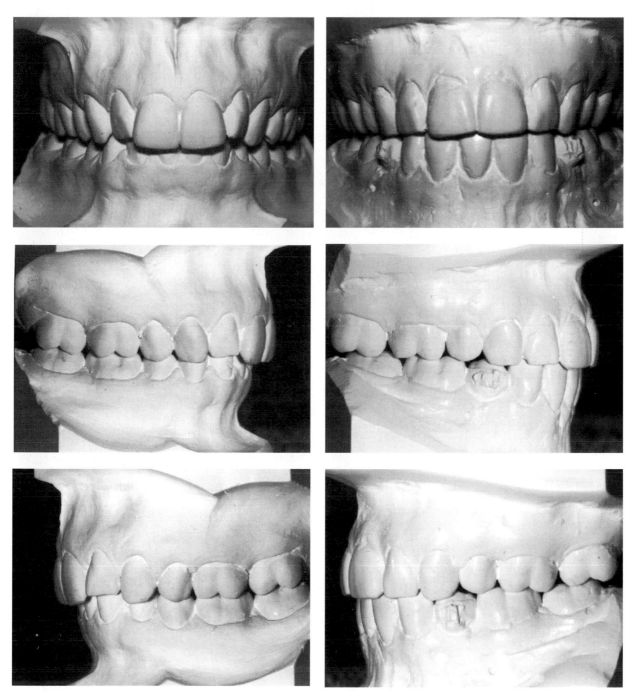

FIG. 6-106, cont'd

MANDIBULAR ADVANCEMENT WITH ANTERIOR MANDIBULAR SUBAPICAL OSTECTOMY

Contingency statement

When the lower curve of Spee is extreme, maximal advancement of the bony chin is desired, and an increase in the anterior lower face height is to be avoided, surgical leveling of the lower curve of Spee by a subapical ostectomy, as opposed to orthodontic leveling, is to be considered. This combined orthodontic-surgical approach is also most useful when either the orthodontic mechanics to level the excessive curve of Spee are problematic or significant reductions in the treatment time will result from surgically assisted leveling of the curve of Spee. When a mandibular subapical ostectomy is done in the Class II dentofacial deformity with an excessive curve of Spee, the vertical height of bone below the canine root apices must be considered. In general, when a mandibular subapical ostectomy is accomplished, the ostectomy is performed as far inferiorly as possible to optimize the vascular supply to the subapical segment. A minimum of 10 mm of bone inferior to the canine root apices ensures adequate blood supply to the teeth within the mobilized segment.

Patients who require an advancement genioplasty in addition to an anterior mandibular subapical ostectomy must have an adequate amount of bone below the mandibular canine root apices to allow for both the subapical ostectomy and the genioplasty to be performed simultaneously. These decisions are easily made by careful evaluation of the lateral cephalometric radiograph.

If the vertical amount of the available bone below mandibular canine root apices is less than adequate, a combined ostectomy and horizontal osteotomy genioplasty is not practical. In these instances, while it is not ideal, the chin can be augmented with an alloplastic material or done as a secondary procedure by the traditional horizontal osteotomy.

It is important to realize that potential compromise in the blood supply to the mobilized subapical segment during the anterior mandibular subapical ostectomy increases the risk of devitalization of the anterior dentition and the risk of periodontal problems both surrounding the teeth in the mobilized segment and in the teeth adjacent to the ostectomy. As such, *this operation is not a substitute for the routine orthodontic leveling of the curve of Spee.*

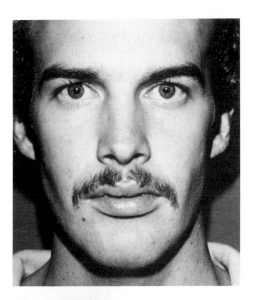

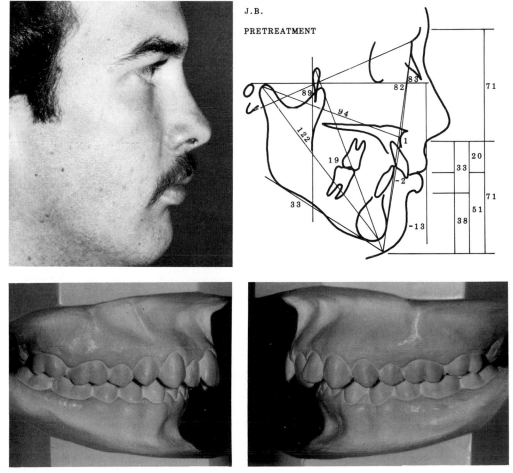

FIG. 6-107

Details of treatment

Presurgical orthodontic treatment

As was the case with the routine Class II, division I, deep bite, the lower curve of Spee is usually the cause of the deep bite in this deformity. The upper arch is treated as previously discussed in this chapter, but the lower arch must be dealt with in an entirely different manner.

The anatomy of the lower curve of Spee is important. There are two general types: (1) the dual plane curve, in which the molars and premolars are essentially on one plane while the canines and incisors are elevated; and (2) the rainbow curve, in which the curve is continuous from molars through central incisors, which are the highest points on the curve (Fig. 6-108). When the rainbow curve

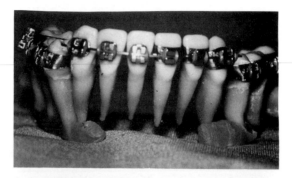

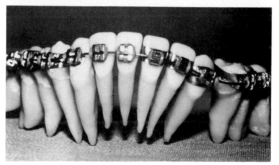

FIG. 6-108

exists, it must first be converted into a dual plane curve by orthodontic treatment before surgical leveling is possible. This is so because the teeth within the segment are not properly related to one another. As such, if the surgeon sets the segment straight down, the canine teeth will be too low (Fig. 6-109). If subsequently

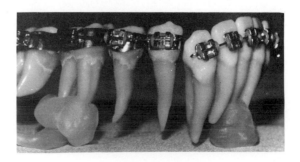

FIG. 6-109

leveled orthodontically, the bone level may create a periodontal problem. Worse yet, if the canines were to ankylose at that level, they are lost to function. If the surgeon "levels" the segment by anterior tipping, a defect is created in the crestal bone distal to the canines and periodontal problems are guaranteed (Fig. 6-110). It makes no difference if premolar teeth are extracted, the problems are the same (Fig. 6-111).

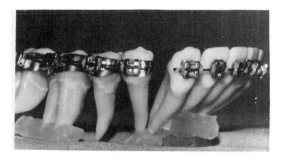

FIG. 6-110

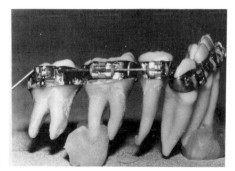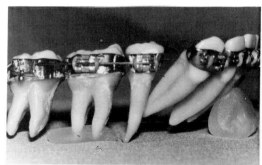

FIG. 6-111

The orthodontic mechanics for treating the lower arch are the same with either type of curve. However, when the dual plane already exists (rarely), treatment time will be significantly reduced since the presurgical treatment objective is to produce a dual plane type of curve. Treatment of the lower arch can begin after any indicated extractions have been done. Appliances are placed on all lower teeth, and sectional archwires are placed beginning with small round wires, or when possible, superflexible square or rectangular wires. Square or rectangular sectional archwires are placed as early as possible because the desired effects cannot be produced by round wires. The sectional archwires run from second molar through the premolar(s) on each side and from canine to canine anteriorly. These archwires are progressively increased in size until ideal rectangular sectional arches can be placed. A 16 × 22 wire in an 0.018 slot is usually large enough to produce all the torque necessary (Fig. 6-112). When control of transverse dimension of the buccal segments is desired, this is easily effected by a removable lingual arch, although this is seldom necessary.

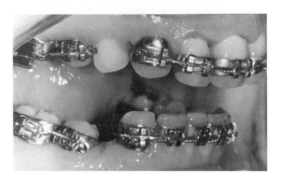

FIG. 6-112

The natural effect of such rectangular sectional archwires is to produce a dual plane curve of Spee (Fig. 6-113). Because of the angulation of the lower incisors, extrusive forces are produced on the canines while intrusive forces as well as labial root torque are acting on the incisors.

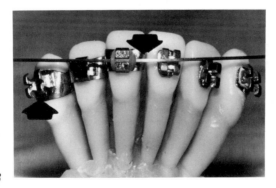 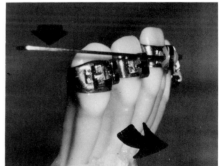

FIG. 6-113

It is important that the three sections of the mandibular teeth fit the maxillary teeth at the time of surgery. Thus, these sectional archwires must be coordinated with the maxillary archwire. This is done by first producing an archwire for the lower teeth that is coordinated with the ideal upper archwire and marking the midline. This wire is then cut distal to the canine brackets, the ends are bent in to avoid irritating the cheeks, and the sectional archwires are placed into the appropriate lower segment (Fig. 6-114).

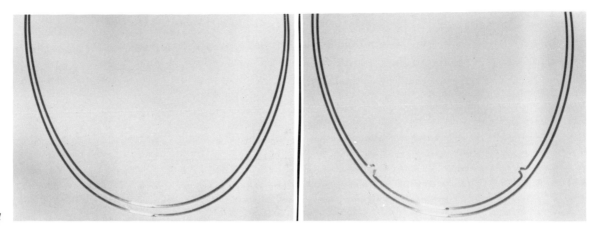

FIG. 6-114

When it appears that the desired orthodontic tooth movement has been achieved, study models are made and feasibility model surgery is done on them to determine if further orthodontic treatment is necessary before surgery. It is important when studying the result of this feasibility model surgery for the orthodontist to be concerned only with whether the patient's occlusion can be perfected from the result obtained. Conversely, the surgeon's concern must be with his/her ability to perform the necessary osteotomies and ostectomies without injury to the adjacent teeth. When feasibility model surgery produces a result that is acceptable to both the surgeon and orthodontist (Fig. 6-115), all archwires are tied with ligature wires, elastic hooks are placed where desired, and the patient is ready for surgery.

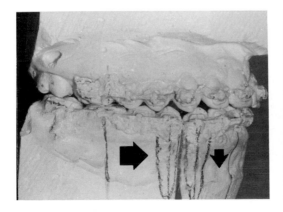 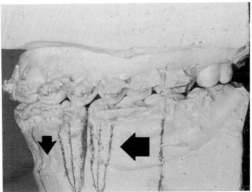

FIG. 6-115

Orthognathic reconstructive surgery

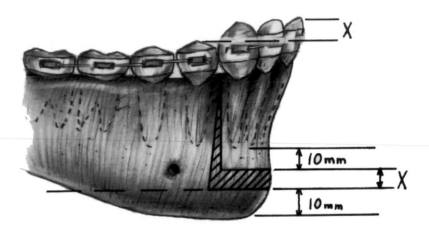

FIG. 6-116

When the anterior mandibular subapical ostectomy is done in concert with sagittal advancement of the mandible, it is performed first, the occlusal splint is wired into place, and then the sagittal ramus osteotomies are done in a routine fashion as described previously in this chapter. In cases requiring an anterior mandibular subapical ostectomy and advancement genioplasty in conjunction with bilateral sagittal split osteotomies the suggested sequence of surgery is: (1) completion of the genioplasty osteotomy without fixation; (2) completion of the subapical ostectomy; (3) stabilizing the subapical segment into the splint; (4) stabilizing the genioplasty segment; and then (5) completing the sagittal split osteotomies in a routine fashion. When this sequence is followed, the occlusal splint must be constructed with sufficient physical strength so it does not fracture. The critical factor in accomplishing these three procedures during a single surgery is the vertical height of available bone below the apices of the mandibular canines. The specifics of the aforementioned surgery are described next.

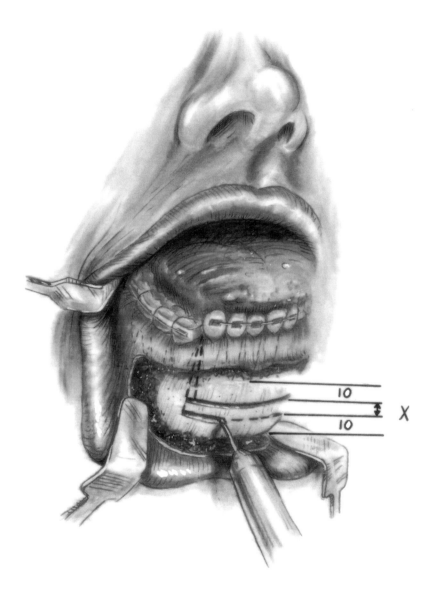

FIG. 6-117

Figure 6-116 depicts the critical measurements and illustrates the necessary osteotomies and ostectomies. The x in the illustrations represents the vertical height of the ostectomy. Figures 6-117 through 6-121 illustrate the subapical ostectomy as an isolated procedure. Comments are integrated during the surgical description of the subapical ostectomy as they pertain to the combined genioplasty/subapical ostectomy procedure.

The inferior horizontal ostectomy is completed first. The superior aspect of this ostectomy is about 10 mm below the apices of the mandibular anterior teeth.

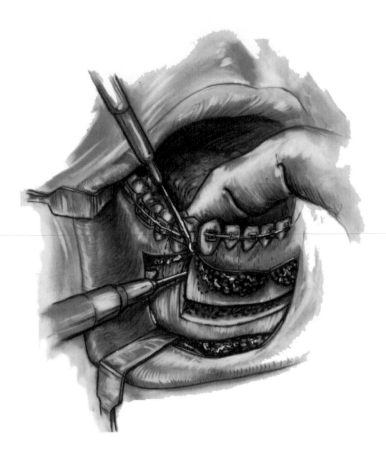

FIG. 6-118

The interdental osteotomies are done following the completion of the horizontal ostectomy. They are begun inferiorly with a fissure bur and are carried superiorly only after identifying the adjacent tooth root eminences. These osteotomies are not carried through the interdental alveolar crestal bone with the bur since removal of this thin bone will generally result in a subsequent periodontal bone defect.

The lingual cortex is osteotomized inferiorly while maintaining a finger in the floor of the mouth to avoid excessive tearing of the lingual mucoperiosteum. The angle of the cutting instrument is carefully maintained at 90 degrees to the buccal cortex while this osteotomy is made to avoid injury to the lingual portions of the adjacent tooth roots.

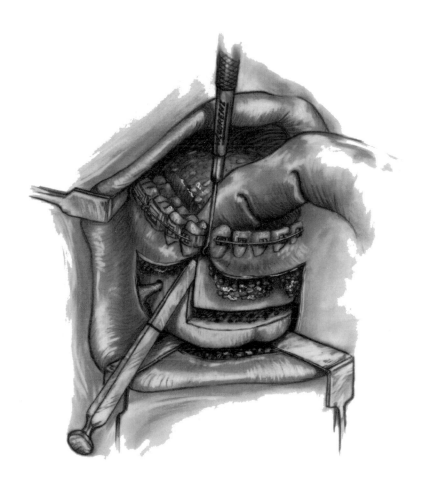

FIG. 6-119

The alveolar crestal bone and any residual lingual cortical bone is osteotomized with a small sharp osteotome. This results in the alveolar crestal bone being split, rather than removed, as would occur if this were osteotomized with a bur. Thus, the potential for resultant periodontal bone loss and pocket formation is minimized.

After the vertical osteotomies are completed bilaterally, the anterior mandibular segment is mobilized by positioning the subapical segment superiorly. If this is not effective, the osteotomies are all checked for completeness with a small straight osteotome.

During the actual mobilization, the lingual soft tissues are maintained maximally attached to the subapical segment. This is achieved by mobilizing the lingual tissues from the adjacent proximal segments with a periosteal elevator as the subapical segment is being progressively mobilized.

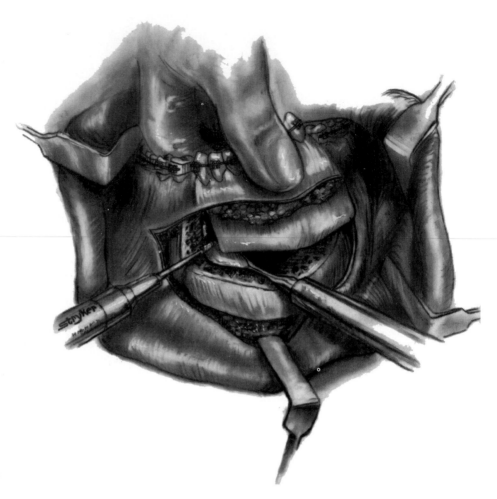

FIG. 6-120

After completion of this sequence of ostectomies and mobilization, an attempt is made to reposition the segment into its desired position as directed by the occlusal splint. When this is not initially possible, the lingual cortices in the vertical portions of the osteotomies are checked because this is generally where the interferences exist that prohibit the proper positioning of the segment. If interferences are detected in this area, their removal is accomplished by superiorly mobilizing the subapical segment and removing them under direct visualization. This process is repeated until proper positioning of the segment can be achieved with passive placement of the subapical segment into the surgical occlusal splint.

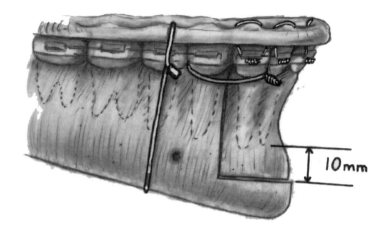

FIG. 6-121

Once the anterior segment is fully mobilized and able to be positioned properly into the splint, the segment is stabilized. The splint is secured to the posterior mandibular dentition with a 22-gauge circummandibular wire placed over the occlusal splint bilaterally in the region between the mandibular first molar and second premolar. The mobilized segment is then secured to the splint by 26-gauge wires passed through holes in the splint and tightened around the orthodontic brackets of the anterior teeth. These wires are important to prevent the segment from becoming displaced inferiorly, especially if any excessive bone has been removed below the root apices.

Plates and/or screw fixation is not recommended for securing a mandibular subapical ostectomy since it would serve to hinder postoperative orthodontic manipulation of the segment. When an occlusal splint and wire fixation is employed as described herein, the dentoosseous segment is adequately secured and early postoperative orthodontic/orthopedic movement can be effected as indicated.

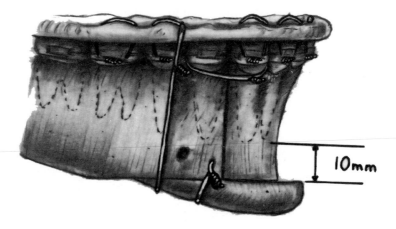

FIG. 6-122

When a genioplasty is performed in conjunction with a mandibular subapical ostectomy, wire fixation is the preferred method of stabilization. The occlusal splint is wired to the mandibular anterior and posterior teeth using 26-gauge stainless steel wire. Next the genioplasty segment is advanced to the planned position and wired with 22-to-24-gauge stainless steel wire as described above. Finally, a 22-gauge stainless steel wire is used to secure the occlusal splint, mandibular subapical, and genioplasty segments as a single unit.

The incision is closed in layers with special care taken to reapproximate the mentalis muscles bilaterally before closure of the mucosa. On completion of the soft-tissue closure, the modified sagittal ramus osteotomies are done as described in detail above. Special considerations for this procedure are also discussed above.

Postsurgical orthodontic treatment

The patient is ideally seen the same day the splint is removed. (Indeed, it may be preferable to have the splint removed by the orthodontist after the circum-mandibular wires are removed.) At this time all archwires are removed, and the appliances are checked for damage. Any loose, broken, or bent appliances are replaced. The upper archwire is checked for shape and repaired or replaced as necessary. The lower sectional archwires are discarded, and a continuous lower arch is made. Since the lower brackets adjacent to the osteotomy are rarely level, the lower arch is usually a 16 × 22 T-loop arch with the loops being placed at the osteotomy sites (Fig. 6-123).

FIG. 6-123

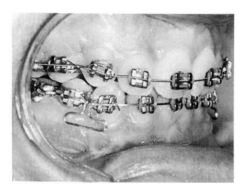 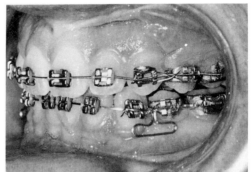

Use of light, flexible wires such as nitenol is *not* recommended, as the effects of such wires are adjacent teeth at different levels is primarily to tip the teeth. If loops are to be avoided then the stiff segmental wires are maintained and a light, flexible archwire is placed over them. This lower archwire is coordinated with the upper archwire before being placed. Figure-8 ligature ties are placed between the teeth adjacent to the osteotomies and cinched as tightly as possible to close any residual spaces or to prevent reopening of any space at these sites. Finally, the occlusion is checked, any elastics that might be deemed appropriate are placed, and the patient is instructed to wear these continuously until the next appointment, except while brushing or eating.

The second postsurgical visit is generally 2 to 3 days later. If the segments in the lower arch are level by this time (they usually are), the lower T-loop archwire is replaced by a plain continuous archwire carefully coordinated with the upper archwire. Again the teeth adjacent to the ostectomies are ligated together with figure-8 ligature wires. The occlusion is checked, and appropriate elastics are prescribed. The patient is seen again in 1 week.

The third postsurgical visit is usually only to check the appropriateness of the adjustments previously made and to check compliance with elastic wear. Adjustments may be made in the archwires, elastic direction, and duration. Frequently elastics will be discontinued by this time. The patient is seen again in 2 weeks when treatment is progressing as expected.

Again elastic wear and archwire adjustments are checked, making corrections as necessary. Finishing procedures are instituted as necessary. If treatment is progressing well, the patient is placed on routine 4-week recall. As a general rule, the longer and the more difficult the postsurgical orthodontic treatment, the poorer the presurgical orthodontic preparation or the surgical procedure. In any instance when treatment is not progressing as well as expected, appropriate records are made to determine the source of the problem so that adequate measures can be taken to correct it (Chapter 5). The earlier the problem is recognized, diagnosed, and treated, the better the overall result will be.

From this point to the completion of treatment, all visits are routine. Details such as root parallelism, marginal ridge leveling, and torque control are perfected, the appliances are removed, and retainers are placed.

Factors affecting stability of treatment
Orthodontic factors

In addition to the factors governing success in patients who require mandibular advancements (see above), four additional factors must be considered when a mandibular anterior subapical procedure is part of the treatment. This discussion pertains only to the stability of the anterior mandibular subapical ostectomy.

ADEQUATE ROOM TO PERFORM THE INDICATED SURGERY

It is the orthodontist's responsibility to ensure, and the surgeon's to reaffirm, that there is adequate space between the roots of the teeth adjacent to the interdental osteotomy sites for adequate bone removal. The surgeon will advise regarding the necessity to produce more space, and the orthodontic appliances are adjusted to produce more space if necessary. When inadequate space exists, the subapical segment will be poorly repositioned at surgery or adjacent tooth roots will be injured. Either of these may result in poor attainment of the proposed occlusal result. This will necessitate more extensive postsurgical orthodontic treatment, which is generally less stable than when both the teeth and the supporting bone are placed into the proper relation at surgery.

TEETH PROPERLY RELATED WITHIN THE SUBAPICAL SEGMENT

When a rainbow curve of Spee is present, the subapical ostectomy cannot be successfully done because the teeth within the segment are not properly related to one another (for example, roots are not parallel or torque is not normal) (Figs. 6-109 to 6-111). When the subapical ostectomy is attempted, either the canine teeth will be repositioned too far inferiorly, creating the need for possibly unstable extrusion of these teeth, or bone contact at the alveolar crest will be poor, creating probable periodontal problems and making orthodontic space closure impossible to retain (see "Surgical Factors: Excessive Ostectomies," below). An adequate subapical procedure cannot be done until the orthodontist produces a dual plane curve of Spee in which all teeth within each segment are properly related (Fig. 6-124).

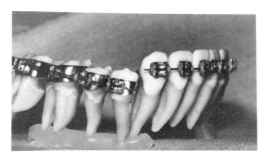
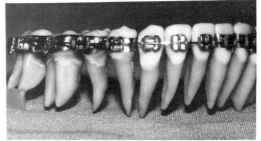
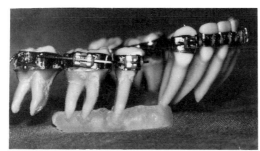
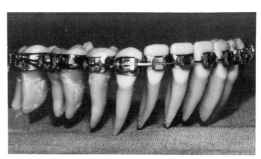

FIG. 6-124

PROPER ARCH SHAPE

Care must be taken so that the curvature of the buccal and anterior mandibular segments matches that of the maxillary arch and that any tooth mass discrepancies have been eliminated. When this is not done, the teeth cannot fit properly at surgery and more postsurgical orthodontic treatment will be required to correct

Details of treatment

Presurgical orthodontic treatment

Appropriate notation is made in the chart that this patient is to be treated by an orthodontic-surgical approach. It is most common for this procedure to be done without segmentalization of the mandibular dentoalveolus. When such is the case, the upper and lower teeth are aligned and leveled either with or without extractions.

When segmentalization of the mandibular dentoalveolus is made necessary because of leveling difficulties or the desirability of closing preexisting spaces within the lower arch, the presurgical orthodontic objectives are essentially the same as when a lower anterior subapical ostectomy combined with a mandibular advancement will be done (see above).

Since this presurgical orthodontic treatment is essentially the same as discussed previously in this chapter (see fourth adjunctive approach) it is not repeated here. The upper teeth must be placed both anteroposteriorly and vertically as determined from the prediction tracing, with or without extractions and mechanics designed to achieve this goal. When there are transverse (arch width) problems in the maxilla, the maxilla can generally be expanded orthopedically in the patient under age 18 years or it may be necessary to do combined orthodontic-surgical expansion (see above). The lower arch is treated segmentally to produce a dual plane curve of Spee. Aside from aligning the teeth within the alveolar bone, there are no anteroposterior, vertical, or transverse considerations within the lower arch, since the lower teeth will be placed surgically to conform with the upper. For this reason it is imperative that the upper teeth be in their ideal position presurgically and that any tooth mass problems be corrected during the presurgical phase of treatment.

If there is insufficient space for the interdental surgical osteotomies or ostectomies to be made, the orthodontist must provide this space by tipping the teeth adjacent to the proposed interdental osteotomy (ostectomy) site to allow access. The surgeon must assist in making the decision regarding when this is necessary.

Placing a removable lingual arch following surgery to effect cross-arch control is often desirable. Such an arch is capable of producing controlled movements in all three planes of space. Thus, in all cases when an arch is to be segmentalized and all segments are moved surgically (this applies in the maxilla as well), a horizontal lingual sheath is placed on either the first or second molars (Fig. 6-128).

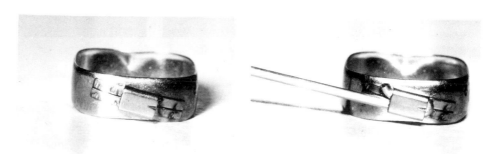

FIG. 6-128

While the lingual arch may not be necessary, it is much easier to provide such an attachment at the initial banding than to have to remove bands, weld an attachment, and recement the bands following surgery.

When it appears that the desired presurgical orthodontic result has been achieved, study models are made and feasibility model surgery is done on them to determine if further orthodontic treatment is necessary before surgery. It is important when viewing the result of this feasibility model surgery for the orthodontist to be concerned primarily with whether the patient's occlusion can be subsequently perfected from the results obtained (Fig. 6-129). Rarely if ever will segmental total lower subapical surgery produce a lower arch that will require little or no postsurgical orthodontic treatment. *When the model surgery produces a result that is acceptable to the orthodontist and is feasible to achieve by the surgeon,* all archwires are tied with ligature wires, elastic hooks are placed where appropriate, and the patient is ready for surgery.

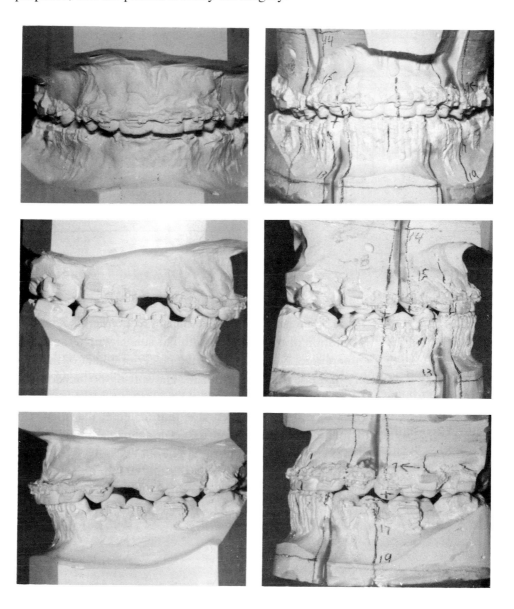

FIG. 6-129

Surgical factors

This operation is performed far less frequently than the others discussed in this book for correction of Class II dentofacial deformities, and no detailed studies in a large series of these operations have been done. However, follow-up evaluation of patients treated by this surgical approach has revealed several important things regarding stability. These will be discussed as they relate to (1) anteroposterior stability, (2) vertical stability, and (3) vascular compromise.

ANTEROPOSTERIOR STABILITY

The generally excellent anteroposterior stability of this procedure is most certainly because of the fact that the basic musculoskeletal portion of the mandible, including the condyle, is not repositioned or anatomically altered. This means that once the total subapical segment is properly mobilized and stabilized, there are minimal forces acting on it to cause relapse. Inadequate soft-tissue mobilization, which requires the segments being forced into the splint, is the only force that will adversely affect anteroposterior stability. If adequate mobilization of the subapical segments is not achieved after completion of all ostectomies, the surgeon can distract the condyles anterioinferiorly from their fossas as the subapical segment is advanced and intermaxillary fixation established. This condylar distraction will inevitably induce relapse, as was discussed earlier in this chapter for mandibular advancement surgery.

VERTICAL STABILITY

This operation is also used on occasion to increase lower face height by the incorporation of an interpositional bone graft in the region of the subapical osteotomy. In such instances this vertical correction is not optimally stable, and relapse of up to 50% will occur. This relapse is minimized by the combined use of (1) cortical bone blocks to position the proximal mandible inferiorly, (2) autogenous cancellous bone packed liberally into the osteotomy site to effect maximal osteogenesis and rapid bone union, and (3) skeletal stabilization with or without bone plates.

VASCULAR COMPROMISE

Virtually the entire vascular supply to the total subapical segment(s) is from the lingual soft tissues. Indeed, the tongue and suprahyoid muscles and their associated entering nutrient vessels are the single most important source of blood supply to the mobilized segment(s). This fact mandates that the actual subapical osteotomies be made as inferiorly lingually as possible so that maximum amount of soft tissue will remain attached to the mobilized segment(s). Careless stripping or tearing of the lingual pedicle will decrease the vasculature supply to the segment(s) and result in delayed bony union or possible avascular necrosis with loss of teeth and/or bone. On removal of fixation at 6 weeks, the segment(s) will still be mobile and will tend to relapse when moderate reduction of blood supply has occurred. If significant mobility is noted on release of fixation, fixation is reapplied and removed when the segments exhibit clinical stability.

Age-related factors

No definitive studies have been done on a series of patients who have undergone this procedure during active facial growth. Yet the several individuals observed have not demonstrated subsequent abnormal skeletal growth or relapse of the occlusal result achieved with the orthodontic-surgical treatment described in this section. This is most likely predicated on the fact that after age 12 to 14 years most mandibular growth occurs in the condyle ascending ramus area.

Results of treatment

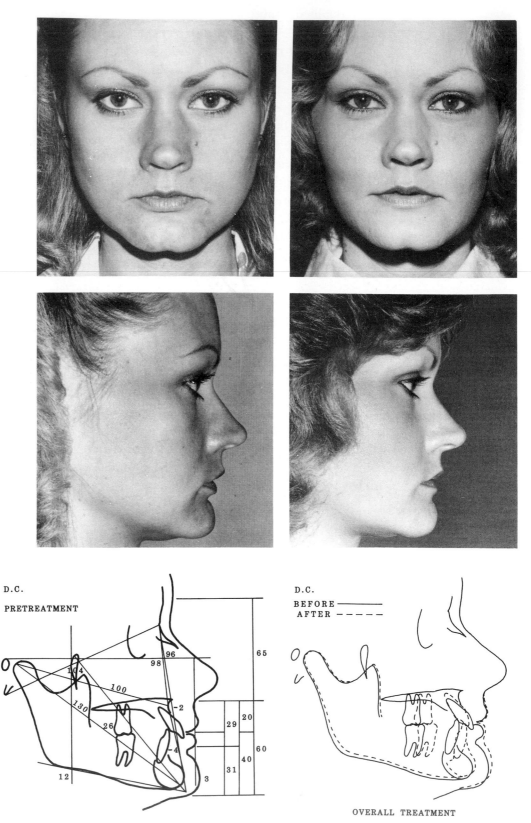

FIG. 6-137

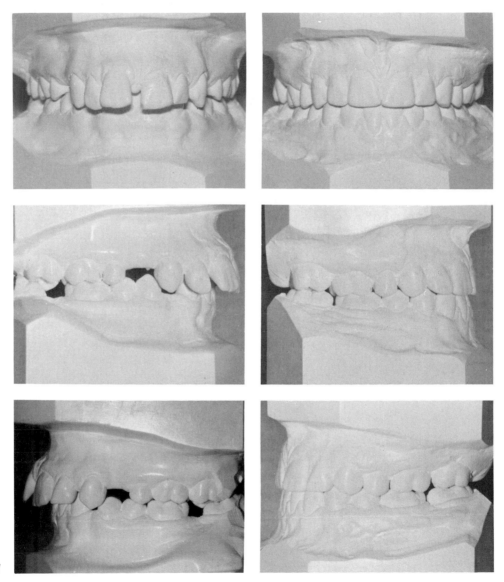

FIG. 6-137, cont'd

INFERIOR REPOSITIONING OF THE MAXILLA WITH MANDIBULAR ADVANCEMENT

Contingency statement

There are several conditions that sometimes coexist in the Class II dentofacial deformity that may cause the clinician to consider inferior repositioning of the maxilla in concert with mandibular advancement. These conditions are (1) a very short lower third facial height, (2) the upper incisors are positioned superiorly such that the upper lip covers them in repose and sometimes even during smiling, and (3) an extreme reverse curve of Spee exists in the maxillary dental arch, which if leveled orthodontically would result in an unacceptable decrease in the exposure of the maxillary incisors. In such cases, if the patient desires improvement in facial balance and in upper tooth-to-lip esthetics, consideration must be given to simultaneous maxillary inferior repositioning and mandibular advancement. It is emphasized that this operation is not frequently indicated in Class II patients, since the vertical height of the maxilla is usually within normal limits or excessive (Chapters 7, 8, and 9) as determined by esthetic and cephalometric criteria.

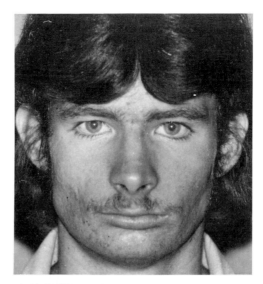

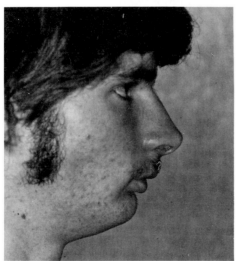

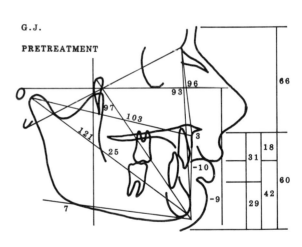

G.J.

PRETREATMENT

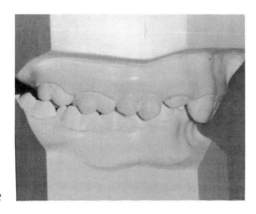

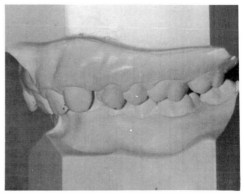

FIG. 6-138

Orthognathic reconstructive surgery

When simultaneous mobilization of both jaws is to be performed, the recommended surgical sequence is as follows. The mandibular sagittal split osteotomies are completed and the splits are initiated *but are not completed*. This is important as it allows the clinician to determine that appropriate splits will occur before proceeding with the remaining surgical procedures.

The maxillary osteotomies are next completed and the maxilla is repositioned with the routine use of an intermediate splint and stabilized by the placement of suspension wires and/or bone plates. The sagittal splits are completed, the mandibular distal segment is advanced, and the teeth are interdigitated into the final occlusion. When maxillomandibular fixation is required, it is accomplished with skeletal stabilization by placing an intermediate wire from the circummandibular wire to the piriform rim wires. Bone screws are now employed to secure the proximal segments into their appropriate position. If rigid fixation is being used in both the maxilla and the mandible, the intermaxillary fixation is removed after final placement of all screws and plates and the occlusion is carefully checked. The operative sites are then irrigated and closed.

This surgical sequencing both minimizes the need to load, and thereby, potentially displace the repositioned maxilla during the sagittal ramus osteotomies, and reduces the possibility of inadvertent inferior alveolar nerve injury as a result of either distraction of the mandible or crushing the nerve within the splits during the maxillary surgery. Blood loss is also reduced, since less oozing occurs when the sagittal splits are not completed until after the maxillary surgery is completed.

The details of the sagittal split ramus osteotomies for mandibular advancement have been described and illustrated previously. The surgical technique for inferior repositioning of the maxilla is described in detail in Chapter 11.

Intermaxillary fixation, when used, is maintained for 3 to 4 weeks. On release of fixation, jaw physiotherapy begins as discussed previously. No chewing is permitted for approximately 2 to 3 additional weeks. (Normal chewing begins at about 6 weeks postoperatively.) During this time the patient is periodically checked to make certain that the mandibular teeth bite perfectly into occlusion with the maxillary teeth. After normal range of asymptomatic jaw function has returned, the skeletal suspension wires may be removed under local anesthesia with or without light sedation. Postsurgical orthodontic treatment is now begun. The patient now begins to chew very soft food and gradually returns to normal dietary consistency over the next 2 weeks (approximately 8 to 10 weeks after the maxillary inferior repositioning procedure).

Postsurgical orthodontic treatment

When the arches have not been segmentalized, the first appointment, within 48 hours of splint removal, consists of removing the archwires, checking and repairing the appliances as necessary, and checking archwire coordination. The patient is instructed to wear elastics, if appropriate, and is seen again in 2 to 3 days. The patient is seen more frequently than usual for 1 month, and adjustments are made in both archwires and elastic wear to perfect the occlusion. The patient is instructed to wear any elastics that are appropriate to "finish" the occlusion, as if no surgery has been done.

When one or both arches have been segmentalized, it is preferable that the patient be seen as soon as possible following removal of the occlusal splint, usually later that same day. All archwires are removed, and the appliances are checked for damage and are repaired as necessary. Continuous coordinated archwires are then placed with loops at the osteotomy sites where additional archwire flexibility is desirable (Fig. 6-140). An alternate approach is to leave the rigid sec-

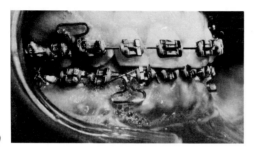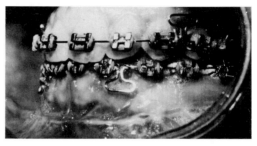

FIG. 6-140

tional archwires and place one of the superflexible wires "piggyback" on top of these wires. Using only the superflexible wires will cause leveling of the teeth in adjacent segments by tipping, which is usually undesirable as this tipping must subsequently be resolved by placing heavier and heavier archwires, thereby increasing postsurgical treatment time. Cross-arch stabilization may be desired, and when this is so, it is produced by a lingual arch (Fig. 6-141).

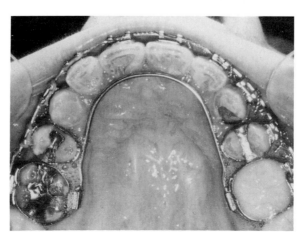

FIG. 6-141

When the arches have been segmentalized, the orthodontist must realize that there will often occur not only movement of the teeth but, to some extent, of the bony segments as well. (Segmentalization frequently precludes rigid fixation due to technical difficulties. When skeletal stabilization is used, some mobility will usually exist between the osteotomized segments. Conversely, if rigid fixation is used for one or more segments, these will be immobile and the teeth therein can be moved only in a more traditional orthodontic time frame.) As such, movement will be rapid, and any errors in the postsurgical mechanics will be expressed equally rapidly. Thus, the importance of taking great care in archwire and lingual arch fabrication cannot be overemphasized. The patient is instructed in the wearing of any elastics that are appropriate and is seen again in 2 to 3 days.

Since movement generally occurs very rapidly, the effect of the mechanics must be thoroughly checked at the second postsurgical appointment. Necessary adjustments are made in both the archwires and the elastics. Loops in the archwires especially are checked, and when they are no longer necessary, new archwires are made without them. The patient is seen again in 4 to 5 days.

Progress is checked at each subsequent visit. Adjustments are made in the archwires and in direction, force, and duration of elastic wear. These appointments are scheduled at intervals of 1 week and then 2 weeks, after which the usual 4-week intervals are resumed. Once the desired occlusal result has been obtained, the appliances are removed and retainers are placed in the usual manner.

In any instance in which satisfactory progress is not being made postsurgically, new records are made and a critical evaluation is made of all postsurgical records to determine the source of the problem. Once this is done, it is possible to correct the difficulty and finish the treatment (Chapter 5).

Factors affecting stability of treatment
Orthodontic factors

In the case of whole-arch surgery, the same principles that were discussed following the usual approach earlier in this chapter are operative and will not be reiterated here. It is sufficient to note that when the accepted principles of good orthodontic techniques are adhered to, orthodontic-related relapse will not be expected to occur. Particularly, there is little if any tendency for return of the deep bite in these patients. This is true regardless of the method of arch leveling that has been used, be it surgical, orthodontic intrusion of the anterior teeth, or orthodontic extrusion of the teeth in the buccal portion of the arch.

When segmental surgery is done, several unique situations occur and must be understood. These pertain to the interdental surgical osteotomies and ostectomies, proper relation of the teeth within the segments, and immediate postsurgical orthodontic control of the occlusion.

ROOM TO DO THE PROPOSED SURGERY

When segmental surgery will be done, there must be sufficient space for the interdental surgical osteotomies or ostectomies to avoid root damage and possible subsequent tooth ankylosis. When sufficient space is not available, the surgical result will be compromised, requiring more postsurgical orthodontic treatment.

Specifically, when the canine roots are tipped back too far, either the segments will not be able to be placed into good contact at the alveolar crest, resulting in possible periodontal defects and inability to close the residual space orthodontically, or the segments will be placed so that the arches are not level, in which case postsurgical leveling is subject to all the factors that can cause orthodontic relapse in nonsurgically treated patients.

RELATION OF THE TEETH WITHIN THE SEGMENTS

Overall stability is enhanced when the surgically moved segments fit well at the time of surgery because major orthodontic changes are avoided following surgery. In this regard, it becomes important that the teeth are properly related to each other within each segment with regard to level and torque. Segment shape and tooth mass are carefully matched before surgery to avoid the necessity for major arch shape changes following surgery.

IMMEDIATE POSTSURGICAL ORTHODONTIC CONTROL

Possibly the most important consideration is immediate postsurgical orthodontic control following the release of fixation. By so doing, the orthodontist can take advantage of any mobility of the segments, thus aligning not just teeth but the bony segments before their becoming completely immobilized by solid bony union. Accordingly, minor irregularities are rapidly resolved, and these effects become quite permanent once complete bone union has occurred. Indeed, the stability of the overall result is increased by the extent to which any immediate postsurgical adjustments in the occlusion are produced by movement of the dentoosseous segments. Furthermore, when an osteotomy or ostectomy has been done between teeth, the teeth adjacent to the osteotomy are to be ligated together tightly to prevent the formation of fibrous tissue in this area. Doing so helps to avoid problems with space opening in this area following treatment.

Surgical factors

MANDIBULAR ADVANCEMENT STABILITY

The stability of mandibular advancement has been discussed in detail previously in this chapter and will not be reiterated here. However, it must be appreciated that all of the factors that cause relapse in the instance of isolated mandibular advancement will be magnified when simultaneous mobilization of the maxilla is done. Thus, the importance of achieving stability of the mandibular surgery is critical, as any significant forces applied to the maxilla will now act to displace the entire maxillary-mandibular complex (relapse). Importantly, with simultaneous mandibular advancement and inferior repositioning of the maxilla the direction of acute relapse (during fixation) will be such that the maxillary-mandibular complex is displaced downward and backward. The accompanying esthetic results would be exhibited clinically as lengthening of the lower third face with excessive exposure of the upper incisors, lip incompetence, and retrusion of the chin. If this is not avoided, as discussed below, it may be clinically very significant.

MAXILLARY INFERIOR REPOSITIONING

Both biologic factors and technical factors are important in understanding the stability of maxillary inferior repositioning.

BIOLOGIC FACTORS. The two biologic factors that most profoundly affect the stability of maxillary downgrafts are parafunctional habits and the preexisting dentofacial deformity. Parafunctional habits such as clenching and bruxing may prematurely load the downgraft, delay skeletal union, and promote relapse. Patients with a low angle Class I or II dentofacial deformity predictably have a supernormal bite force that may also load the downgraft before complete healing and predispose the patient to relapse.

When inferior repositioning of the maxilla is not accompanied by mandibular ramus surgery, the muscles of mastication load the maxilla and it relapses superoanteriorly. This relapse tendency is minimized when simultaneous mandibular ramus surgery is done. The loads on the maxilla and bone grafts are now reversed and relapse during the period of intermaxillary fixation tends to occur in an inferoposterior direction.

It is the authors' contention that patients who exhibit parafunctional habits, a low-angle Class I or II dentofacial deformity, or both, have incorporated into their treatment plan a means of reducing the effect of the bite force on the maxillary downgraft. This is most predictably done by performing bilateral sagittal split ramus osteotomies and deliberately stripping the masseter and medial pterygoid muscles from the ramus. In addition, intentionally rotating the proximal segments approximately 5 degrees counterclockwise will shorten the pterygomasseteric sling to further decrease bite force. Such rotation is planned on the cephalometric prediction tracings.

TECHNICAL FACTORS. The interpositional grafts used in the lateral maxillary walls must have sufficient structural integrity to enable them to stabilize the maxilla in the proper position. Hydroxylapatite blocks provide a very stable, noncompressible interpositional material. However, *they must be used in conjunction with autogenous bone.* When only allogeneic or autogenous cortical interpositional grafts are used, there is a definite tendency for superoanterior relapse of the entire maxillary-mandibular complex after release of intermaxillary fixation. This relapse is due to the masticatory loading of the graft before a stable bony union can be produced by the slow, physiologic replacement of the graft with new living bone. Fresh autogenous cancellous graft material must be overlaid on the graft site to promote osteogenesis and a more rapid, stable bony union. Thus, the optimal bone graft is a composite one: hydroxylapatite blocks to provide structural integrity and fresh autogenous cancellous bone to provide osteogenesis essential for a rapid bony union.

The bone plating method of stabilizing the downgrafted maxilla described previously provides excellent stability for the time it takes to allow consolidation of the bone graft. Importantly, no single factor can be safely relied on to produce stable results in maxillary downgraft procedures. Both understanding the biologic and technical factors of relapse and applying the methods of offsetting them as described herein are important to produce the most stable result possible.

Age-related factors

Insufficient data with long-term documentation exist to provide definitive recommendations regarding the effect of early combined surgical inferior maxillary repositioning with simultaneous mandibular advancement on subsequent growth because of the relatively uncommon nature of this specific treatment approach in the Class II dentofacial deformity.

Results of treatment

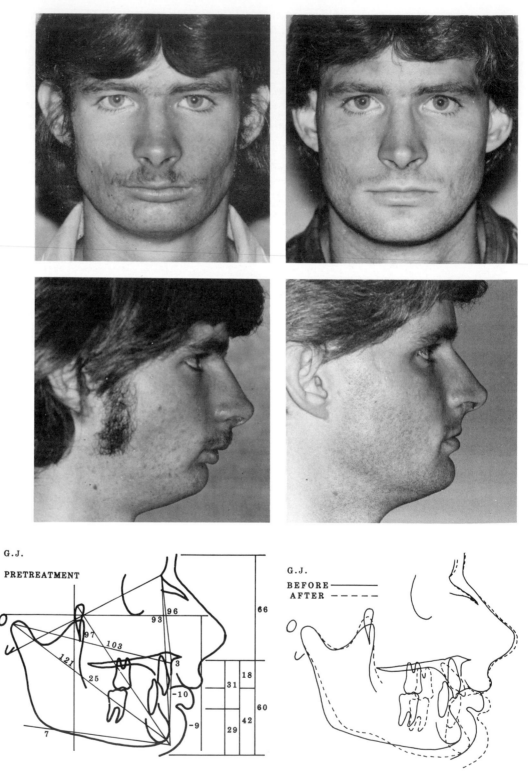

FIG. 6-142

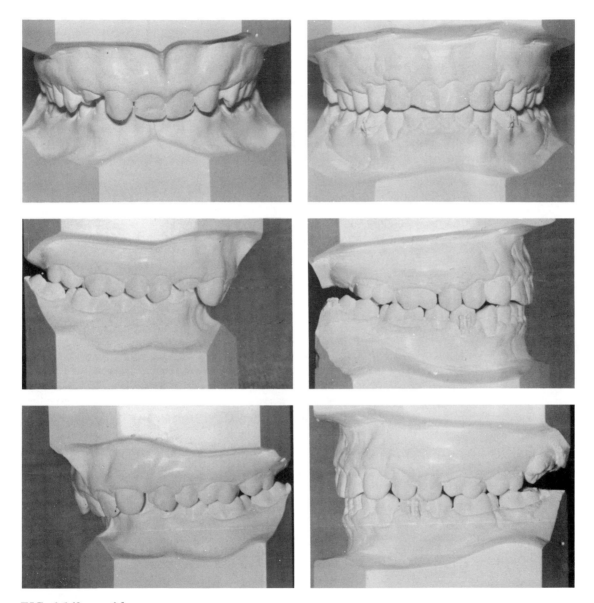

FIG. 6-142, cont'd

REFERENCES

Abeloos, J. De Clercq, C, and Neyt, L.: Skeletal atability following miniplate fixation after bilateral sagittal split osteotomy for mandibular advancement, J. Oral Maxillofac. Surg. **91**(4):624, 1993.

Aragon, S.B., and Van Sickels, J.E.: Mandibular range of motion with rigid/nonrigid fixation, Oral Surg. Oral Med. Oral Pathol. **63**(4):408, 1987.

Arnett, G.W., and Tamborello, J.A.: Temporomandibular joint ramification of orthognathic surgery. In Bell, W.H. (ed): Modern practice in orthodontic and reconstructive surgery, vol 1, Philadelphia, 1992, W.B. Saunders Company.

Bjork, A., and Skiller, V.: Facial development and tooth eruption: and implant study at the age of puberty, Am. J. Orthod. **62**:39, 1972.

Bjork, A., and Skiller, V.: Growth in width of the maxilla studied by the implant method, Scand. J. Plast. Reconstr. Surg. **8**:26, 1977.

Carlson, D.S., Ellis, E., and Dechow, P.C.: Adaptation of the suprahyoid muscle complex to mandibular advancement surgery, Am. J. Orthod. Dentofac. Orthop. **92**:134, 1987.

Ellis, E. III., and Hinton, R.J.: Histologic examination of the temporomandibular joint after mandibular advancement with and without rigid fixation: an experimental investigation in adult Macaca mulatta, J. Oral Maxillofac. Surg. **49**(12):1316, 1991.

Ellis, E., and Gallo, W.J.: Relapse following mandibular advancement with dental plus skeletal maxillomandibular fixation, J. Oral Maxillofac. Surg. **44**:509, 1986.

Ellis, E., Reynolds, S., and Carlson, D.S.: Stability of the mandible following advancement: a comparison of three postsurgical fixation techniques, Am. J. Orthod. Dentofac. Orthop. **94**:38, 1988.

Epker, B.N., and Wylie, A.: Control of the condylar-proximal mandibular segments after sagittal split osteotomies to advance the mandible, Oral Surg. **62**:613, 1986.

Ewing, M., and Ross, R.B.: Soft tissue response to mandibular advancement and genioplasty, Am. J. Orthod. Dentofac. Orthop. **101**(6):550, 1992.

Flynn, B., Brown, D.T., Lapp, T.H., et. al.: A comparative study of temporomandibular symptoms following mandibular advancement by bilateral sagittal split osteotomies: rigid versus nonrigid fixation, Oral Surg. Oral Med. Oral Pathol. **70**(3): 372, 1990.

Foley, W.L., Frost, D.E., Paulin, W.B., and Tucker, M.R.: Internal screw fixation: comparison of placement pattern and rigidity, J. Oral Maxillofac. Surg. **47**:720, 1989.

Foley, W.L., Frost, D.E., Paulin, W.B., and Tucker, M.R.: Uniaxial pullout evaluation of internal screw fixation, J. Oral Maxillofac. Surg. **47**:277, 1989.

Gassmann, C.J., Van Sickels, J.E., and Thrash, W.J.: Causes, location, and timing of relapse following rigid fixation after mandibular advancement, J. Oral Maxillofac. Surg. **48**(5):450, 1990.

Goddio, A.S.: Suction lipectomy: the gold triangle at the neck, Aesthet. Plast. Surg. **16**(1):27, 1992.

Isaacson, R.J., et al.: Extreme variations in vertical facial growth and associated variations in skeletal and dental relations, Angle Orthod. **41**:219, 1971.

Kirkpatrick, T.B., Woods, M.G., Swift, J.Q., and Markowitz, N.R.: Skeletal stability following mandibular advancement and rigid fixation, J. Oral Maxillofac. Surg. **45**:472, 1987.

Krekmanov, L., and Kahnberg, K.E.: Soft tissue response to genioplasty procedures, Br. J. Oral Maxillofac. Surg. **30**(2):87, 1992.

Leira, J.O., and Gilhuus-Moe, O.T.: Sensory impairment following sagittal split osteotomy for correction of mandibular retrognathism, Int. J. Adult Orthodont. Orthognath. Surg. **6**(3):161, 1991.

Mayo, K.H., and Ellis, E.: Stability of the mandible after advancement and use of dental plus skeletal maxillomandibular fixation: an experimental investigation in Maca mulatta, J. Oral Maxillofac. Surg. **45:**243, 1987.

Moenning, J.E., Bussard, D.A., Lapp, T.H., and Garrison, B.T.: Comparison of relapse in bilateral sagittal split osteotomies for mandibular advancement: rigid internal fixation (screws) versus inferior border wiring with anterior skeletal fixation, Int. J. Adult Orthodont. Orthognath. Surg. **5**(3):175, 1990.

Mottura, A.A.: Liposuction: more curettage than aspiration, Aesthet. Plast. Surg. **15**(3):209, 1991.

O'Ryan, F., and Epker, B.N.: Deliberate surgical control of mandibular growth: a biomechanical theory, J. Oral Surg. **53:**2,1982.

Phillips, C., Medland, W.H., Fields, H.W. Jr., et al.: Stability of surgical maxillary expansion, Int. J. Adult Orthodont. Orthognath. Surg. **7**(3):139, 1992.

Polido, W.D., de Clairefont, R.L., and Bell, W.H.: Bone resorption, stability, and soft-tissue changes following large chin advancements, J. Oral Maxillofac. Surg. **49**(3):251, 1991.

Profitt, W.R., Phillips, C., and Turvey, T.A.: Stability after surgical-orthodontic corrective of skeletal Class III malocclusion: combined maxillary and mandibular procedures, Int. J. Adult Orthodont. Orthognath. Surg. **6**(4):211, 1991.

Ricketts, R.M., et al.: Bioprogressive therapy, book 1, Denver, 1979, Rocky Mountain Orthodontics.

Sillman, J.H.: Dimensional changes in the dental arches: longitudal study from birth to twenty-five years, Am. J. Orthodont. **50:**824, 1964.

Snow, M.D., Turvey, T.A., Walker, D., and Proffit, W.R.: Surgical mandibular advancement in adolescents: postsurgical growth related to stability, Int. J. Adult Orthodont. Orthognath. Surg. **6**(3):143, 1991.

Stoller, A.E.: The universal appliance, St. Louis, 1971, The C.V. Mosby Company.

Thomas, P.M., Tucker, M.R., Prewitt, J.R., and Profitt, W.R.: Early skeletal and dental changes following mandibular advancement and rigid internal dixation, Int. J. Adult Orthodont. Orthognath. Surg. **3:**171, 1986.

Thurow, R.C.: Atlas of orthodontic principles, St. Louis, 1970, The C.V. Mosby Company.

Van Sickels, J.E.: A comparative study of bicortical screw and suspension wires versus bicortocal screws in large mandibular advancements, J. Oral Maxillofac. Surg. **49**(12):1293, 1991.

Van Sickels, J.E., Larsen, A.J., and Thrash, W.J.: Relapse after rigid fixation of mandibular advancement, J. Oral Maxillofac. Surg. **44:**698, 1986.

Vedtofte, P., Nattestad, A., Hjrting-Hansen, E., and Svendsen, H.: Bone resorption after advancement genioplasty: pedicled and non-pedicled grafts, J. Craniomaxillofac. Surg. **19**(3):102, 1991.

Wertz, R., and Dreskin, M.: Midpalatal suture opening, a normative study, Am J. Orthodont. **71:**367, 1977.

Will, L.A., and West, R.A.: Factors influencing the stability of sagittal split osteotomy for mandibular advancement, J. Oral Maxillofac. Surg. **47:**813, 1989.

Zimmer, B., Schwestka, R., and Kubein-Messenburg, D.: Changes in mandibular mobility after different procedures of orthognathic surgery, Eur. J. Orthodont. **14**(3):1988, 1992.

Class II dentofacial deformities secondary to vertical maxillary excess

Introduction

There are two surgical decisions to be made in planning for treatment of vertical maxillary excess: Is simultaneous mandibular advancement required? and What basic surgical technique will be used to superiorly reposition the maxilla?

A majority of individuals with Class II vertical maxillary excess can be treated with isolated superior repositioning of the maxilla with or without advancement genioplasty. This determination is made by integrating clinical esthetic findings—nose size, paranasal configuration, and nasolabial angle—with a cephalometric prediction tracing, which uses only superior repositioning of the maxilla and mandibular autorotation to correct both the vertical esthetic discrepancy and the Class II malocclusion. When this prediction is done in the Class II individual, some posterior movement of the maxilla is almost always required. This posterior maxillary movement is usually small and produces almost no visible effect in most patients. In other patients, it can produce a positive change.

Nevertheless, there exists a patient population who have facial esthetic features that will be worsened by any posterior movement of the maxilla. When the prediction tracing shows the maxilla will require several millimeters of posterior repositioning to correct the Class II occlusion *and* the individual in question has either a large nose, a concave paranasal configuration, and/or an obtuse nasolabial angle, facial esthetics would be worsened by isolated maxillary superior repositioning. The posterior maxillary movement in such an individual will make the nose appear more prominent, further flatten the paranasal area and make the already obtuse nasolibial angle even more so. Accordingly, simultaneous superior repositioning of the maxilla and advancement of the mandible is preferred for such a patient.

Conversely, for the more usual patient whose nose is normal, the paranasal area is convex, and the nasolabial angle is acute, this same posterior movement of the maxilla will produce favorable esthetic changes, and isolated superior repositioning of the maxilla is indicated. This chapter discusses the patient population requiring isolated superior repositioning with or without an advancement genioplasty. Chapter 8 discusses the much smaller patient population who require both maxillary superior repositioning and simultaneous mandibular advancement.

There are two *basic techniques* for superior repositioning of the maxilla: (1) the LeFort I maxillary ostectomy and (2) the total maxillary subapical ostectomy. Either technique can be done with or without segmentalization. When esthetics permit, it is preferable to move the entire maxilla superiorly and posteriorly enough to correct the Class II molar relation. However, when the distance from the upper second molar to the pterygoid plates is very small, sufficient posterior movement may not be possible because of the difficulty of removing sufficient bone in this area. When this is so, maxillary premolars are extracted, the maxilla is segmentalized, a Class II molar–Class I canine relation is established, and the need to remove large quantities of bone in the retromolar area is avoided. (When this situation is determined to exist during treatment planning, upper premolars are extracted and the upper arch is idealized by the presurgical orthodontic treatment, thus avoiding segmentalization of the maxilla when doing so is preferable.)

The LeFort I is the most commonly used surgical procedure for maxillary superior repositioning. However, there exist several *relative* indications for the total subapical superior repositioning procedure: (1) the maxilla is to be maximally (> 7 mm) superiorly repositioned; (2) major movement of multiple segments is to be done (that is, simultaneous expansion, removal of premolars and closure of these spaces, and/or an anterior maxillary midline osteotomy to increase intercanine distance); (3) the lateral maxillary walls are excessively horizontal; and (4) the patient's palatal vault is excessively deep. Because these are relative indications, if only one exists in a given case, it is a marginal indication for the use of the total subapical superior repositioning of the maxilla. If two or more exist, the total subapical, though technically more difficult, may be the procedure of choice.

The usual orthodontic surgical approach:
LE FORT I SUPERIOR REPOSITIONING OF THE MAXILLA AND ADVANCEMENT GENIOPLASTY

Outline of treatment

Presurgical orthodontic treatment

1. Place appliances—align and level
2. Coordinate arch forms
3. Elastics as necessary to place the lower incisors in the proper anteroposterior position

Immediate presurgical planning

1. Cephalometric prediction tracing
2. Model surgery
3. Splint construction (when indicated)

Orthognathic reconstructive surgery

1. LeFort I superior repositioning of the maxilla
2. Advancement genioplasty

Postsurgical orthodontic treatment

1. Repair appliances as necessary
2. Check archwire coordination
3. Routine finishing procedures
4. Retain

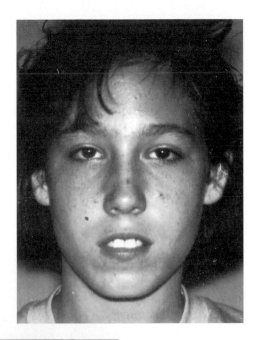

H. E.

PRETREATMENT

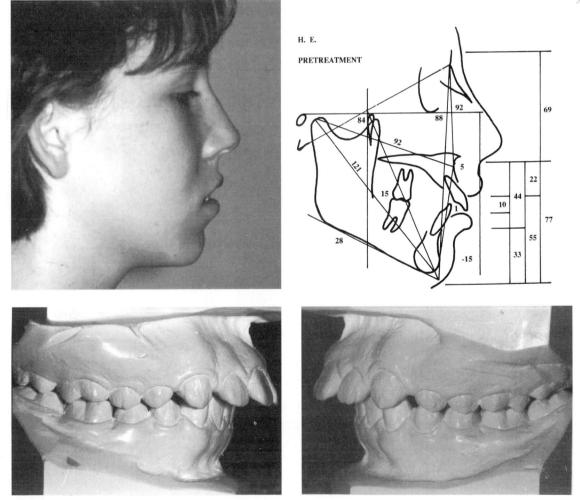

FIG. 7-1

Details of treatment

Presurgical orthodontic treatment

Of all the dentofacial deformities treated by combined orthodontics and surgery, vertical maxillary excess can be treated with little or no presurgical orthodontic treatment more frequently than any other deformity. Some patients can have orthodontic appliances placed and undergo maxillary surgery immediately thereafter as either a single piece or a segmentalized procedure with or without extraction of the upper first premolars. This is so if the occlusion thus produced can easily be finished postsurgically by routine orthodontic treatment (Fig. 7-2).

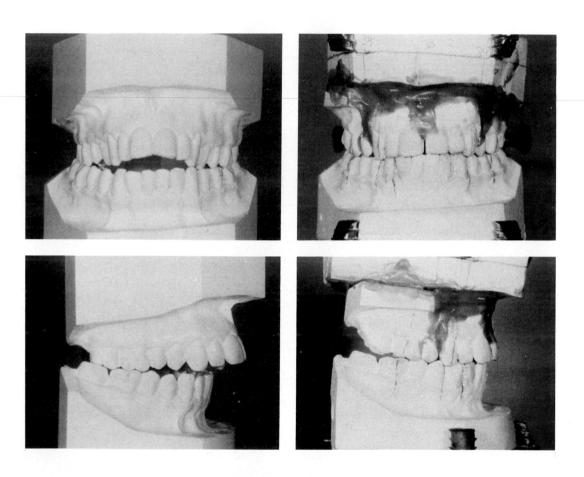

FIG. 7-2

More commonly the dental arches will need to be prepared for surgery by presurgical orthodontic treatment. Most of the attention during the presurgical orthodontic treatment for this deformity is directed toward the lower arch because the lower arch is the "target" for placing the upper arch when surgery is done. The anteroposterior and transverse positions of the lower teeth at the time of surgery are critical because they determine the upper tooth-to-lip relationships both in projection and symmetry. Since the anteroposterior projection of the upper teeth determines the nasolabial angle and lip drape, it is imperative that a prediction tracing be done to plan the orthodontic tooth movement desired in the lower arch

(Fig. 7-3). When the desired tooth movements are known, the orthodontic mechanics to produce this result can be determined and carried out. *All too frequently, simultaneous two-jaw surgery is made "necessary" by poorly planned or poorly executed presurgical orthodontic treatment of the lower arch.*

PRESENT POSITION ————————

DESIRED POSITION — — — —

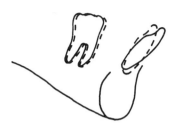

FIG. 7-3

The frequency of extraction versus nonextraction treatment in these patients is nearly equal. From the orthodontic viewpoint, the need for extractions depends on what is to be done in the lower arch to achieve the desired anteroposterior position of the incisors. This can be determined only by a well-done cephalometric tracing (Chapter 2). To avoid repetition, treatment wherein the maxilla is not segmentalized is discussed in this chapter while the mechanics used for maxillary segmentalization are discussed in Chapter 9. In either instance the lower dentition is orthodontically placed in its optimal position relative to the mandible and the upper dentition is aligned orthodontically and surgically placed into the desired occlusal and vertical relation.

When a Class II occlusion is to be made Class I by superior maxillary repositioning, the maxilla will usually require some amount of posterior movement for full correction. If there exists considerable room between the distal of the upper second molar and the pterygoid plates this movement can be accomplished with relative ease. However, when little room exists in this area, the surgeon may require premolar extraction in the upper arch so that a Class II molar–Class I canine relation is produced surgically, thus avoiding the potential difficulties involved with bone removal in this area. If such is the case (example patient), the maxilla can be treated segmentally as described in Chapter 9 or the extraction space closed orthodontically and the upper arch idealized by the most expeditious method, as anchorage is not a consideration.

The presurgical orthodontic treatment for the nonextraction patient when whole-arch surgery is to be done is straightforward. Once proper notation has been made on the patient's chart that treatment is to be by combined orthodontics and surgery so that both the clinician and the staff are alerted to this fact, the upper and lower appliances are placed and both arches are aligned and leveled *independently*. Progressively larger archwires are placed until the desired archwire size is achieved to produce arch form coordination. Once the arches are coordinated, a progress cephalometric radiograph is made to check the anteroposterior position of the *lower* teeth. Appropriate elastics (usually Class III) are then worn until the proper position of the lower teeth is achieved. Once the lower arch is in its desired anteroposterior position and feasibility model surgery shows that a reasonable occlusion can be produced by surgery, the archwires are tied with ligature wires to prevent inadvertent disengagement during surgery and the patient is referred for surgery.

When extractions are necessary the desired amount of lower incisor and molar movement is determined from the prediction tracing. When maximal retraction of the lower incisors is required, the mechanics described in the first usual approach in Chapter 6 are applicable for the lower arch. Less retraction of the lower incisors is provided by using en mass retraction of the six lower anterior teeth and still less is provided by extracting lower second premolars.

As in the nonextraction regimen, the upper arch is treated independently or can be used to supplement the lower anchorage by use of Class III elastics before surgery. The extractions chosen for the upper arch are largely dependent on the inclination of the upper incisors and the tooth mass considerations. When the upper incisors are too upright or the upper second premolars are extremely small, extraction of upper second premolars is the treatment of choice to correct the tooth mass or allow some labial tipping of the upper incisors during aligning of the teeth. If the upper incisors are tipped labially excessively before treatment, extraction of the first premolars will allow them to be uprighted during space closure.

One factor that must be understood regarding the presurgical treatment of the maxillary arch is that *there is no anchorage requirement in the maxilla since the maxilla will be surgically repositioned relative to the mandibular dentition.* Thus, the lower arch is critical to success as described previously, and the maxillary teeth need only be aligned and leveled within the confines of the alveolar bone. The maxillary arch should not be inadvertently expanded by the presurgical orthodontic treatment or intentionally expanded beyond the limits of good technique as determined by the age of the patient and the inclination of the posterior teeth. Expansion, when necessary, is best provided surgically for reasons of stability.

Three conditions deserve further comment due to their importance. These are the symmetry of the lower dental arch, the tooth mass, and presurgical arch coordination.

The lower dental midline must be coincident with the facial midline and the lower canines must be equal in their anteroposterior position. If this condition is not achieved during the presurgical orthodontic treatment, the maxillary teeth will assume the same asymmetry as the mandibular teeth when the maxilla is surgically repositioned (Fig. 7-4). Thus, when mandibular dental asymmetry exists (as opposed to skeletal, see Volume III, Section VII), it is necessary to correct this before maxillary surgery by unilateral extraction, asymmetric extractions, or appropriate elastic therapy. The clinician need not be concerned about producing some asymmetry of the maxillary dentition presurgically by using elastics to correct the lower arch, as any dental asymmetry thus produced will be corrected when surgery is done.

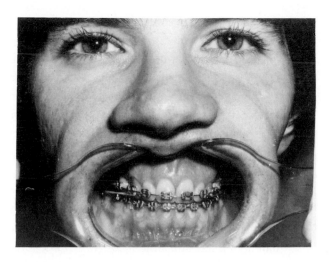

FIG. 7-4

When the mandibular dental asymmetry is too severe to correct by these methods, it is necessary to align the lower teeth segmentally and correct it surgically, most frequently by an anterior subapical procedure, at the same time the maxillary surgery is done (Fig. 7-5).

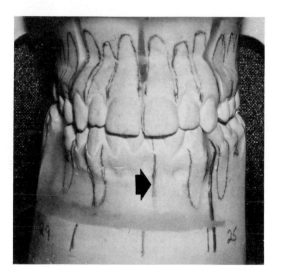

FIG. 7-5

The second condition requiring special consideration is the tooth mass. It is essential that patients who have tooth mass problems have these corrected *before* surgery or a satisfactory occlusion and proper overbite-overjet relationship cannot be produced at surgery. Correction is most frequently possible by dental recontouring, but some instances require extraction of a lower incisor tooth or opening spaces in the maxillary arch in anticipation of correction by restorative dentistry after completion of the orthodontic-surgical treatment.

The third condition is arch coordination. Patients with vertical maxillary excess frequently have a narrow, V-shaped maxillary arch and a broader, more U-shaped mandibular arch even when no posterior crossbite exists before treatment. When this is so, considerable expansion may be necessary in the canine and premolar areas of the maxillary arch to coordinate the arch forms orthodontically. In such instances the maxillary arch shape is best changed by surgery. Segmental mechanics are used in the maxilla presurgically (see Chapter 9), with the teeth being aligned in two segments (left and right), three segments (left and right molars and premolars, and canine to canine), or four segments (left and right molars and premolars, and canine to central incisor left and right). Four segments are usually preferred whenever the maxillary intercanine width must be expanded to such an extent that doing so by orthodontic means could jeopardize the periodontal tissues labial to the canine teeth (Fig. 7-6).

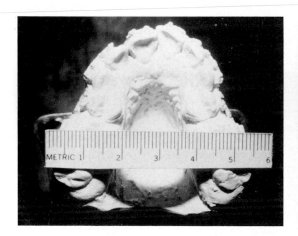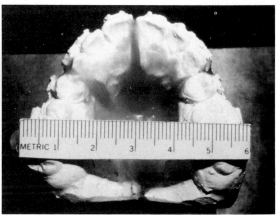

FIG. 7-6

Immediate presurgical planning

SURGICAL CEPHALOMETRIC PREDICTION TRACING FOR SUPERIOR REPOSITIONING OF THE MAXILLA WITH ADVANCEMENT GENIOPLASTY

Unlike the combined orthodontic-surgical prediction tracings discussed in Chapter 2, the surgeon is bound by the position of the teeth that has been produced by the presurgical orthodontic treatment. As such, the surgical cephalometric prediction tracings are more simply and directly done. These prediction tracings provide much of the essential information required to perform the surgery properly. Furthermore, by superimposing the prediction tracing on the cephalometric radiograph obtained immediately following surgery the accuracy of the surgical changes can be studied. Significant discrepancies between the predicted and actual result may warrant additional surgical intervention before the patient leaves the hospital (Chapter 5).

The primary surgery is superior repositioning of the maxilla to correct both the Class II dental relation and the upper tooth-to-lip relationship. In addition, a determination is made regarding the need for and, if necessary, the magnitude of an advancement genioplasty.

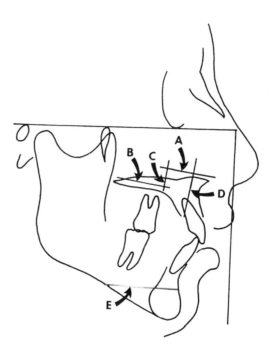

FIG. 7-7

All usual structures are traced from the presurgical cephalometric radiograph. Frankfort horizontal and subnasale perpendicular are constructed on this tracing for purposes of determining the need for and magnitude of a genioplasty. A maxillary reference line is constructed on this tracing that closely approximates the planned ostectomy. The anterior component of this line (*A*) is 35 mm above the cusp tip of the maxillary canine (occlusal plane), and the posterior component (*B*) is 25 mm above the cusp tips of the maxillary first molar. These lines are made parallel to the maxillary occlusal plane and are joined by a vertical line (*C*) perpendicular to the occlusal plane and just mesial to the first molar. An anterior vertical reference line (*D*) is placed perpendicular to the maxillary occlusal plane approximately at the position of the cusp tip of the maxillary canine. When an advancement genioplasty is anticipated, an additional reference line (*E*) is constructed on this tracing to correspond to the location of the horizontal osteotomy for the genioplasty (see Chapter 6 for a detailed description of the genioplasty technique). This is referred to as the ***tracing*** (black line).

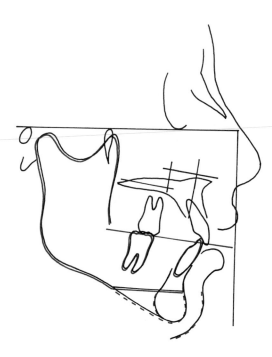

FIG. 7-8

The **prediction** (red lines) is begun by tracing the mandible, condyle, mandibular teeth, and occlusal plane on a new piece of tracing acetate overlaid on the **tracing**. (Note: In all instances when lines are being traced from the **tracing** to the **prediction**, superimpositions are shown slightly offset to better show which lines are being traced.) The genioplasty line is traced and a dashed line is used to indicate the present position of the bony chin below this line and the soft-tissue chin.

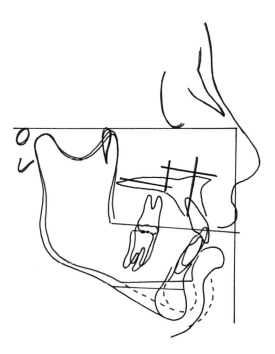

FIG. 7-9

The ***prediction*** is rotated counterclockwise about the condyle head,* until the mandibular occlusal plane is positioned 1 to 2 mm below the upper lip on the ***tracing.*** (This occlusal plane position provides approximately 2 to 3 mm of upper incisor exposure below the upper lip. When more tooth exposure is desired, the occlusal plane is placed further below the upper lip). The "fixed structures" and the maxillary osteotomy reference lines (*A* to *D*) are traced onto the ***prediction*** while this superimposition is held.

---

*The center of rotation is not exactly about the condyle. Rather, it is located posteriorly and inferiorly somewhere in the mastoid area. While this difference is of academic interest, it is not *clinically* significant in the vast majority of patients undergoing this surgical procedure.

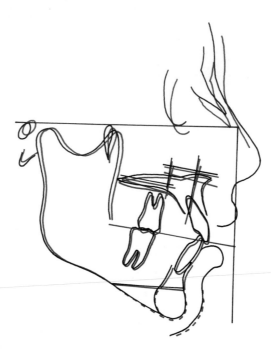

FIG. 7-10

The ***prediction*** is repositioned on the ***tracing*** such that the maxillary dentition is placed into an ideal occlusal relationship with the mandibular dentition. The palate, maxillary alveolus, maxillary teeth, and reference lines (*A* to *D*) for the maxilla are now traced.

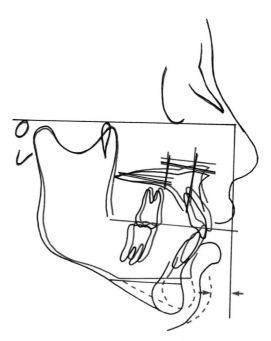

FIG. 7-11

The fixed structures of the ***prediction*** are now superimposed on those of the ***tracing***. The position of the dashed line at soft-tissue pogonion on the ***prediction*** is now evaluated noting its distance from subnasale perpendicular on the ***tracing***. If a genioplasty is necessary, it is planned and added as described in Chapter 6. The soft-tissue structures are traced as described in detail in Chapter 2.

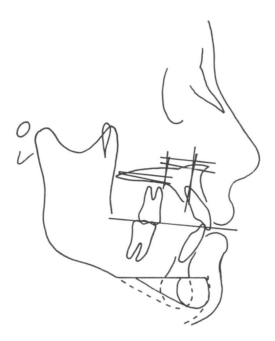

FIG. 7-12

The completed prediction tracing is illustrated in Fig. 7-12. The changes in the skeletal reference marks indicate the size of the lateral wall ostectomy (horizontal references) and the amount of anteroposterior repositioning of the maxilla (vertical references) that is to be achieved at surgery. When whole-arch maxillary superior repositioning is being done, these references are definitive. However, when segmentalization or asymmetric movements are required, references taken from the definitive model surgery are more precise because three-dimensional movements are being done that are not seen or well illustrated in a two-dimensional cephalometric prediction tracing.

382   *Class II Dentofacial Deformities*

MODEL SURGERY FOR SUPERIOR REPOSITIONING OF THE MAXILLA

When isolated, symmetric, nonsegmentalized maxillary surgery is to be performed, the model surgery should provide precisely the same information as the definitive cephalometric prediction tracing. As such, some may consider it unnecessary, yet it serves as an excellent method to check the accuracy of the prediction. Certainly when the model surgery and prediction tracing are at variance, the clinician must determine which is in error and correct the error *before* going to surgery. In this way several postsurgical complications directly related to surgical planning are avoided.

The definitive immediate presurgical model surgery for LeFort I with superior repositioning is described. When doing so, the authors prefer to use a semiadjustable anatomic articulator with a face-bow transfer. While this may be unnecessary when isolated, symmetric, nonsegmentalized maxillary surgery is to be performed and an accurate cephalometric prediction tracing has been done, the time and energy spent in doing model surgery as described can expedite surgery and help prevent postsurgical complications.

FIG. 7-13

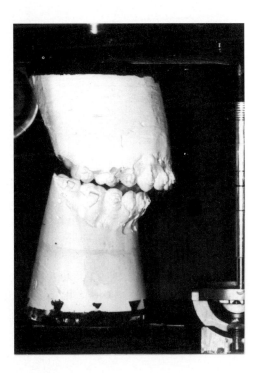

Step 1. The models are mounted on a semiadjustable anatomic articulator by a face-bow transfer. The mounted models are trimmed to simulate the actual skeletal anatomy of the maxilla and mandible.

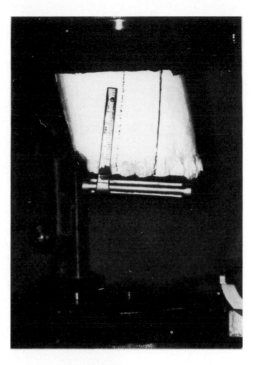

FIG. 7-14

Step 2. The models are marked as follows:

a. Vertical reference lines (perpendicular to the occlusal plane) are drawn from the mounting ring of the maxillary model to the first molar and canine teeth bilaterally using the maxillary reference device.* These vertical maxillary reference lines are then extended inferiorly onto the mandibular casts.

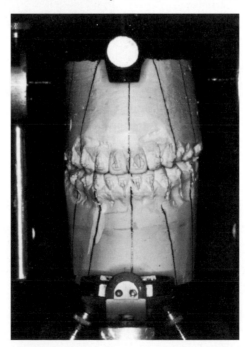

FIG. 7-15

b. The facial midline is drawn on the maxillary cast. The line is extended onto the mandibular dentition and down through the mandibular symphysis.

---

*Walter Lorenz Instrument Company, Jacksonville, FL.

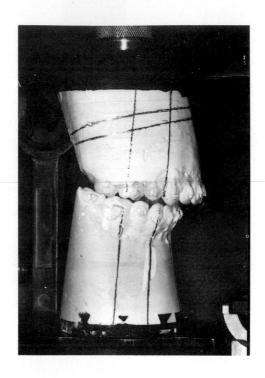

FIG. 7-16

    c. A horizontal line is drawn on the models beginning approximately 35 mm above the maxillary canine cusp tip and tapering posteriorly to 25 mm above the maxillary first molar cusp tips. This line marks the point at which the saw cut is made to section the maxillary model from its base and simulates the location of the most inferior aspect of the lateral maxillary wall ostectomy to be made at surgery. A second horizontal line is drawn on the maxillary model 2 to 3 mm farther above the first line than the anticipated vertical movement as determined from the prediction tracing. This line approximates the superior extent of plaster removal for the model surgery.

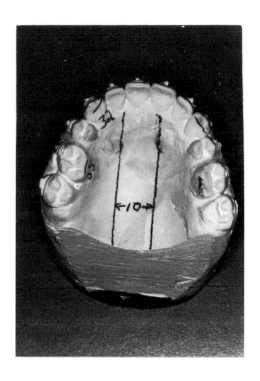

FIG. 7-17

d. If maxillary expansion is to be performed, parallel lines 10 mm apart are drawn on the midpalate. Changes in this measurement illustrate the magnitude of bony width change at the height of the palatal vault, which may be substantially different from changes at the occlusal level when tipping of the maxillary segments occurs.

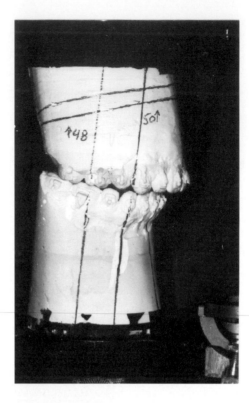

FIG. 7-18

Step 3. The following numerical measurements are made and recorded on the models:

a. The distance from the maxillary mounting ring to the first molar and canine cusp tips bilaterally. This measurement is made along the previously drawn reference lines.

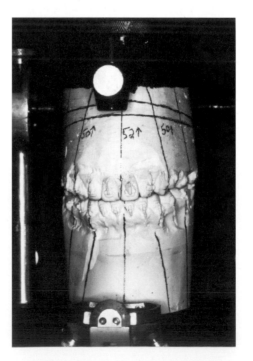

FIG. 7-19

b. The distance from the maxillary mounting ring to the incisal edge of the maxillary central incisors (recorded adjacent to the upward pointing arrow).

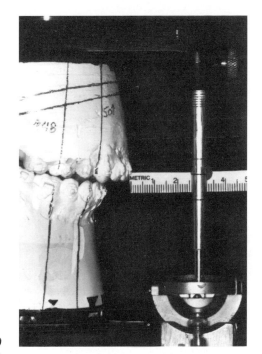
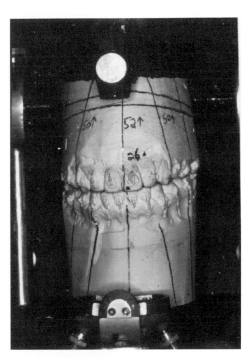

FIG. 7-20

c. The horizontal distance from the maxillary central incisal edge to the incisal guide pin of the articulator (recorded adjacent to the dot on the central incisor).

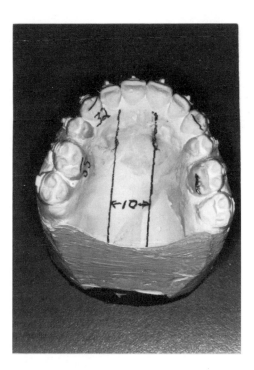

FIG. 7-21

d. The intercanine, interpremolar, and intermolar distances are recorded if midline maxillary expansion is to be performed.

Step 4. After all reference lines and measurements have been placed on the maxillary and mandibular models, the maxillary model is sectioned from its base at the level previously marked. Following this, plaster is removed from the base until the second horizontal reference line is reached.

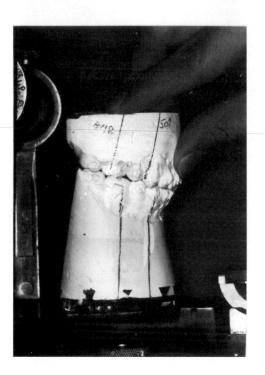
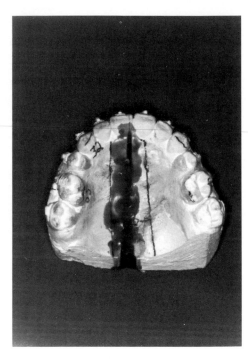

FIG. 7-22

Step 5. In instances in which a midline split with widening is planned in conjunction with LeFort I superior repositioning, the maxillary cast is separated in the midline by sawing downward from the base of the cast toward the teeth. Once the saw is near the contact point of the maxillary incisors, the model is broken apart so that no tooth material is lost between the incisors. The two halves of the maxilla are held together with a soft wax, while the teeth are placed into their optimal occlusion with the intact mandible, and luted to the opposing dentition with a light application of sticky wax. Once the optimal occlusion is achieved, the maxillary segments are consolidated into a "single" unit with a heavy application of sticky wax.

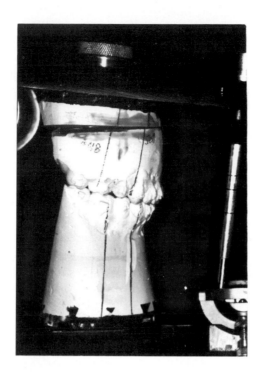

FIG. 7-23

Step 6. The maxilla-mandible complex is now autorotated into its desired position. This is done by loosening the set screw of the incisal guide pin and permitting the upper component of the articular with the attached mounting ring to rotate inferiorly. As the upper component rotates inferiorly, the distance between the mounting ring and the upper central incisor edges is measured. Once the proper vertical position of the incisors is reached (i.e., the distance from mounting ring to central incisor has been decreased by the amount of superior repositioning desired), the set screw on the incisal guide pin is tightened. The repositioned maxilla is provisionally joined to the maxillary base with soft wax and all measurements are checked.

Step 7. Once the maxilla is determined to be in its desired location, a heavy application of sticky wax is used to secure the maxilla to the base. The vertical location of the maxillary incisor is rechecked for accuracy and the vertical changes at the canines and first molars are recorded. These vertical changes will determine the geometry of the maxillary ostectomy at surgery.

OCCLUSAL SPLINT CONSTRUCTION

An occlusal splint is constructed when either the maxilla is segmentalized or the occlusal interdigitation is equivocal. If maxillary widening is to be performed with a midline split of the maxilla, the splint is made with a palatal bar to increase its transverse rigidity and is made to interdigitate deeply with the maxillary teeth since there is a tendency for the segments to tip at the time of surgery. While a splint frequently is not necessary for LeFort I whole-arch surgery, a detailed discussion of splint fabrication is provided here for the times when one is necessary.

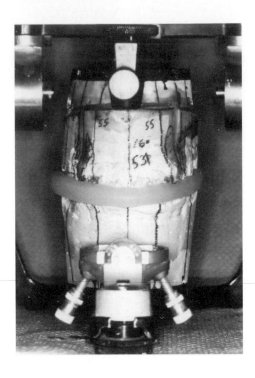

FIG. 7-24

The acrylic surgical occlusal splint with a palatal bar is constructed on the articulated models. To fabricate such a splint, the occlusal portion is first completed by coating the occlusal surfaces of the models with a separating medium and using self-curing acrylic rolled into a cylinder and placed between the maxillary and mandibular models. The models are closed into the soft acrylic and then are gently opened and closed to prevent the acrylic from becoming locked into any undercuts in the models while it cures. After the acrylic fully cures, the splint is trimmed such that the maxillary dentition is maximally interdigitated into the splint to permit optimal positioning of the maxillary segments at the time of surgery. When these interdigitations are not discrete, there is a tendency for the segments to be tipped arbitrarily, either buccally or palatally, at the time of surgery. The splint does not extend past the terminal molars. The mandibular occlusal interdigitations are definite, but shallow, to preclude occlusal interferences when the intermaxillary fixation is released and the patient begins to initiate jaw function (physiotherapy) with the splint left attached to the maxillary dentition. Importantly, this is not to be a functional splint from the standpoint that the patient can masticate with it in place. Rather, it is to permit hinge-axis closure of the mandible so that the patient's occlusion can be checked periodically after release of intermaxillary fixation to make certain the surgical result is stable.

After the splint is properly trimmed, holes are drilled just lateral to each interproximal space. The occlusal portion is now polished.

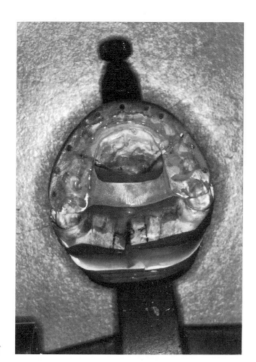 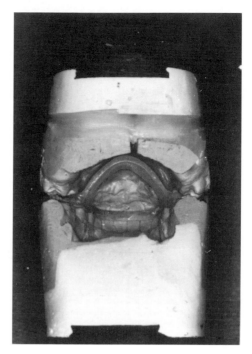

FIG. 7-25

Once the occlusal portion of the splint has been completed, it is lightly sticky waxed to the maxillary model and one layer of thin pink base plate wax is applied to the palatal vault between the maxillary first molars to provide relief for the palatal bar. A strip of acrylic, approximately 2 to 3 mm thick, and 10 mm wide is placed on the wax relief and is connected to the splint in the area of the maxillary first molar with a thin layer of acrylic.

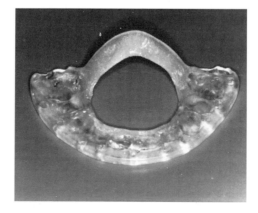

FIG. 7-26

After the palatal bar has been completed, the splint is polished. The completed splint is shown in Fig. 7-26.

Orthognathic reconstructive surgery

When performing a LeFort I superior maxillary repositioning and advancement genioplasty, the surgical sequence preferred is to complete the genioplasty and then the LeFort I. This section discusses the surgical procedure for LeFort I superior repositioning only. The technique for advancement genioplasty is presented on pages 251–259 in Chapter 6.

LEFORT I

The maxillary vestibule is injected with 2% lidocaine with 1:100,000 epinephrine 5 to 10 minutes prior to beginning the maxillary surgery. This injection is carried posteriorly on each side into the pterygoid maxillary recess to effect a second division block.

Prior to incising maxillary tissues, base-line measurements from the medial canthus of the eyes to the orthodontic brackets of the maxillary central incisors are made with a large caliper. This external vertical reference is recorded and the change in it is checked at the completion of the maxillary repositioning to further indure the accurate vertical positioning of the maxillary central incisors.

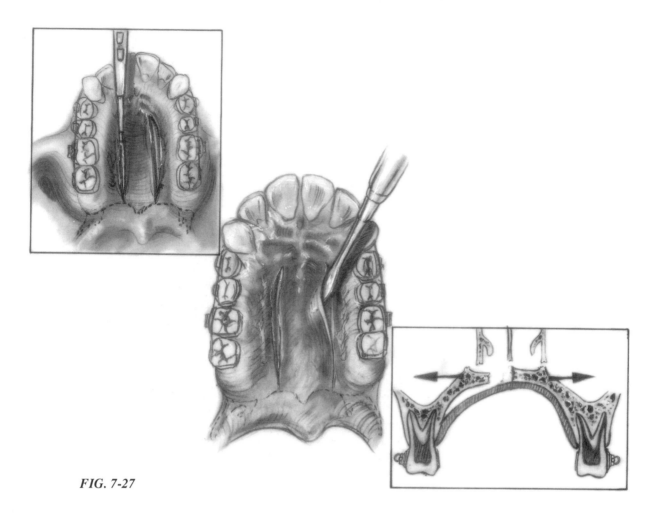

FIG. 7-27

If more than 4 or 5 mm of maxillary expansion is planned as a part of the surgery, the first stage of surgery is to make two parasagittal soft-tissue palatal incisions with a diathermy knife. These incisions are made just medial to the greater palatine neurovascular bundles from the posterior edge of the hard palate anteriorly to the premolar region. No local anesthetic is injected palatally. The mucoperiosteum between the two incisions is completely undermined subperiosteally. This flap is generally about 12 to 15 mm wide. Care is exercised not to tear either end of the flap, especially the posterior, because this will compromise its primary vascular source. This flap permits the maxilla to be surgically expanded without resistance from the palatal mucoperiosteum, and prevents both a midline palatal mucosal tear and/or stripping of the important palatal pedicles (blood supply) from the lateral maxillary segments during expansion.

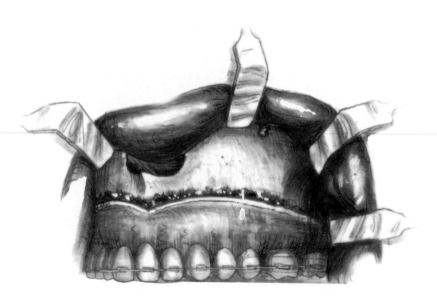

FIG. 7-28

An incision is made in the depth of the maxillary vestibule using a diapthermy knife. The incision is made down to bone and initially extends from the mesial aspect of the first molar on one side to the midline. This diathermy incision is made in layers with progressive retraction so that tissues that have been incised are not repeatedly cauterized. After this incision has been completed, a periosteal elevator is used to reflect the mucoperiosteal flap superiorly to expose the infraorbital nerve. Next, the dissection is carried posteriorly in the subperiosteal plane first into the area of the malar prominence and then posteriorly to the region of the pterygoid maxillary junction. Finally, the nasal mucoperiosteum is carefully elevated from the piriform rim and is dissected free of the inferior-lateral nasal wall posteriorly about 15 to 20 mm.

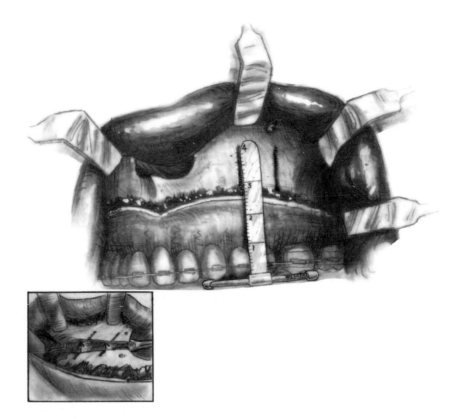

FIG. 7-29

The maxillary reference device used during the definitive model surgery is now interdigitated onto the maxillary dentition. Vertical reference lines are scored with a 701 bur on the lateral maxillary walls in positions similar to those made during the definitive model surgery—perpendicular to the occlusal plane in the area of the maxillary canine and first molar bilaterally.

Vertical reference lines made differently at surgery from those that were made on the model surgery will only serve to deceive the surgeon rather than aid him/her. A straight superior movement of the maxilla may appear as if the maxilla has been moved posteriorly as illustrated in the inset of Fig. 7-29. If the vertical reference lines were canted in the opposite direction, the maxilla would appear to have moved anteriorly with a straight superior movement.

Next the *level and width* of the planned ostectomy is marked. Bur reference marks are made 35 mm above the cusp tips of the maxillary canines and 25 mm above the cusp tips of the maxillary first molar in the region of the zygomatic buttress to mark the *inferior* extent of the ostectomy. These reference marks are joined as described below to form a line with three segments. The anterior segment parallels the occlusal plane and extends from the piriform rim to the zygomatic buttress at the level of the anterior reference mark. The posterior segment parallels the occlusal plane and extends from the mesial of the first molar to the most distal root of the second molar at the level of the posterior reference mark. The third segment, perpendicular to the occlusal plane and just mesial to the first molar, joins the first two lines.

The superior extent of the lateral wall ostectomy is marked in a similar manner with a second line above the first reference line. The distance between these lines is determined by the amount of superior repositioning desired as previously determined by the esthetic considerations of the patient with regard to upper tooth exposure in repose. This distance is the same as that shown to occur on the model surgery and prediction tracing as part of the definitive presurgical planning, and permit making the ostectomy similar to that on the models and cephalometric prediction tracing.

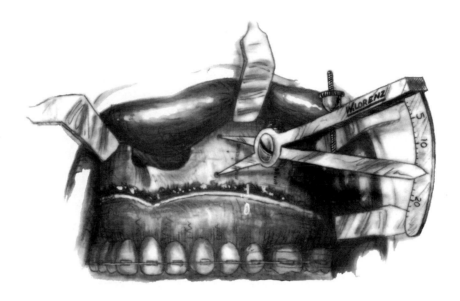

FIG. 7-30

Internal reference marks—bur holes approximately 15 mm apart and on either side of the proposed LeFort I ostectomy (reference lines described above) in the area of the maxillary canines—are next placed using a caliper and a 701 bur. By directly measuring the change in these internal reference marks after the maxilla has been repositioned, the clinician can easily and accurately determine if the vertical change that occurred during the model surgery and cephalometric prediction tracing has been accurately reproduced at surgery.

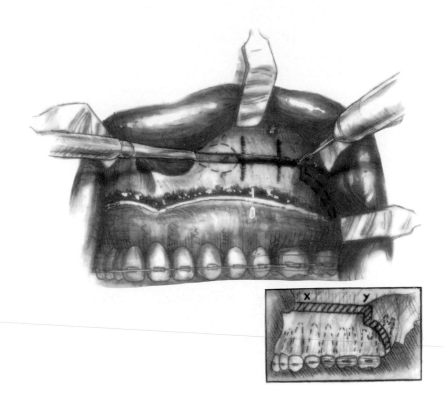

FIG. 7-31

The lateral maxillary wall ostectomy is begun in the region of the piriform rim approximately 35 mm above the maxillary canine tip, and continues posteriorly, parallel to the maxillary occlusal plane, to a point just mesial to the first molar. Here it is stepped down with a vertical osteotomy, perpendicular to the occlusal plane, to a level approximately 25 mm above the first molar cusp tips. A periosteal elevator is inserted beneath the nasal mucoperiosteum to protect it while the lateral and medial maxillary ostectomies are performed. The magnitude and geometry of these ostectomies were determined from the cephalometric prediction tracing and definitive model surgery. In the inset of Fig. 7-31, *X* represents the magnitude of superior repositioning in the canine area and *Y,* the magnitude of ostectomy in the molar area.

Posterior to the step, the lateral maxillary ostectomies are carried posteriorly and tapered sharply inferiorly just distal to the tooth-root apices of the terminal molar. Tapering the ostectomy inferiorly in the retromolar area makes the subsequent down-fracturing easier and decreases the chance of pathologic fracture of the pterygoid plates and/or perpendicular portion of the palatine bone. (Avoiding pathologic fractures of these bones greatly decreases the chance of serious vascular sequelae.)

When an impacted third molar is present it is ignored. During the lateral maxillary wall osteotomy it is cut through and removed after down-fracturing the maxilla.

The tuberosity-pterygoid maxillary area is sectioned with a curved osteotome, attempting to cut through the retromolar bone and medial portion of the pterygoid bone (Fig. 7-33, *right inset*).

The lateral nasal wall is osteotomized with a curved osteotome while the nasal mucoperiosteum is protected with a periosteal elevator. This lateral nasal wall osteotomy is carried approximately 30 mm posteriorly. The location of the greater palatine canal and its enclosed nerve and vessels is approximately 35 mm posterior to the piriform aperture of the nose. By stopping short of the perpendicular plate of the palatine bone the potential for troublesome bleeding from the vessel before actual down-fracture is avoided, the vascular supply to the mobilized maxilla is maximized, and the loss of sensation to the palatal, buccal, and maxillary periodontal soft tissues is minimized.

Similar soft-tissue incisions, subperiosteal dissection, bone marking and ostectomies are completed on the opposite side.

In cases requiring maxillary expansion by a maxillary midline osteotomy, a subperiosteal dissection is accomplished labially to the maxillary central incisors beginning superiorly and proceeding down to the level of the attached gingiva. A skin hook is then used to engage the mucoperiosteum in the region of the central incisor roots to provide direct visualization of the proposed midline osteotomy.

A thin osteotome is placed near the anterior nasal spine and is malleted posteriorly along the palatal plane. Next it is reinserted more inferiorly to divide the crestal bone. An index finger is placed on the palate to help prevent the osteotomies from piercing the palatal mucosa. Complete separation of the midline is not accomplished until the subsequent down fracture is completed.

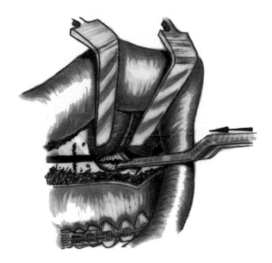

FIG. 7-32

Finally, the nasal septum is separated from the maxilla. To minimize disruption of the nasal mucoperiosteum while doing so, the anterior cartilaginous nasal septum is first reflected from its groove in the nasal crest of the maxilla. Next, the anterior nasal crest of the maxilla is removed with an osteotome to improve direct visualization for reflection of the nasal mucoperiosteum from the nasal floor and to make it easier to direct the septal osteotome properly in the nasal floor, thus sectioning the bony nasal septum *at its base* and avoiding unnecessary tearing of the nasal mucoperiosteum. While using the nasal septal osteotome, it is helpful to place one finger on the posterior nasal spine as a target toward which the osteotome is directed.

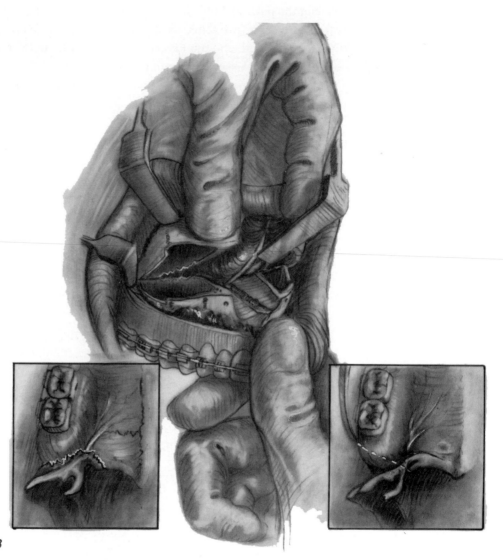

FIG. 7-33

The maxilla is down-fractured by manually applying an inferior force. This is most readily done by forcing the maxilla inferoposteriorly with one hand while stabilizing the superior midface structures with the opposite hand. When the osteotomies are all performed as described, the greater palatine neurovascular bundles are preserved because the fractures occur through the sutures *around* the greater palatine canals.

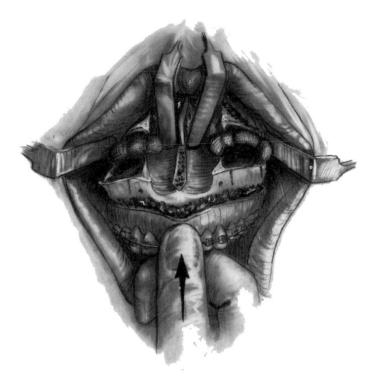

FIG. 7-34

Upon down-fracturing, any nasal mucoperiosteum still attached to the floor of the nose is elevated under direct visualization. Moist gauze packs are inserted firmly into the posterior floor of the nose and into the distal most portions of the lateral wall osteotomies. This aids both hemostasis and subsequent mobilization of the posterior maxilla. After placement of these packs, the anterior maxilla is forced *superiorly* to mobilize the posterior maxilla inferiorly by using the gauze packs as fulcrums.

With the maxilla in the down-fractured position all osteotomies are rechecked for completeness and the level of the fracture in the area of the perpendicular plate of the palatine bone is checked. It is best if this fracture is visible and low. If the fracture is not easily seen or appears high, it is prudent to make osteotomies to establish this "fracture" in a more inferior, visible location.

The maxilla is retracted inferiorly and all irregular bone edges and probable bony interferences are removed. Interferences are most likely to be found in the following areas: (1) the nasal septum, (2) the lateral nasal walls, (3) the palatine bones, (4) the pterygoid plates, and (5) the maxillary tuberosities. *Complete removal of all interferences in the latter areas (3 to 5) is critical to successful completion of this operation since the maxilla will be repositioned not only superiorly, but also somewhat posteriorly to correct the Class II occlusion.*

The nasal septal area is relieved first by removing any remaining septum from the nasal floor of the maxilla using a rongeur. A groove several millimeters deep is then made in this area with a medium-sized round bur. If this is insufficient to permit the desired amount of superior repositioning, a portion of the inferior *bony* nasal septum is removed with rongeurs. Although the inferior aspect of the cartilaginous nasal septum is exposed *no cartilaginous nasal septum is removed at this time*. Refinement of the amount of bony and cartilaginous nasal septum removed is accomplished first when the maxilla is being rotated superiorly to check on interferences to its superior repositioning and finally after the maxilla has been stabilized in its superior position. These refinements are described later in this section.

The lateral nasal walls are generally very thin and are easily removed with rongeurs. While doing this, care is taken not to transect the greater palatine neurovascular bundles. Deliberate, sequential removal of bony interferences due to the posterior lateral nasal walls enables the greater palatine neurovascular bundles to be readily exposed and preserved.

After the septal and lateral nasal wall ostectomies have been completed, the posterior interferences in the palatine, pterygoid, and maxillary tuberosity areas are removed. If impacted third molars are present, they are removed by exposing them from the superolateral approach and elevating them posteriorly. After this is done, or if a third molar is not present, several millimeters of bone are removed across the retromolar area in the line of the fracture with a medium-large round bur or a small curved osteotome. Finally the bone directly inferior and distal to the greater palatine neurovascular bundle is removed with a small osteotome and/or round bur.

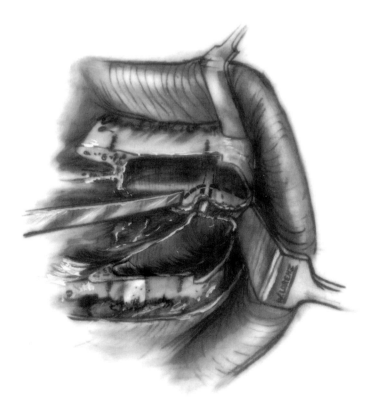

FIG. 7-35

If the maxilla must be repositioned posteriorly by more than the amount of bone that can be safely removed from the retromolar area without jeopardizing the second molar roots, additional bone is removed from the anterior aspect of the pterygoid plates with either a round bur or an osteotome.

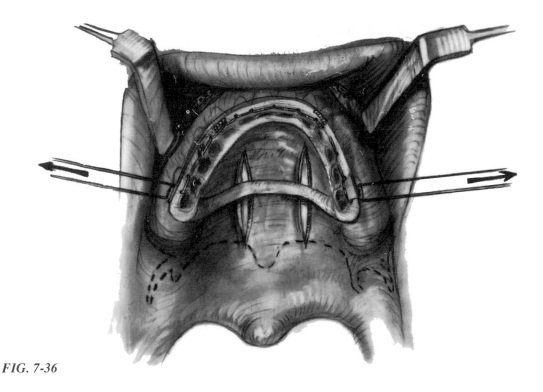

FIG. 7-36

When maxillary expansion is planned, a straight osteotome is reinserted into the midline of the palate at the level of the palatal plane, and levered to initiate the physical separation. (The posterior dental alveolus may be "pinched" by the thumb and index finger to ensure completeness of the midline osteotomy.) A 24-gauge stainless steel wire is then looped through each maxillary first molar buccal tube to aid in the slow, deliberate expansion of the two maxillary segments. Lateral mobilization of the two halves of the maxilla is accomplished by grasping these wires and pulling the halves of the maxilla apart slightly more than the needed expansion. The tension is then released and the mobilization is checked. This process is repeated with slightly more separation each time until the segments fit *passively* into the splint. Once this is so, the segments are wired into position.

Tears in the nasal floor mucosa that may have occurred during surgery are identified and repaired at this time with 4-0 chromic gut. Generally, these will have occurred primarily in the area of the nasal septum. The nasal mucosa is not sutured across the midline since some cartilaginous nasal septum may need to be trimmed on the caudal aspect when the maxilla is placed in its final superior position.

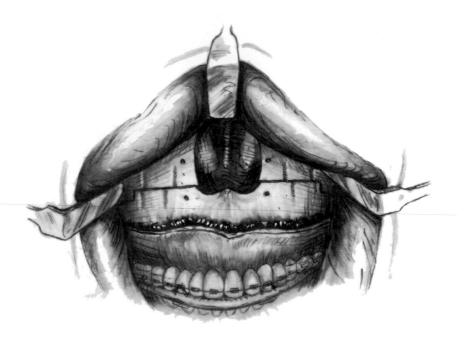

FIG. 7-37

When an occlusal splint is required, it is wired to the maxillary dentition. The maxilla, with or without splint, is now secured to the mandibular dentition using interdental fixation. The entire complex—maxilla, splint (if used), and mandible—is now rotated superiorly until the internal reference marks are the correct distance apart. If any bony interferences are encountered at this time, they are located and removed so that the maxilla can be repositioned the predetermined amount without the use of force. Once the maxilla can be rotated to its desired position, the cartilaginous nasal septum is checked for deviations and is judiciously trimmed when necessary, but only enough to prevent deviations. Final refinement of the septum is done with regard for nasal esthetic considerations only after stabilization of the maxilla. Both the internal and external vertical reference measurements are now checked to ensure that the appropriate amount of superior repositioning of the maxilla has been accomplished. In Fig. 7-31 *inset, X* represents the amount of the maxillary superior repositioning.

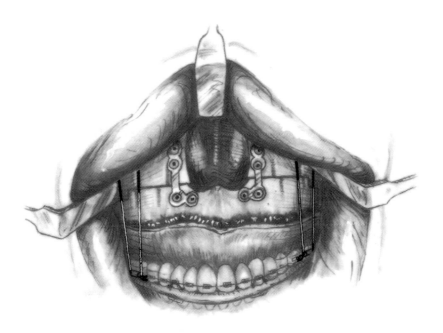

FIG. 7-38

Suspension wires are now placed from the buttress area and passed through the buccal tube of the first or second molar bracket and are gently tightened. These posterior suspension wires must have an appropriate vector. If a straight superior vector is desired, care is taken both in placing the bone hole in a proper anteroposterior location and in choosing which orthodontic bracket is best for securing the wire.

With the maxillary and mandibular complex secured by the posterior suspension wires, two L bone plates are adapted anteriorly and screwed to the mobilized maxilla. The intermaxillary fixation wires are now removed and, while applying an upward force in the region of the gonial angles, the occlusion is checked, paying particular attention to any evidence of an anterior open bite. When it is determined the occlusion is proper, the bone plates are attached to the stable superior portion of the maxilla.

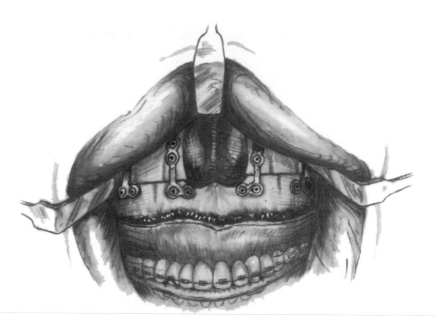

FIG. 7-39

If bone contact is poor in the posterior maxilla, bone plates may be placed in the zygomatic buttress area for added stability.

In all cases, there is deliberate control of alar base width and upper lip esthetics as discussed in the following section on adjunctive esthetic procedures. After attention to the nasal esthetics, the maxillary incision is closed in the appropriate manner and attention is then directed to the chin.

The mentalis muscle and mucoperiosteum are not closed until the end of the surgery so that the magnitude and symmetry of the chin advancement can be reevaluated following the maxillary surgery. Once the chin is determined to be as desired, the genioplasty incision is closed as described in Chapter 6.

If an occlusal splint is required or the immediate postoperative occlusion is not tight, it is recommended that the patient be placed in intermaxillary fixation for 1 to 3 weeks. Regardless of the presence or absence of intermaxillary fixation, *no chewing is permitted for 3 weeks*. Three weeks after surgery (all patients are out of intermaxillary fixation by this time), the patient is given written and verbal instruction with regard to diet, physical therapy, and monitoring of his/her occlusion as discussed in Chapter 6.

The occlusal splint, when used, may be removed 1 week after release of intermaxillary fixation in one-piece LeFort I cases if the patient bites repeatedly into the splint. When a midline split and expansion has been done, it is prudent to keep the splint wired to the maxillary dentition for a total of 4 to 6 weeks and for the patient to see the orthodontist the day the splint is removed for placement of a new archwire and a lingual arch to maintain the surgically achieved maxillary expansion.

About 3 to 5 weeks after surgery, normal range of asymptomatic jaw function has returned, the skeletal suspension wires (if used) have been removed under local anesthesia, the patient has begun to chew soft foods, and active postsurgical orthodontic treatment is begun. The patient gradually returns to an unlimited dietary consistency over the next 2 weeks—approximately 5 to 7 weeks following the maxillary surgery.

Adjunctive esthetic maxillofacial procedures

Unpredictable and highly variable alterations of the nose and upper lip occur during total maxillary surgery. Unesthetic cheek fullness can also become evident. These unfavorable changes can be avoided and, in many instances, esthetic improvement in these relations can be achieved with proper attention to certain details of surgical technique. The specific techniques used to control the nasal tip, alar base width, upper lip fullness, upper lip length, upper lip vermilion exposure, and excessive fullness of the cheeks are sequentially discussed. The decision to use the procedures discussed herein must be made on an individual basis by careful preoperative assessment of each of the areas and the desirability of change therein. For a given patient, all of the following procedures may be indicated; for another patient, none may be indicated.

NASAL TIP CONTROL

In maxillary surgery the nasal tip projection is controllable, to the greatest extent, by alterations in the support of the cartilaginous nasal septum. Thus, the relation of the nasal floor to the cartilaginous nasal septum must be routinely examined after stabilization of the maxilla.

When it is desirable to avoid additional nasal tip projection (supratip break), the cartilaginous nasal septum must rest *passively* on the anterior nasal floor after the maxilla had been superiorly repositioned. (This may likewise be important to avoid deviation of the septum and possibly the nasal tip.) If it does not rest passively in the midline, as evidenced by the fact that a periosteal elevator can be passed between it and the nasal floor with little or no resistance, deliberate excision of the inferior edge of the cartilaginous septum is done until this situation exists.

Conversely, if additional nasal tip projection is desired, the septum is made to rest on the anterior nasal floor as firmly as possible after surgery, but *without producing significant deviation of the nasal septum or nasal tip*. Optionally, a septal cartilaginous columella strut may be placed.

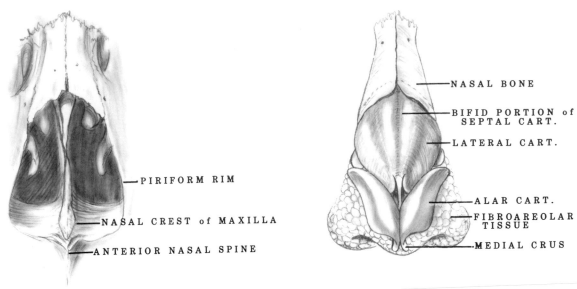

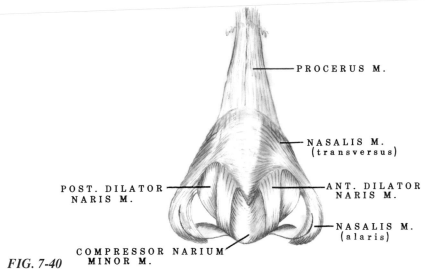

FIG. 7-40

ALAR BASE WIDTH CONTROL

Alar base width and shape is determined by: (1) the anatomy of the osseous support for the attached and overlying soft tissues, (2) the cartilaginous structures of the caudal aspect of the nose (primarily the lower lateral cartilages), and (3) the facial muscles directly related to the nose. The width and projection of the piriform rims of the nose provide the support for the alar bases, both by indirect support for the alar cartilages and by providing the areas for attachment to the nasalis muscles. Accordingly, the intricate interaction of alterations in these osseous-cartilaginous-muscle relations must be conjointly considered in maxillary surgery. The means of controlling alar base esthetics is discussed herein, with particular attention to the factors that determine alar base esthetics.

The width and symmetry of the alar bases are evaluated and recorded as part of the clinical patient evaluation (Chapter 1). Before surgery, and with the patient's input, it is decided what changes, if any, are desired in the alar base esthetics. At surgery, these esthetic desires are accomplished as described below.

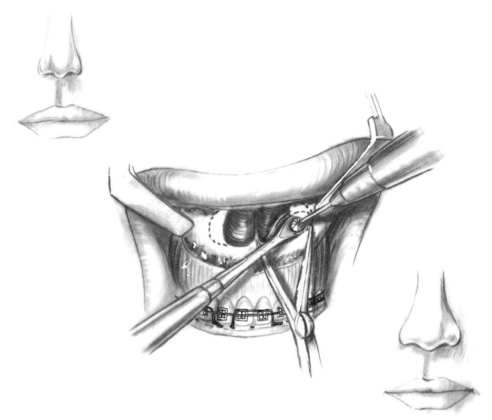

FIG. 7-41

WIDENING NARROW ALAR BASES. In many instances the alar bases are excessively narrow and the widening that usually occurs with maxillary superior repositioning is favorable. If not deliberately controlled, the amount of widening that occurs is highly variable. In some instances the widening is minimal and additional widening is esthetically desirable. Alar base widening may even be desired in select individuals when maxillary surgery is not planned. In either instance, intentional widening can be achieved by symmetric enlargement of the piriform apertures on each side from 4 to 8 mm. Approximately 1 mm of alar base widening occurs with each 2 mm of bony piriform aperture widening. Importantly this procedure is not a substitute for skeletal nasal base augmentation (Chapter 10), which is performed when it is desirable to produce *both* widening of the alar bases and reduction of the relative prominence of the nose in profile by converting the concave paranasal areas to convex.

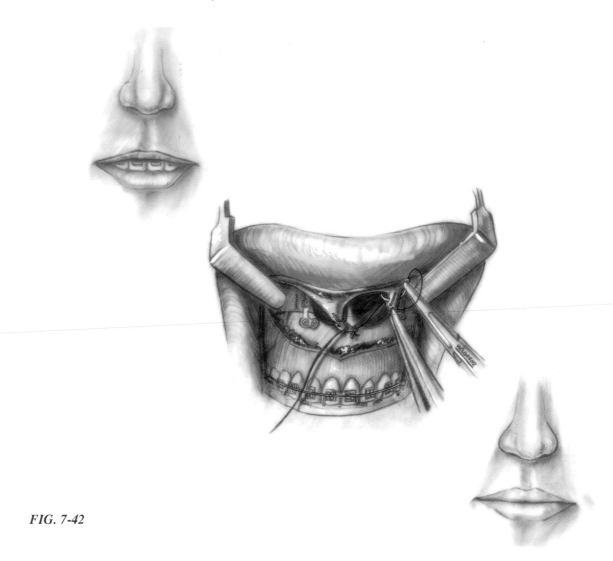

FIG. 7-42

PREVENTING EXCESSIVE WIDENING OF THE ALAR BASES OR PRODUC-ING SLIGHT NARROWING OF THE ALAR BASES. The possibility of excessive widening of the alar bases exists with all total maxillary surgery. Excessive widening produces an unesthetic result that is more objectionable than a failure to achieve optimal widening. *Excessive widening of the alar bases can occur when the maxilla is repositioned in any direction* and the preexisting alar base width is narrow, normal or slightly excessive. *Thus, deliberate control of alar base width must be considered in virtually all maxillary surgical procedures.*

Before surgery the alar base width is measured and recorded. A deliberate decision is made with the patient's input with respect to the *desired* alar base width. At the completion of all surgery except for closure of the maxillary vestibular incision, deliberate control of the alar bases is routinely performed as described below.

The "alar base tissues" are identified within the vestibular incision. This is done by placing the forefinger facially directly over the ala of the nose, retracting the lip with the thumb, and grasping that tissue directly beneath the forefinger with tissue pickups. Anatomically, these tissues are the nasalis muscles and the associated fibroareolar connective tissues that are attached superiorly to the alar cartilages. Occasionally, accessory alar cartilages are also present in this area. When the alar base tissue is grasped, the alar base can be rotated medially almost to the columella, as observed facially. It is essential to identify these specific tissues, and it may be necessary to grasp the tissues in this area several times until the correct tissues are located. Once identified, a 2-0 permanent suture is passed in a figure-8 fashion through them and through a bur hole placed in the region of the anterior nasal spine. This is repeated on the opposite side. Each suture is tightened independently, while maintaining symmetry, until the desired alar base width is attained, as confirmed facially by measurement with calipers.

While the alar base width may appear satisfactory at the completion of maxillary surgery, it may widen considerably during the immediate postoperative period because of edema. Such widening may become permanent. Thus, intentional control of alar width is routinely used during maxillary surgery, except when very narrow alar bases exist preoperatively.

If some narrowing of the original alar base width is desired, the above "alar cinch" procedure is done to overcorrect the actual width as much as possible. When the *primary* objective is to narrow very wide alar bases significantly, an external alar rim excisional approach must be considered.

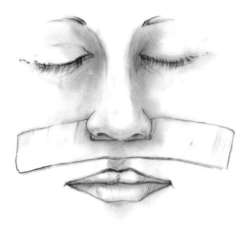

FIG. 7-43

An external support tape dressing is routinely placed and left for 2 to 3 days to reduce edema. The tape is made to hold firmly by coating the skin with tincture of benzoin. The dressing is replaced if it becomes soiled. In addition, the cheeks are routinely taped from the region of the lower eyelids to the inferior mandibular borders with 1/2-in. paper tape. These dressings are left in place for 48 hours, and the patient is instructed to remove them after soaking them in the shower.

When the alar base width is prevented from widening by this technique, the upper lip length is essentially unchanged from its preoperative to postoperative state. This is an important consideration in treatment planning with regard to the precise magnitude of the superior repositioning of the maxilla.

UPPER LIP FULLNESS

When total maxillary repositioning is done and the conventional circumvestibular incision is closed by suturing only the mucosa, the upper lip predictably thins anteroposteriorly. This may be a desirable result in certain individuals with excessively full or thick lips. However, in others it is undesirable. When no thinning of the upper lip is desired, a two-layered closure, periosteum and mucosa, is performed.

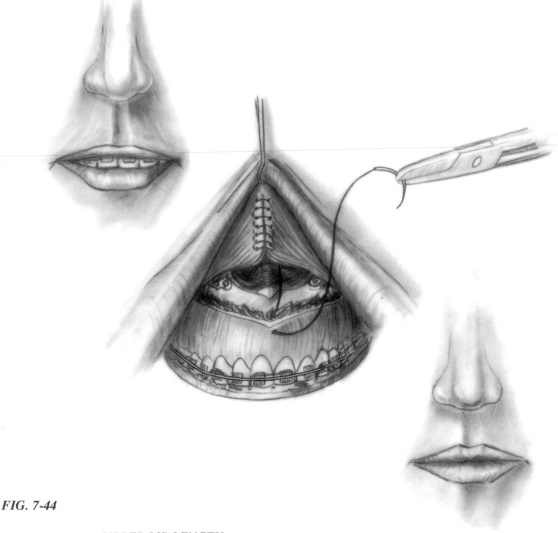

FIG. 7-44

UPPER LIP LENGTH

When both an increase in length and prevention of thinning are desired, the periosteum is first sutured in the routine manner and the mucosa is then closed using the V-Y advancement principle.

More commonly, especially in individuals with vertical maxillary excess, the appearance of the upper lip vermilion is somewhat diminutive or "gull-winged": (1) A concave appearance of the inferior aspect of the lip vermilion from commissure to commissure, (2) the absence of a philtral tubercle, and (3) a decreased exposure of the lip vermilion laterally. When this characteristic appearance of the upper lip exists in individuals for whom superior repositioning of the maxilla is to be done, routine horizontal closure of the maxillary vestibular incision often worsens upper lip appearance by accentuating the gull-winged appearance and further reducing the already inadequate exposure of the vermilion.

Whenever it is desired to increase the upper lip vermilion exposure, closure of the vestibular mucosal incision by using the V-Y advancement principle is indicated. The mucosa of the lip must be rather extensively undermined to increase the vermilion exposure. Such undermining must extend almost to the wet line anteriorly and a comparable distance posteriorly. In addition, the incision must be closed with a 15- to 25-mm vertical line to increase vermilion exposure. (Maintenance of vermilion exposure is achieved with a 10- to 15-mm vertical line.) This closure improves all aspects of the gull-winged upper lip and makes it appear more normal. This procedure will actually lengthen the *midportion* of the upper lip 1 to 2 mm and must therefore be taken into consideration in treatment planning for maxillary superior repositioning.

BUCCAL LIPECTOMY

Buccal lipectomy may be used as an isolated procedure but is more often performed in conjunction with orthognathic surgical procedures. The primary indication for cosmetic buccal lipectomy is clinical evidence of buccal lipomatosis with lack of cheek definition. In patients with buccal lipomatosis, reduced cheek prominence is not secondary to actual absence of the malar eminence, but due to the confluence of the malar eminence with the inferior border of the mandible as a result of a relatively large buccal process of the buccal fat pad. For example, the eminence of the cheek from a frontal prospective is in a relatively normal location in relation to the lateral canthus (1 cm lateral, and 1.5 cm inferior, see Fig. 1-5). In spite of this normal position, the malar eminence lacks definition.

Patients with vertical maxillary excess who have buccal lipomatosis and are undergoing a superior maxillary repositioning will predictably have this cheek fullness worsen. In such cases, the body and buccal process of the buccal fat pad can be removed through the same incision made to accomplish the maxillary surgery.

SURGICAL ANATOMY OF THE BUCCAL FAT PAD. Classically the buccal fat pad has been described as consisting of a body and four processes—buccal, temporal, pterygopalatine, and pterygoid. Since only the body and buccal process of the buccal fat pad are removed during cosmetic buccal lipectomy, only the anatomy of these two processes are described.

In the adult, the body or main mass of the buccal fat pad rests directly on the maxillary periosteum of the tuberosity region and is superior to the maxillary insertion of the buccinator muscle. The only vital structures found in the mass of the body is the buccal nerve, a sensory branch of V3.

The buccal process of the buccal fat pad is located at the anterior border of the masseter muscle deep to the superficial musculoaponeurotic system, and is covered with a thick fibrous connective-tissue capsule. When the buccal process is exposed from the intraoral approach, it can be easily separated from the surrounding capsule. No vessels or nerves can be seen within the buccal process of the buccal fat pad.

SURGICAL TECHNIQUE. The traditional approach for cosmetic buccal lipectomy has been through a transoral incision in the region of the first molar or zygomatic alveolar crest from the depth of the maxillary vestibule down to the region of the attached gingiva. However, when performing buccal lipectomy simultaneously with maxillary orthognathic surgery, the lipectomy is easily done after the maxillary surgery is completed by either sharp or blunt dissection through the periosteum and buccinator muscle in the region just posterior to the zygomatic buttress.

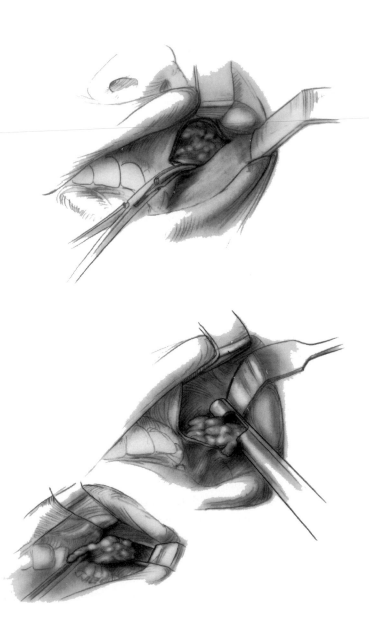

FIG. 7-45

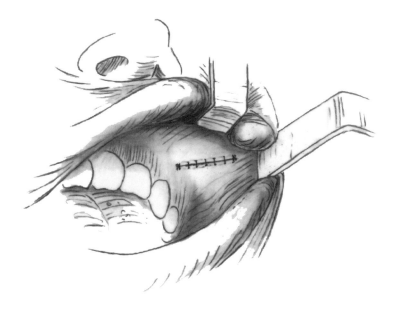

FIG. 7-45, cont'd

Only the buccal fat pad body and buccal process are removed using a combination of suction extirpation and forcep delivery (Fig. 7-45).

When the body and buccal processes of the buccal fat pad are carefully extirpated by suction and forcep technique, there will be no perforation of the lateral capsule of the buccal fat pad, and therefore, no damage to the overlying facial nerve. After the buccal fat pad is extirpated, a pressure dressing—three cotton rolls overlaid with paper tape—is placed on the patient's face just beneath the zygomatic arch. This dressing obliterates the potential dead space created by the fat removal and prevents hematoma and seroma formation that would decrease the definition between the bony malar eminence and the inferior aspect of the cheek.

The results of buccal lipectomy are not as dramatic as those of a number of other cosmetic maxillofacial procedures, and therefore patient expectations of this procedure must be realistic. The patient must clearly understand that when this cosmetic procedure is done in conjunction with maxillary superior repositioning its primary purpose is *to prevent untoward changes* in cheek cosmetics that would predictably have occurred. When this cosmetic procedure is properly performed it will create several generally desirable facial changes. The most obvious of these changes are an increase in cheek bone definition and a decrease in the "roundness" of the face. The patient in Fig. 7-46 illustrates these improvements.

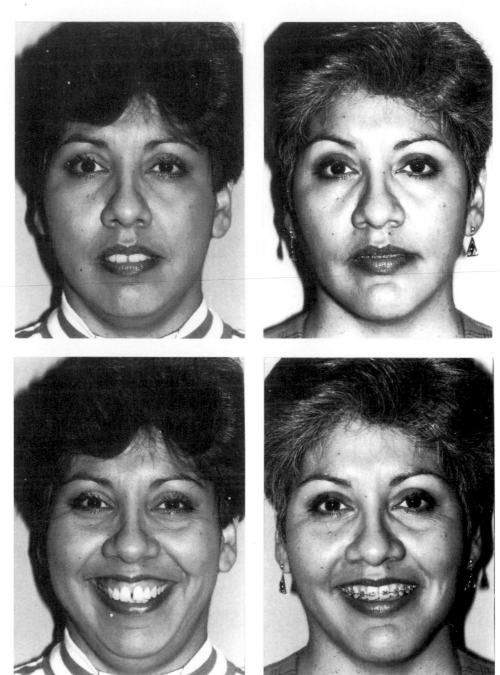

FIG. 7-46

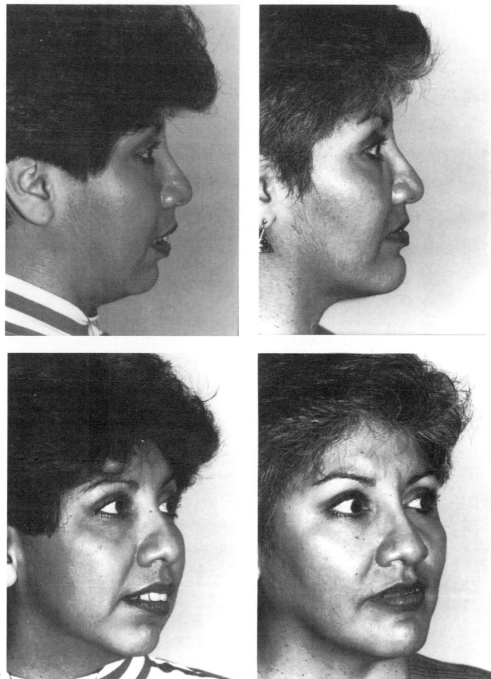

FIG. 7-46, cont'd

Postsurgical orthodontic treatment

When no segmentalization of the maxilla was done, the patient is seen within 48 hours after release from the surgeon's care. (This is generally after removal of the splint, if used, and reestablishment of normal asymptomatic jaw function.) At this time the appliances are checked for damage and repaired as necessary, archwires are checked for coordination and adjusted if necessary, and appropriate elastic therapy is begun as if no surgery had been done. Photographs of the patient's occlusion are routinely made at this and subsequent appointments to record objectively the progress being made. In any instance when progress is not as expected, these photographs help to document the problem. The patient is seen again in 2 to 3 days.

The second appointment is to check the adjustments made previously and to review the elastic therapy, changing it if necessary. Future appointments are at 1 week and 2 weeks. The usual 4-week intervals are then resumed. The usual adjustments are made in the archwires and elastic wear until the desired occlusal result is achieved, at which time the appliances are removed and retainers are placed in the usual manner.

With the exception of the frequency of appointments immediately following the resumption of orthodontic treatment, there are no special considerations in the postsurgical phase of treatment. Indeed, any and all procedures are implemented that are used to "finish" the occlusion of the nonsurgical patient.

When the maxilla has been expanded, the patient is ideally seen the same day the splint is removed; the maxillary segmental archwires are replaced at the first appointment with a continuous, coordinated archwire with loops between the central incisors if necessary; the maxillary central incisors are ligated together; and a removable lingual arch is placed to maintain any surgically achieved expansion. Movement of any segment stabilized at surgery by rigid fixation (plates & screws) cannot be produced by orthodontic means. Rather, the teeth within the segment are moved in the usual manner. This is in direct contrast to the segments not so stabilized, wherein movement of the entire segment may be produced by orthodontic forces. This movement of entire segments may be extremely rapid so that great care must be exercised in forming the archwires to produce exactly the desired movements. Segmentalization is discussed in more detail in Chapter 9.

If the occlusion is not rapidly and predictably perfected during the postsurgical phase of treatment, new records are obtained and compared with those made after surgery. A diagnosis of the specific cause of the problem is made and appropriate therapy is then done to correct it (Chapter 5).

Factors affecting stability of treatment
Orthodontic factors

The following specific orthodontic factors may contribute to relapse in the correction of the Class II vertical maxillary excess deformity.

INAPPROPRIATE VERTICAL MECHANICS

Specifically, extrusion of anterior teeth or intrusion of posterior teeth presurgically and extrusion of anterior teeth postsurgically must be avoided. Most frequently this problem is encountered when a patient with open bite has had orthodontic treatment attempted with vertical elastics used to close the open bite. If such a patient subsequently has a surgical procedure to correct the vertical maxillary excess, the vertical correction done orthodontically is subject to relapse postsurgically, thus reopening the bite (Fig. 7-47). When such treatment has been done before surgery, postsurgical orthodontic relapse can be avoided by placing light (.012), segmental wires in both upper and lower arches to maintain alignment and rotation while allowing any vertical changes to take place before surgery. Vertical relapse is measured at each monthly appointment until no change is noted for a 2-month period. The segments can then be coordinated as necessary and the patient referred for surgery without concern of postsurgical vertical instability.

PRESURGICAL ORTHO   SURGERY   ORTHO RELAPSE AFTER SURGERY

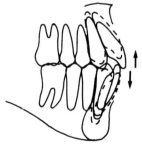

FIG. 7-47

EXPANSION OF THE MAXILLA

When vertical maxillary excess is to be corrected in the adult by either a LeFort I or total subapical surgery in the maxilla, presurgical orthodontic maxillary expansion is contraindicated. Any relapse of such expansion will produce a cusp-to-cusp occlusion posteriorly and such cuspal interferences will frequently open the bite anteriorly by causing a downward and backward rotation of the mandible (Fig. 7-48). When maxillary expansion is desirable, as it frequently is, it can most simply and stably be done as part of the surgery.

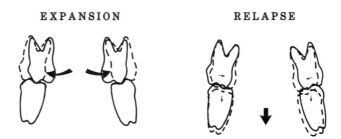

EXPANSION   **RELAPSE**

FIG. 7-48

Surgical factors

Two primary surgical factors have been identified as directly contributing to relapse after superior maxillary respositioning. These are (1) condylar distraction, resulting from improper repositioning of the maxilla and (2) poor bone contact. The former generally results in an acute Class II open-bite "relapse" after removal of fixation. The later results in relatively slow superior relapse and unesthetic "hidden" upper anterior teeth.

CONDYLAR DISTRACTION

Condylar distraction is the result either of errors in treatment planning or technical errors at the time of surgery.

When either the preoperative records are not taken in true centric and/or the reference marks from the cephalometric prediction tracing and definitive model surgery are not accurately transferred to the patient at the time of surgery, relapse can occur secondary to imprecise repositioning of the maxilla. If the patient's treatment is planned using an inaccurate (habitual) centric relation and the surgery is executed precisely as planned, the condyles will be distracted by the amount of error in the centric relation. This emphasizes the need for using cephalometric radiographs taken in true centric and models accurately mounted on a hinge-axis articulator. In addition, accurately transferring *meaningful* reference marks from the treatment planning to the patient is essential to avoid inaccurate maxillary positioning at surgery.

Whenever the maxilla is improperly placed at surgery, relapse will occur. When no intermaxillary fixation is used relapse is noted soon postoperatively. When dental intermaxillary fixation is used, skeletal relapse will occur during the period of intermaxillary fixation with accompanying extrusion and tipping of the teeth and will be noted as occlusal changes after release of intermaxillary fixation. When skeletal intermaxillary fixation is used, skeletal relapse will occur after release of fixation. If the condyles are distracted primarily inferiorly, relapse will produce a Class I anterior open bite. When the condylar distraction is both downward and forward, the relapse will produce a Class II open bite. If the condyles are forced posteriorly (rarely) there is a tendency for a Class III occlusion postsurgically.

In nearly all Class II vertical maxillary excess patients, straight superior maxillary repositioning with autorotation of the mandible is usually not sufficient to produce correction of the Class II occlusion. Rather, the maxilla is repositioned both superiorly and posteriorly. If insufficient bone is removed at the posterosuperior aspect of the maxilla, the maxilla this excess posterior bone. Thus, the mandibular condyles are distracted from their fossas as the suspension wires are tightened. This is avoided at surgery by following the sequence of locating and removing any posterior interferences *before* applying the fixation.

POOR BONE CONTACT

When the LeFort I ostectomy is used to reposition the maxilla superiorly, lack of adequate bone contact will result in superior relapse of the maxilla. This may be clinically insignificant if it is 1 or 2 mm, yet it can result in so much unplanned superior movement of the maxilla that the maxillary anterior teeth are ultimately located above the lip embrasure. This results in the patient experiencing an unesthetic edentulous appearance. In addition, lack of adequate bone contact may produce an unstable maxilla due to a nonunion or fibrous union and may result in the inability of the patient to masticate. Both problems occur primarily because little or no bone contact exists when the maxilla is moved superiorly by a LeFort I ostectomy and the lateral maxillary walls are atypical of vertical maxillary excess (that is, more horizontal in nature) (Fig. 7-49). If and when this occurs at the time of surgery four bone plates and possibly even bone grafting must be used to prevent this serious problem.

LEFORT I: **SUPERIOR REPOSITIONING**

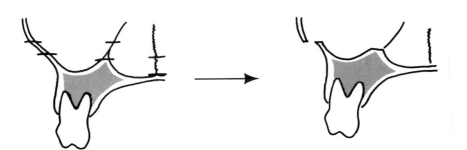

FIG. 7-49

The existence of atypical vertical maxillary excess can be recognized presurgically by careful palpation of the lateral maxillary walls and evaluation of presurgical posteroanterior cephalometric radiographs. Once diagnosed, the problem is avoided by (1) performing the actual ostectomies *after* mobilization and attempted repositioning, (2) using the total subapical maxillary procedure, or (3) using four miniplates and placing a bone graft.

Age-related factors

The age at which the maxilla can be successfully superiorly repositioned is a question that has been widely and somewhat emotionally debated, with many authorities thinking that this surgery is best delayed until all growth is completed. This view is not supported by our studies and long-term experience. Indeed, it is possible successfully and stably reposition the maxilla superiorly once the maxillary canines and second molars are sufficiently erupted to allow the surgery to be done (usually between the ages of 12 and 14 years).

To address the relationships of age, growth, and stability, two essential questions must be answered. First, what effect will maxillary superior repositioning have on the subsequent growth? Second, what effect will this subsequent growth have on the result attained by the surgery?

EFFECT OF MAXILLARY SUPERIOR REPOSITIONING ON SUBSEQUENT FACIAL GROWTH

Considerable concern has been expressed about possible untoward effects of early maxillary surgery on subsequent maxillary growth. Indeed, rather extensive clinical and research literature document that early surgical resection of the nasal septum in animals can adversely influence subsequent maxillary growth. Detailed experimental work in primates reveals that while septal resection does influence the growth of the face, the effects depend on the amount of septum resected and the age at which resection occurs. Indeed, some cartilaginous nasal septal resection can be accomplished without producing undesirable growth effects. Therefore, when considering superior repositioning of the maxilla during growth, the surgeon must consider performing the total subapical repositioning procedure (see Chapter 9), since this procedure involves minimal surgery on the nasal septum.

The growth in animals and humans following isolated superior repositioning of the maxilla has been studied. Observations reveal that continued growth is expressed in the normal downward and forward direction for both maxilla and mandible. In animals, less vertical maxillary growth occurs than occurred in control animals. In patients with Class II vertical maxillary excess dentofacial deformity the vector of growth is more favorable—less vertical maxillary growth occurs—than would be predicted to occur without surgery.

EFFECT OF SUBSEQUENT GROWTH ON THE SURGICAL RESULT

Because growth was observed to be essentially normal following surgery and that there was less than normal vertical maxillary growth when these patients were operated on before completion of growth, the continued facial growth does not result in clinically significant effects on either the esthetic or occlusal result attained at surgery. During the postsurgical orthodontic treatment and retention, no more growth-related problems have been observed or occur in these patients than occur in the nonsurgically treated orthodontic population.

In summary, isolated superior maxillary repositioning during growth appears to produce a favorable effect on the subsequent vector of facial growth (relocation) and results in a stable occlusal result.

Results of treatment

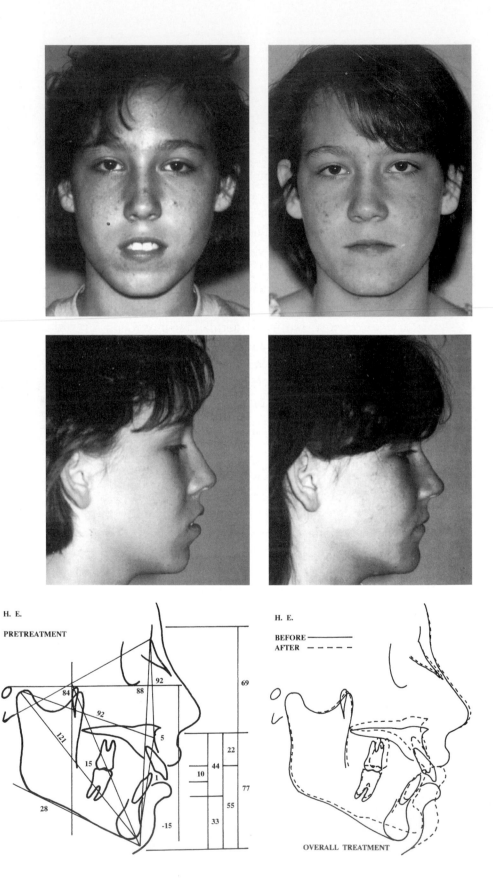

FIG. 7-50

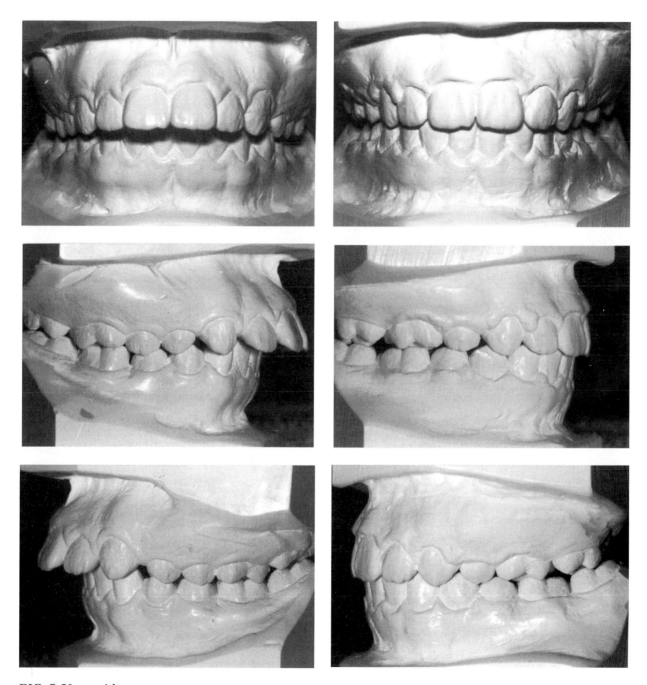

FIG. 7-50, cont'd

Alternative orthodontic-surgical approaches:
* *SEGMENTAL LE FORT I MAXILLARY SUPERIOR REPOSITIONING*
* *TOTAL SUBAPICAL MAXILLARY SUPERIOR REPOSITIONING*
* *SEGMENTAL TOTAL SUBAPICAL MAXILLARY SUPERIOR REPOSITIONING*

Contingency statement

The three alternative surgical approaches listed here are all valuable methods of superiorly repositioning the maxilla. The total subapical procedure (whole arch) is least used due to technical difficulty and rarity of indication. Perhaps its only indication is to avoid compromising the nasal airway (turbinates) when superior movement over 6 mm is desired and then only when there is no open bite due to a dual occlusal plane and no accompanying transverse discrepancy (cross bite). Fortunately, the larger the superior movement, the less technically difficult is this operation. The more superior movement desired, the larger is the size of the buccal "windows" through which the palatal ostectomies are accomplished. The whole-arch total subapical surgical procedure is not discussed in this book. Rather, the more useful segmental modification is described in Chapter 9.

Segmental treatment of the maxilla may be indicated to correct simultaneously arch shape and size (transverse deformity), dentoalveolar protrusion (anteroposterior deformity), arch symmetry, missing maxillary teeth, and open bite (vertical deformity). Again, the total subapical procedure is primarily useful when the superior repositioning is to be 6 mm or more, more than 5 mm of expansion is anticipated, and/or significant movement of several segments is to be done. Since both the LeFort I and total subapical segmental techniques for superiorly repositioning the maxilla are most commonly used in conjunction with correction of an open bite, the reader is directed to Chapter 9 for detailed discussions of these techniques.

REFERENCES

Bishara, S.E., Chu, G.W., and Jakobsen, J.R.: Stability of the LeFort I one-piece maxillary osteotomy, Am. J. Orthodont. Dentofac. Orthop. **94**(3):184, 1988.

Bjork, A: Skieller, V.: Growth in width of the maxilla studied by the implant method, Scand. J. Plast. Reconstr. Surg. 8:26–33, 1974.

Collins, P., and Epker, B.N.: Alar base cinch: a technique for prevention of alar base flaring secondary to maxillary surgery, Oral Surg. **53**:549, 1982.

Epker, B.N., and Schendel, S.A.: Total maxillary surgery, Int. J. Oral Surg. **9**:1, 1980.

Epker, B.N., Schendel, S.A., and Washburn, M.: Effects of early surgical superior repositioning of the maxilla on subsequent growth. III. Biomechanical considerations. In McNamara, J., Carlson, D., and Ribbens, K., editors: The effects of surgical intervention on craniofacial growth, monograph no. 12, Ann Arbor, MI, 1982, Center for Human Growth and Development, University of Michigan.

Epker, B.N.: Superior surgical repositioning of the maxilla: long-term results, J. Maxillofac. Surg. **9**:199, 1981.

Fish, L.C., Wolford, L.M., and Epker, B.N.: Surgical-orthodontic correction of vertical maxillary excess, Am. J. Orthodont. **73**:241, 1978.

Herbosa, E.G., Rotskoff, K.S., Ramos, B.F., and Ambrookian, H.S.: Condylar position in superior maxillary repositioning and its effect on the temporomandibular joint, J. Oral Maxillofac. Surg. **48**(7):690, 1990.

Lanigan, D.T., Hey, J.H., and West, R.A.: Aseptic necrosis following maxillary osteotomies: report of 36 cases, J. Oral Maxillofac. Surg. **48**(2):142, 1990.

Nanda, R., et al.: Effect of maxillary osteotomy on subsequent craniofacial growth in adolescent monkeys, Am. J. Orthodont. **83**:391, 1983.

Nanda, R., et al.: Mandibular adaptations following total maxillary osteotomy in adolescent monkeys, Am. J. Orthodont. **83**:485, 1983.

Newman, J.: Re: buccal fat pad excision: aesthetic improvement of the midface, Ann. Plast. Surg. **28**(5):502, 1992.

O'Reilly, M.T.: A longitudinal growth study: maxillary length at puberty in females, Angle Orthodont. **49**:234, 1979.

O'Ryan, F., and Epker, B.N.: Surgical-orthodontics and the temporomandibular joint. I. Superior repositioning of the maxilla, Am. J. Orthodont. **83**:407, 1983.

Profitt, W.R., Phillips, C., and Turvery, T.A.: Stability following superior repositioning of the maxilla by LeFort I osteotomy, Am. J. Orthodont. Dentofac. Orthop. **92**(2):151, 1987.

Sarver, D.M., and Weissman, S.M.: Long-term soft tissue response to LeFort I maxillary superior repositioning, Angle Orthodont. **61**(4):267, 1991.

Sassouni, V., and Nanda, S.: Analysis of dentofacial vertical proportions, Am. J. Orthodont. **50**:801, 1964.

Savara, B.S., and Singh, I.J.: Norms of size and annual increments of seven anatomical measures of maxillae in boys from three to sixteen years of age, The Angle Orthodontist, **38**:104–20, 1968.

Schendel, S., et al.: The long face syndrome: vertical maxillary excess, Am. J. Orthodont. **70**:398, 1976.

Schendel, S.A., et al.: Superior repositioning of the maxilla: stability and soft tissue osseous relations, Am. J. Orthodont. **70:**663, 1976.

Seal, W.M.: Facial growth changes from 8 to 18 years, Master's Thesis, University of Washington School of Dentistry, Seattle, Washington, 1957.

Siegel, M.L.: Mechanisms of early maxillary growth: implications for surgery; J. Oral Surg. **34:**106, 1976.

Sillman, J.H.: Dimensional changes of the dental arches: longitudinal study from birth to 25 years, Am. J. Orthodontics 50:824–42, 1964.

Singh, I.J., and Savara, B.S.: Norms of size and annual increments of seven anatomical measures of maxillae in girls from three to sixteen years of age, The Angle Orthodontist, **36:**312–24, 1968.

Walker, G.F.: Prediction and simulation of craniofacial growth, Biometrics Laboratory, Dental Research Institute, Ann Arbor, Michigan, 1975.

Wertz, R., and Dreskin, M.: Midpalatal suture opening, a normative study, Am. J. Orthodont. **71:**367, 1977.

Wessberg, G.A., et al.: Autorotation of the mandible: effect of surgical superior repositioning of the maxilla on mandibular resting posture, Am. J. Orthodont. **82:**465, 1982.

Wessberg, G.A., et al.: Neuromuscular adaptation to surgical superior repositioning of the maxilla, J. Oral Maxillofac. Surg. **9:**73, 1981.

CHAPTER 8   *Class II dentofacial deformities secondary to vertical maxillary excess and mandibular deficiency*

Introduction

With proper treatment planning and presurgical orthodontic treatment, isolated superior maxillary repositioning, with or without advancement genioplasty, is possible in a majority of patients with Class II vertical maxillary excess. However, isolated maxillary superior repositioning is *not* the preferred treatment in some Class II vertical maxillary excess dentofacial deformities. *When the facial esthetics are such that the maxilla must be moved superiorly and anteriorly— a downturned nasal tip, a large nose relative to other midface structures, retrusive upper lip, an obtuse nasolabial angle, and/or recessive paranasal areas—simultaneous mandibular advancement is indicated.* This determination is made by careful study of both the facial esthetics and cephalometric prediction tracings. The decision to simultaneously advance the mandible with maxillary superior repositioning *is independent of chin position.* Inadequate chin projection is most simply corrected by advancement genioplasty.

A cephalometric prediction tracing in which the maxilla is repositioned and the mandible is autorotated (with or without genioplasty) is always done first for all patients for whom treatment is planned for correction of a Class II vertical maxillary excess dentofacial deformity. This permits an accurate assessment of both the amount of the posteroanterior movement of the maxilla that would occur with single-jaw surgery and the esthetic effects of this maxillary movement. This cephalometric prediction tracing may demonstrate that it is necessary to move the maxilla excessively posteriorly, creating unesthetic changes in the nose, upper lip, and paranasal area. When this is true, simultaneous mandibular advancement is indicated with superior and/or anterior repositioning of the maxilla. This specific patient population is discussed in this chapter.

The usual orthodontic-surgical approach:

SUPERIOR REPOSITIONING OF THE MAXILLA WITH MANDIBULAR ADVANCEMENT

Outline of treatment

Presurgical orthodontic treatment

1. Place appliances
2. Align and level lower arch with or without extractions; align and level upper arch or segments
3. Elastics as necessary to place the lower incisors in their proper position
4. Coordinate arches or segments
5. Impressions for feasibility model surgery

Immediate presurgical planning

1. Surgical cephalometric prediction tracing
2. Model surgery
3. Splint construction

Orthognathic reconstructive surgery

1. LeFort I ostectomy with superior-anterior repositioning
2. Bilateral sagittal split ramus osteotomy with advancement
3. Advancement genioplasty (optional)

Postsurgical orthodontic treatment

1. Check appliances; repair as necessary
2. Continuous, coordinated archwires; stabilizing lingual arch
3. Elastics as necessary
4. Routine in finishing procedures
5. Retain

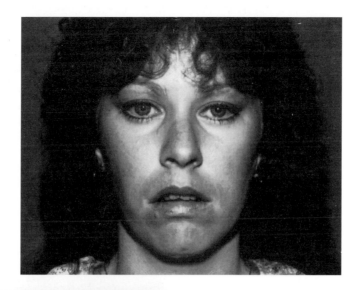

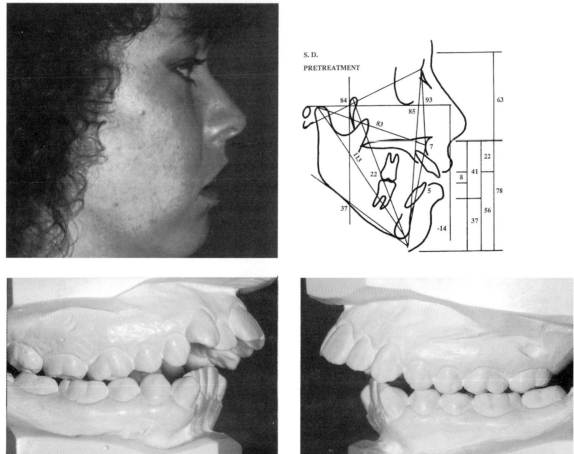

FIG. 8-1

Details of treatment
Presurgical orthodontic treatment

The presurgical orthodontic treatment can greatly affect the surgical result. The possibilities are too numerous to mention; however, the following general principle must be understood. The more the lower dentition is retracted, the further the maxilla will need to be posteriorly repositioned at surgery to correct the Class II relation. Thus, in some instances the need for two-jaw surgery may be avoided by leaving the lower teeth more protrusive and adding a larger genioplasty. Figure 8-2 illustrates this principle. Certainly, there are limitations to this approach. Nevertheless, before electing to do simultaneous mandibular advancement, this possibility should be considered.

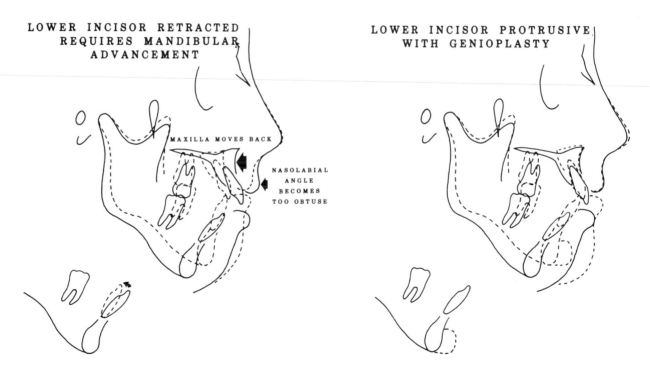

FIG. 8-2

When simultaneous maxillary superior repositioning and mandibular advancement are to be done, the presurgical orthodontic treatment is done as described for when only the maxilla is to be moved superiorly. A carefully done cephalometric prediction tracing is necessary to determine the effect of autorotation and the amount of mandibular advancement desired (Chapter 2). Once these factors are known, a decision regarding extractions and anchorage requirements in the lower arch can be made and treatment instituted to produce the desired changes in the lower arch. There are no anchorage considerations in the upper arch since it will be aligned, leveled, and coordinated with the lower arch either as a whole arch or segmentally, and surgery will place the arch or segments into the desired position.

The need to segmentalize the maxillary arch is primarily predicated on vertical and transverse considerations. When maxillary expansion is necessary beyond that which is predictably and stably achieved by orthodontic means alone— 2 mm bodily movement or uprighting lingually tipped teeth—segmentalization with surgical expansion is the method of choice. When an open bite exists due to an excessive maxillary curve of Spee (dual plane of occlusion) such that orthodontic leveling of the upper arch would require extrusion of the anterior teeth, segmentalization with surgical leveling of the plane of occlusion is again the method of choice.

There is more room for error in the presurgical orthodontic treatment when simultaneous mandibular surgery is to be done (perhaps one reason for its great popularity), since the anteroposterior position of the lower dentition no longer dictates the ultimate anteroposterior position of the upper teeth. Excess anchorage loss can be rectified by decreasing the amount of mandibular advancement and adding a genioplasty, or making one already planned larger, to produce more chin projection. However, lower arch symmetry, width, and form are still critical to the overall result. If the lower teeth are asymmetrically placed in a symmetric mandible, either the mandible may be asymmetrically advanced to straighten the dental midlines and the chin point will become asymmetric, or the mandible may be symmetrically advanced and the dental midlines will remain asymmetric. In addition, if the lower arch width and form are not carefully controlled, the long-term stability may be compromised.

When an open bite exists before treatment it is important to avoid bite-closing mechanics during the presurgical orthodontic treatment. Indeed, it is preferable actually to open the bite more before surgery. When this occurs it is considered positive, since any orthodontic relapse will help to maintain the bite closed after treatment. When the open bite is observed to have become less severe during the presurgical orthodontic treatment, it is important to determine why this occurred and carefully to assess the potential stability of such before surgery (see Chapter 9).

With the aforementioned principles in mind, see Chapter 7 for a detailed description of the presurgical orthodontic treatment wherein the maxilla is not segmentalized, or Chapter 9 for a discussion of the presurgical orthodontic treatment for the patient wherein the maxilla is to be segmentalized.

Immediate presurgical planning

SURGICAL CEPHALOMETRIC PREDICTION TRACING FOR
SIMULTANEOUS SUPERIOR MAXILLARY REPOSITIONING AND
MANDIBULAR ADVANCEMENT

Unlike the combined orthodontic-surgical prediction tracings discussed in Chapter 2, the surgeon is bound by the position of the teeth that has been produced by the presurgical orthodontic treatment. As such, the surgical cephalometric prediction tracings are more simply and directly done. These prediction tracings provide much of the essential information required to perform the surgery properly. Furthermore, by superimposing the prediction tracing on the cephalometric radiograph obtained immediately following surgery the accuracy of the surgical changes can be studied. Significant discrepancies between the predicted and actual result may warrant additional surgical intervention before the patient leaves the hospital (Chapter 5).

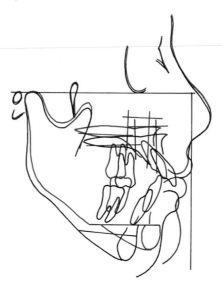

FIG. 8-3

A completed surgical cephalometric prediction tracing illustrating isolated maxillary superior repositioning with mandibular autorotation is shown in Fig. 8-3 for the patient presented herein. The resulting unfavorable skeletal and soft-tissue changes that would occur with isolated superior maxillary repositioning are thus illustrated. With isolated maxillary superior repositioning it is necessary to reposition the maxilla 4 to 6 mm posteriorly to correct the Class II occlusion. Doing so will clearly worsen the facial esthetics by making the nose appear larger, increasing the already obtuse nasolabial angle, and making the paranasal area even flatter. (*Note*: Chin projection is *not* a consideration, as it is easily normalized in this prediction by addition of a genioplasty of average size.)

Careful study of the movement of the *maxilla* in the above prediction makes clear the need for simultaneous mobilization of both maxilla and mandible for this patient. The method of producing the surgical prediction for simultaneous maxillary superior repositioning and mandibular advancement and of obtaining meaningful information therefrom is described in the following paragraphs.

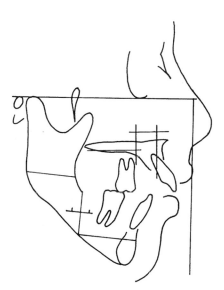

FIG. 8-4

Cephalometric prediction tracing for simultaneous maxillary superior repositioning and mandibular advancement is a combination of those procedures previously described in Chapters 6 and 7. All usual structures are traced from the presurgical cephalometric radiograph. The reference lines described in Chapter 7 for maxillary superior repositioning are constructed on this tracing. The reference lines and marks described in Chapter 6 for mandibular advancement are also constructed on this tracing. Additionally, since a genioplasty is most often indicated, the horizontal reference for this osteotomy is included at this time. This is called *tracing* (black line).

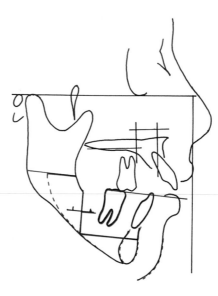

FIG. 8-5

The ***prediction*** (red line) is begun by tracing the distal mandible, mandibular teeth, and associated reference lines on a new piece of acetate overlaid on the ***tracing***. (Note: in all instances when lines are being traced from the ***tracing*** to the ***prediction***, superimpositions are shown slightly offset to better show which lines are being traced.) The mandibular functional occlusal plane is constructed and extended far enough anteriorly that its relation to the upper lip can be clearly established. The condyle is referenced (the authors prefer light dots that are easily erased or ignored later) to serve as the center of rotation for the superior repositioning of the functional occlusal plane. The bony chin below the genioplasty line and the soft-tissue chin are traced with dashed lines at this time as a genioplasty is frequently required.

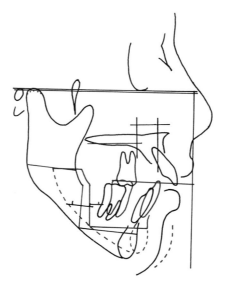

FIG. 8-6

The **prediction** is rotated counterclockwise with the condyle as the center of rotation until the mandibular functional occlusal plane lies 1 to 2 mm below the upper lip on the **tracing**.* Only the Frankfort horizontal plane is traced onto the **prediction** while this superimposition is held. The desired vertical position of the dentition (occlusal plane) has now been established.

---

*In rare instances this rotation may produce an unfavorable angulation of the occlusal plane relative to Frankfort horizontal—angled upward anteriorly rather then downward. If this occurs, the authors suggest that the rotation be disregarded, the original angulation of the occlusal plane be maintained, and the distal segment of the mandible be moved superiorly, without rotation, until the occlusal plane lies in its ideal vertical position relative to the upper lip.

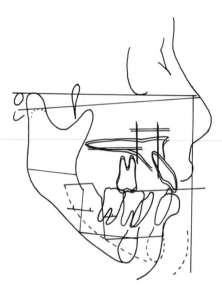

FIG. 8-7

The ***prediction*** is repositioned on the ***tracing*** until the maxillary teeth of the ***tracing*** are placed in their ideal relation to the mandibular teeth and the occlusal plane of the ***prediction***. The maxilla, maxillary teeth, and maxillary reference lines are traced onto the ***prediction*** while holding this superimposition. (If segmental maxillary surgery is planned to level the maxillary occlusal plane, the anterior portion of the maxilla and its associated reference lines are traced first, followed by repositioning the ***prediction*** on the ***tracing*** to trace the posterior maxilla and its associated reference lines (see Chapter 7).

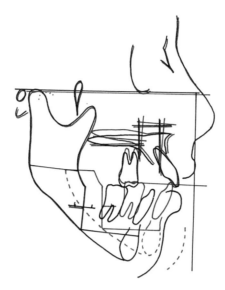

FIG. 8-8

The ***prediction*** is now superimposed on the ***tracing*** on Frankfort horizontal. While keeping Frankfort horizontal superimposed, the ***prediction*** is moved forward (or backward) until the maxilla is in its optimal anteroposterior position. This is predicted primarily on facial esthetics—nasal prominence, paranasal configuration, alar base anatomy, upper lip drape (nasolabial angle), and upper lip position. The amount of anterior maxillary repositioning is based on the amount of change desired in the aforementioned structures and is determined by observing the anterior movement of both the incisor edge and the anterior maxilla. The soft tissues advance approximately half of the underlying dentoskeletal advancement; subnasale and the nasal tip are less affected. Once the desired anteroposterior changes are produced by repositioning the ***prediction***, this superimposition is maintained while the "stable" structures and their associated reference marks are traced onto the ***prediction***. The skeletal reference lines are essential because they determine the specific size of the lateral maxillary ostectomies (horizontal references) and the amount of anteroposterior repositioning (vertical references). By duplicating the changes in these references at the time of surgery, the surgeon can precisely duplicate the predicted objectives.

After tracing the above structures and while holding this superimposition, the projection of the soft-tissue chin is studied relative to the subnasale perpendicular line on the original ***tracing***. So doing allows determination of the need for and, if necessary, the amount of a genioplasty. In the rare instances when the maxilla is advanced sufficiently to effect a *significant* change in subnasale (approximately 1 mm of advancement of subnasale for every 3 to 4 mm of advancement of the anterior nasal spine), one may wish to reconstruct subnasale perpendicular to account for this anticipated change before evaluating the chin projection. When a genioplasty is required, it is added to the ***prediction*** as described in Chapter 6.

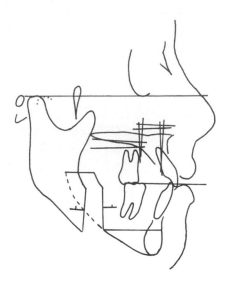

FIG. 8-9

The soft tissue of the nose, upper lip, and lower lip are traced onto the ***prediction*** as described in detail in Chapter 2. The finished ***prediction*** is illustrated.

MODEL SURGERY FOR SUPERIOR MAXILLARY REPOSITIONING AND MANDIBULAR ADVANCEMENT

Regardless of the need to segmentalize the maxilla, model surgery for simultaneous superior repositioning of the maxilla and mandibular advancement is routinely performed on models mounted on a semiadjustable anatomic articulator by a face-bow transfer. A duplicate mandibular model is also anatomically mounted on the articulator to allow the fabrication of an intermediate splint. (The use of an intermediate splint is discussed in the next section of this chapter.)

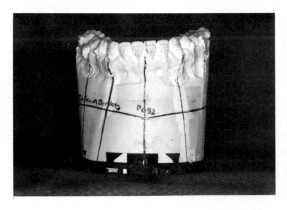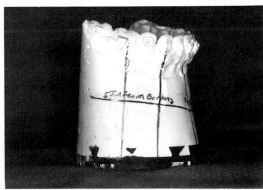

FIG. 8-10

Model mounting and marking is done as described for isolated superior repositioning of the maxilla in Chapter 7. In addition, the approximate location of the inferior border of the mandible and the approximate vertical position of pogonion is indicated on the mandibular model base from measurements made on the cephalometric radiograph.

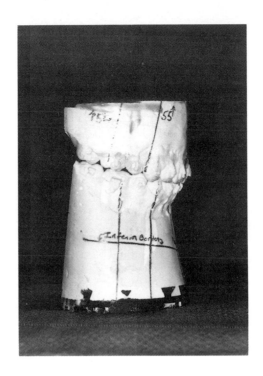

FIG. 8-11

The maxilla is removed along a line approximating the level of the inferior aspect of the planned ostectomy at surgery and if necessary, it is segmentalized as described in Chapter 9. An adequate amount of plaster is removed from the superior aspect of the base to permit the planned superior repositioning.

When the maxilla is segmentalized, the maxillary segments are placed into the best possible occlusion with the mandibular teeth and are stabilized with soft wax or a light application of sticky wax between the maxillary and mandibular teeth. (When there is no segmentalization and the entire maxillary dentition can be placed into ideal occlusion with the mandibular dentition, proceed to the next step.) Once optimal occlusion is achieved with the mandible, the segments are consolidated into a single unit with a heavy application of sticky wax. The consolidated "single-piece" maxilla is now removed from the mandibular dentition to which it was lightly attached and is ready to be placed in its desired surgical position.

SPLINT(S) CONSTRUCTION FOR SIMULTANEOUS SUPERIOR MAXILLARY
REPOSITIONING AND MANDIBULAR ADVANCEMENT

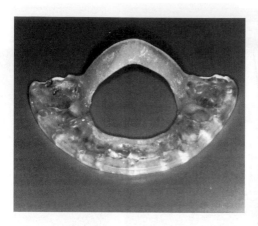
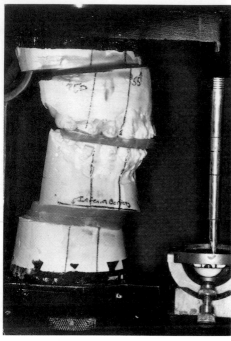

FIG. 8-14

An intermediate splint is helpful in all cases of simultaneous mobilization of the maxilla and mandible. The final surgical occlusal splint, when indicated, is constructed as described in Chapter 7. The completed model surgery and occlusal splint with a palatal bar is illustrated in Figure 8-14. Fabrication of an intermediate occlusal splint is described below.

The intermediate splint is constructed between the repositioned maxilla and the duplicated, anatomically mounted mandibular cast. It helps the surgeon to achieve the desired transverse, anteroposterior, and rotational position of the maxilla by allowing discovery and elimination of the bony interferences that prohibit obtaining the desired maxillary repositioning. *This splint provides no information regarding the proper vertical positioning of the maxilla at surgery.* The vertical position is determined by the internal and external references as discussed in Chapter 7. Once the maxilla is mobilized and placed into the splint, there exists no index with regard to the *amount* the maxillary-mandibular complex should be autorotated. Thus, *this splint is not a substitute for the definitive cephalometric prediction tracing and model surgery, as the measurements taken from these tools, especially the lateral wall reference marks, are necessary to achieve the desired result at surgery.*

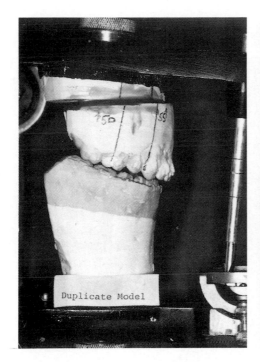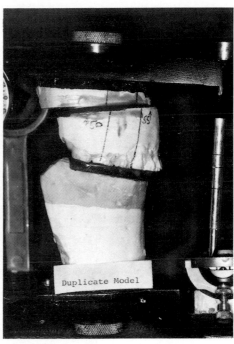

FIG. 8-15

To construct an intermediate splint, the completed maxillary model surgery is mounted opposite the duplicated, uncut, anatomically mounted mandibular model. If a final occlusal splint is not to be used at surgery, the maxillary and mandibular teeth are coated with liquid foil or petroleum jelly and the intermediate splint is fabricated directly between the models.

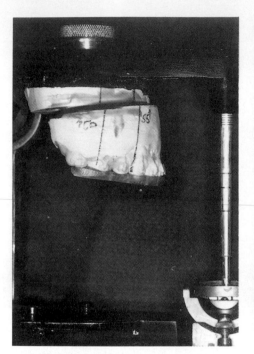 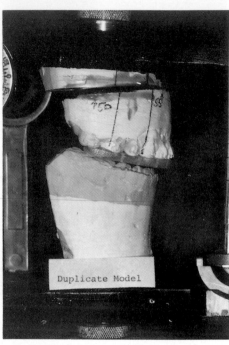

Duplicate Model

FIG. 8-16

More frequently the intermediate splint is fabricated to fit between the final occlusal splint attached to the completed maxillary model surgery and the unaltered mandible. The final occlusal splint—previously completed and polished—is lightly sticky waxed to the maxillary model. Petroleum jelly is liberally applied to the final occlusal splint to prevent its bonding to the intermediate splint during its fabrication, and liquid foil is applied to the teeth on the mandibular model.

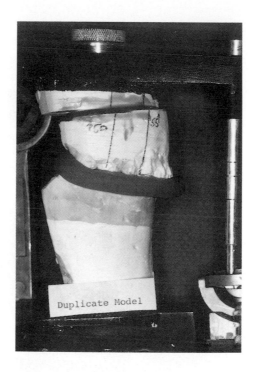

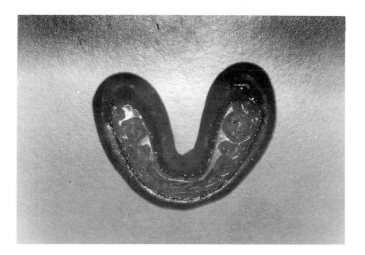

FIG. 8-17

A roll of doughy orthodontic acrylic is placed between the final occlusal splint (attached to the maxillary teeth) and the *uncut, anatomically mounted mandibular model*. The models are now gently tapped together, being careful not to lock the now-hardening intermediate splint acrylic over the final occlusal splint. Both the facial and palatal aspects of the surgical splint are repeatedly examined to prevent the two splints from becoming mechanically inseparable.

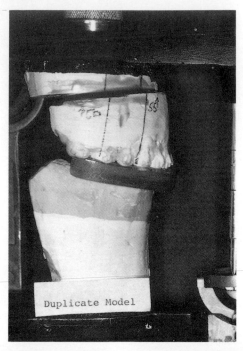

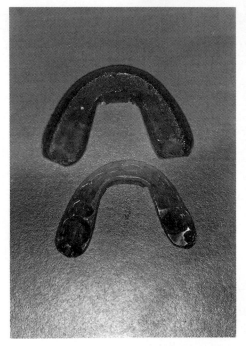
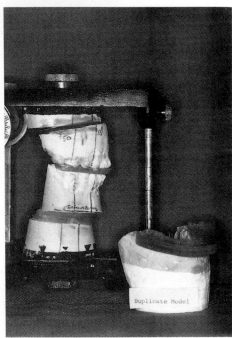

FIG. 8-18

The intermediate splint is trimmed and polished so it fits snugly to the final occlusal splint. Its use during surgery is discussed as part of the surgery sections dealing with simultaneous mobilization of both jaws throughout this book.

Orthognathic reconstructive surgery

The surgical sequence for simultaneous mobilization of the maxilla and mandible with advancement genioplasty is (1) completion of the genioplasty, (2) initiation of the bilateral sagittal ramus osteotomies *without* splitting, (3) completion of the maxillary surgery in its entirety including stabilization, and (4) completing the sagittal splits, mobilization, and mandibular stabilization. The preferred sequence is the same regardless of the method of stabilization—nonrigid or rigid fixation. This surgical sequence avoids intraoperative complications such as displacing a "stabilized" maxilla, unnecessary inferior alveolar nerve injury as a result of either distraction of the mandible or crushing the inferior alveolar neurovascular bundles within the sagittal splits during the maxillary surgery, and excessive blood loss.

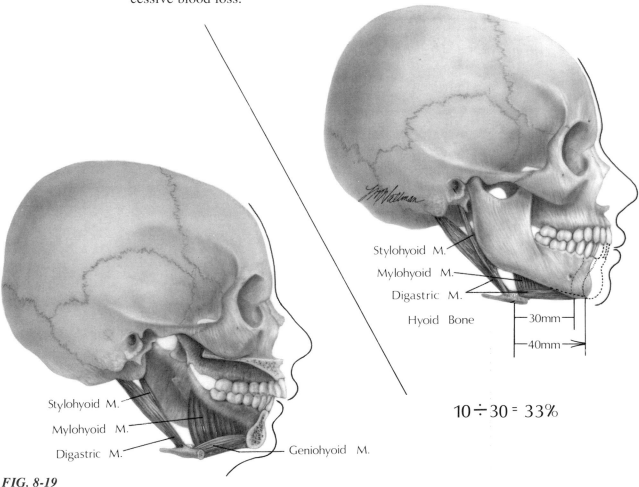

Stylohyoid M.
Mylohyoid M.
Digastric M.
Hyoid Bone

30mm
40mm

Stylohyoid M.
Mylohyoid M.
Digastric M.
Geniohyoid M.

$$10 \div 30 = 33\%$$

FIG. 8-19

The advancement genioplasty is performed to completion and the operative site is packed but not sutured (Chapter 6). This permits the surgeon to reaffirm the symmetry and magnitude of the genioplasty just prior to suturing at the end of surgery. When a suprahyoid myotomy is indicated—the sum of the mandibular advancement and genioplasty produces more than a 30% increase in the distance from the hyoid bone to the lingual aspect of the mandibular symphysis (suprahyoid muscle stretch)—it is performed as part of the advancement genioplasty (Fig. 8-19). The technique for performing suprahyoid myotomies in conjunction with a genioplasty is described in Chapter 9.

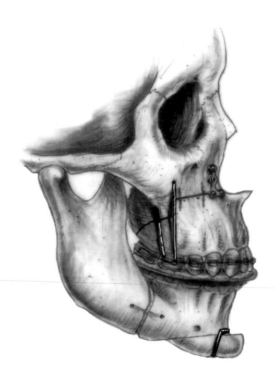

FIG. 8-22

Once the maxilla is confirmed to be in its proper position, it is secured into position with skeletal suspension wires and/or miniature bone plates. It is extremely important that the maxilla be securely held in its desired position when both jaws are mobilized. Thus, the most important factor in determining the optimal method to stabilize the maxilla is the quality of the posterior maxillary bone interfaces. When good posterior bony interfaces are present after the maxilla is repositioned as desired, two posterior suspension wires and two piriform rim plates as described in Chapter 7 are preferred, as they are easily placed and allow more rapid postsurgical orthodontic treatment. When this is not the case, four miniplates are used.

The intermediate splint is removed after the maxilla has been stabilized. Figure 8-22 illustrates this stage of surgery; the maxilla is stabilized, the final occlusal splint is wired in place, the mandibular osteotomies are made but the splits have not been completed, and the occlusion is still Class II. The mandibular sagittal splits are now completed as described in Chapter 6.

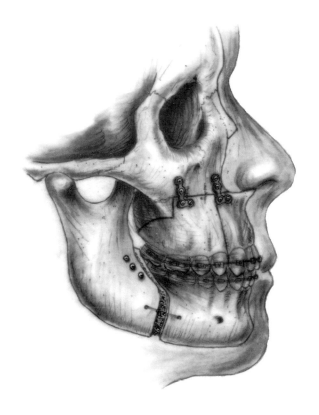

FIG. 8-23

The use of rigid fixation in the mandible is optimal when the amount of mandibular advancement is small (less than 6 mm) and there is no advancement genioplasty. If rigid fixation is to be used to secure the proximal segment to the distal segment, interdental fixation is adequate to stabilize the proximal segment during the surgical phase of screw placement. Triangular wires are placed bilaterally around the upper canines, lower canines, and first premolars to provide a tight Class I canine occlusion. The posterior is then stabilized by bilateral loops around the upper and lower first molars. These four interdental wires provide sufficient stability of the distal segment to allow the proximal segment to be rigidly secured to it by placing three screws as described in Chapter 6. After the mandible is stabilized by the screws, the interdental wires are cut and removed.

As with any rigid fixation case, the patient's diet is restricted to liquids and foods that require no chewing for 4 to 6 weeks. During this time the patient is instructed to observe their bite and, if any change occurs, they are to return immediately to the surgeon. Additionally, the surgeon sees the patient weekly to evaluate the occlusion critically. During this period selective rubber bands are used when necessary to improve the occlusion. After 4 to 6 weeks, the osteotomy and ostectomy sites are stable enough to begin deliberate temporomandibular joint rehabilitation as described in Chapter 4.

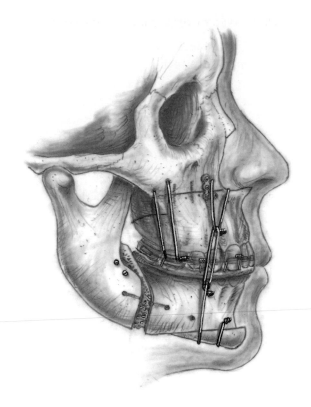

FIG. 8-24

When the advancement of the mandible is large and/or a genioplasty is performed, skeletal maxillomandibular fixation is preferred. Circummandibular wires (22-gauge) are passed bilaterally in the mandibular premolar-canine region and tightened in the interdental embrasure. Next, 22-gauge piriform rim wires are placed and twisted to form a loop in the maxillary vestibule. Intermediate 22-gauge wires are passed bilaterally beneath the circummandibular wires and through the loops in the piriform aperture wires and are then tightened. This provides excellent *skeletal maxillomandibular fixation*. The proximal segments are then stabilized using two screws as discussed in Chapter 6.

When skeletal maxillomandibular fixation is used, the patient is kept in fixation for 3 weeks. After 3 weeks, fixation is released by cutting the intermediate connecting skeletal wires and the centric relation is checked to make certain the patient bites perfectly into the occlusal splint. The splint is left wired to the maxilla. The patient is instructed in jaw exercises (physiotherapy), is not to chew any foods, and is seen again in 24 to 48 hours. (See Chapter 4 regarding the specifics of release of intermaxillary fixation jaw physiotherapy.) At this time the occlusion is checked, and progress with jaw opening is measured. If the patient bites perfectly into the occlusal splint, the same regimen is continued and the patient returns in 5 days for splint and suspension wire removal. The patient is informed that failure to maintain perfect occlusion during this interval warrants an immediate return to the surgeon. The patient is to see the orthodontist within 24 to 48 hours after splint and suspension wire removal to initiate finishing orthodontics.

Postsurgical orthodontic treatment

This patient is treated just as a patient who has had only a mandibular advancement unless the upper arch has been segmentalized or expanded. The patient is seen within 48 hours of splint removal. At this time appliances are checked for damage and repaired as necessary, and archwires are checked for coordination and adjusted if necessary. When the maxilla has been segmentalized, a continuous upper archwire is placed. This archwire, usually a 16 × 22 with T-loops at the site of any osteotomy, should be carefully coordinated to the lower arch before being placed. When there is no problem with bracket alignment on either side of an osteotomy, the T-loops are not necessary. The use of loops to provide flexibility is preferable to using light flexible archwires—nickel titanium, braided rectangular, etc.—because the loop provides flexibility only at the point where it is needed rather than along the entire wire. This provides a more predictable result. Another option for the "wire-bending challenged" is to maintain the sectional archwires placed before surgery and place over these in piggyback fashion, a light flexible archwire. This technique likewise places the flexibility where it is most beneficial without sacrificing rigidity where the teeth are well aligned.

When expansion has been done, a carefully formed removable lingual arch is placed to stabilize this expansion. In either instance, maxilla segmentalized or not, appropriate elastic therapy is begun, if necessary, as if no surgery has been done. Another appointment is scheduled in 2 to 3 days.

The second appointment is primarily to check the adjustments made previously and to review the elastic therapy, changing it if necessary. Future appointments are at 1 week and 2 weeks. The usual 4-week intervals are then resumed. The usual adjustments are made in the archwires and elastic wear until the desired occlusal result is achieved, at which time the appliances are removed and retainers are placed in the usual manner.

With the exception of the frequency of appointments immediately following release of fixation, there are no special considerations in the postsurgical phase of treatment. Indeed, any and all procedures are implemented that are used to "finish" the occlusion of the nonsurgical patient. If any problem arises during the postsurgical phase of treatment, new records are obtained, a diagnosis is made of the specific cause of the problem, and appropriate therapy is done to correct it (Chapter 5).

Factors affecting stability of treatment
Orthodontic factors

The factors affecting stability of this orthodontic-surgical treatment are a composite of those for superior repositioning of the maxilla and for mandibular advancement. These include the following:

1. Avoid inappropriate use of vertical mechanics.
2. Maxillary expansion for the adult is done surgically.
3. Make the occlusion more Class II before surgery.
4. Properly manage tooth mass discrepancies before surgery.
5. Adequately level both upper and lower arches or segments.
6. Appropriately coordinate the lower arch and upper arch segment(s).

The reader is directed to the detailed discussions in Chapter 6 on pages 227–229 regarding mandibular advancement and in Chapter 7 on pages 419–420 regarding maxillary superior repositioning for further information.

Surgical factors

In addition to the specific factors previously discussed in detail in Chapter 6 regarding mandibular advancement surgery and in Chapter 7 regarding isolated maxillary superior repositioning, an additional factor affects stability with the simultaneous superior repositioning of the maxilla and mandibular advancement—the quality and quantity of the posterior maxillary bony interface.

Two problems are encountered with the posterior maxillary bone interfaces: (1) the maxilla is expanded and poor bone contact exists posteriorly, and (2) the posterior bone is thin and structurally does not produce a stable interface. When either of these exists there is a potential for the maxilla to tip during the postoperative healing period, with the posterior portion of the maxilla moving superiorly and the anterior portion moving inferiorly. This tipping is accompanied by a downward, backward movement of the chin (relapse) and/or proximal segment rotation and/or excessive condylar loading. Whenever poor posterior bony interfaces are noted at the time of surgery, four bone plates are used instead of the more usual two anterior plates and posterior suspension wires.

Age-related factors

This orthodontic-surgical approach produces variable effects on facial growth and occlusal stability in the growing individual. This variability is related to the interaction of three factors that can and do result in either some modification of the subsequent growth vector or lack of maintenance of the achieved occlusion. These factors are: (1) alteration of the biomechanics of mastication as it relates to maxillary growth, (2) alteration of the biomechanics of condylar cartilage as it relates to subsequent growth, and (3) possible damage to the condylar cartilage ("growth center").

ALTERATION OF THE BIOMECHANICS OF MASTICATION AS IT RELATES TO MAXILLARY GROWTH

There is a direct relation between the magnitude of vertical maxillary growth and the magnitude of masticatory loading—the greater the masticatory loading, the less the vertical maxillary growth. Since the efficiency of the masticatory mechanism (Class III lever) is decreased as the teeth are advanced (increased distance of the teeth from the muscles of mastication), there theoretically occurs a decreased magnitude of masticatory loading (masticatory efficiency) with mandibular advancement. Although this has not been noted to affect the actual stability of the surgical result, this decrease in masticatory loading tends to result in an increased vertical growth pattern after surgical advancement of the mandible during growth.

Conversely, correction of a Class II dentofacial deformity by isolated superior maxillary repositioning increases the masticatory loading as the maxilla is moved posteriorly to correct the Class II occlusion. This increase is masticatory loading can result in decreased vertical maxillary growth. Thus, when considering simultaneous maxillary superior repositioning and mandibular advancement in growing patients, the less anterior (or more posterior) is the maxillary repositioning, the more favorable the subsequent growth. Despite this, in practice the amount of anterior or posterior maxillary repositioning is based on the existing facial esthetics, not on its potential effect on subsequent growth.

ALTERATION OF THE BIOMECHANICS OF CONDYLAR CARTILAGE AS IT PERTAINS TO SUBSEQUENT GROWTH

Both compressive loading and tensile loading directly influence the rate and direction of articular cartilage growth. With the significant alterations in condylar cartilage loading that occur with simultaneous superior maxillary repositioning and mandibular advancement surgery, it follows that alterations in the magnitude and direction of subsequent condylar cartilage growth can occur. If the resultant loading is either increased or decreased excessively, unfavorable growth (a more vertical than horizontal facial growth pattern) can result (Fig. 8-25). Again, the less anterior maxillary movement the better.

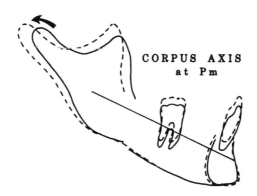

FIG. 8-25

POSSIBLE DAMAGE TO CONDYLAR CARTILAGE

This factor cannot be separated from the previous factor. However, when intermaxillary stabilization is not adequate and skeletal relapse occurs during the period of fixation, the condyles are chronically and forcefully compressed posterosuperiorly into the glenoid fossas during the entire period of fixation. Thus, compressive injury to the condylar cartilages can occur and will likely result in decreased subsequent mandibular growth. This would result in a tendency for the occlusion to become a Class II open bite. This same phenomenon occurs following isolated mandibular advancement surgery.

Similarly, when rigid fixation is used without intermaxillary fixation, the amount of mandibular advancement is great (> 6 to 8 mm), and an advancement genioplasty is done, the soft-tissue tension *will* cause the mandible to be retrodisplaced during the early postoperative period. The result is severe chronic compressive condylar loading with the predictable sequelae.

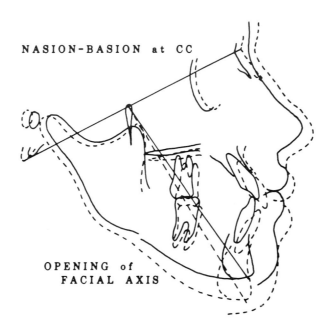

FIG. 8-26

Based on the information in the above discussion, several generalizations are possible that can help to guide the clinician in making surgical decisions and in predicting the probable outcome. For most patients who have undergone maxillary superior repositioning with simultaneous mandibular advancement during growth, the subsequent vector of facial growth (relocation) becomes more vertical than horizontal (Fig. 8-26). The relative magnitude of this vertical growth pattern is most extreme when the maxilla is moved superiorly and anteriorly, thus making the mandibular advancement greater. The combination of the maxilla moving superiorly and anteriorly with a large mandibular advancement predictably decreases the bite force, which may explain the tendency for vertical growth. Conversely, vertical growth is least when the maxilla is moved superiorly and somewhat posteriorly, thus decreasing the magnitude of the mandibular advancement. Accordingly, the most favorable growth occurs when the mandible is minimally advanced. The occlusion and esthetics are not predictably affected adversely by subsequent growth in either instance.

Although hard data are not available, the following observations are noted: (1) the vertical maxillary excess facial appearance seldom returns, although the chin may become noticeably more recessive due to the vertical growth that occurs in some individuals, and (2) the long-term stability of the occlusion is more predictable for the non-open-bite patient than for those who begin treatment with an open bite.

Results of treatment

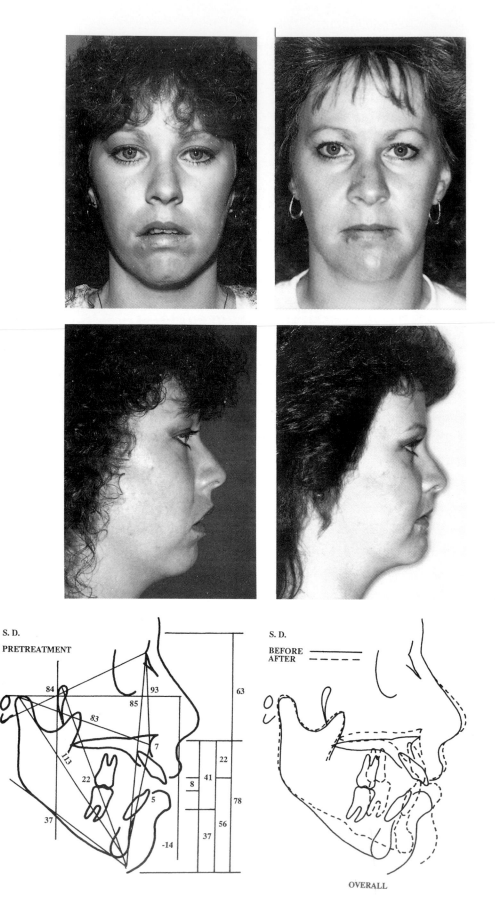

S. D.
PRETREATMENT

84   93
85
83
63
7
113
22   22
41
8
5
78
37
56
37
-14

S. D.

BEFORE ———
AFTER - - - -

OVERALL

FIG. 8-27

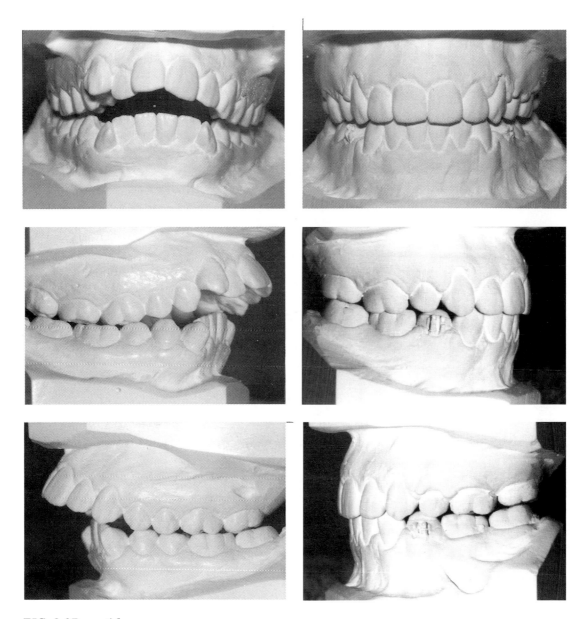

FIG. 8-27, *cont'd*

REFERENCES

Bjork, A., and Skieller, V.: Growth in width of the maxilla studied by the implant method, Scand. J. Plast. Reconstr. Surg. **8:**26, 1977.

Bjork, A., and Skiller, V.: Facial development and tooth eruption: an implant study at the age of puberty, Am. J. Orthodont. **62:**339, 1972.

Epker, B.N., and Fish, L.C.: Superior repositioning of the maxilla: what to do with the mandible? Am. J. Orthodont. **78:**164, 1980.

Epker, B.N., and Wolford, L.M.: Dentofacial deformities: surgical orthodontic correction, St. Louis, 1980, The C.V. Mosby Company.

Epker, B.N., and Wolford, L.M.: Middle third facial osteotomies: their use in the correction of acquired and developmental dentofacial and craniofacial deformities, J. Oral Surg. **33:**491, 1975.

Epker, B.N., Turvey, T.A., and Fish, L.D.: Indications for simultaneous mobilization of the maxilla and mandible for the correction of dentofacial deformities, Oral Surg. **54:**369, 1982.

Epker, B.N., Schendel, S.A., and Washburn, M.: Effects of early surgical superior repositioning of the maxilla on subsequent growth. III. Biomechanical considerations. In McNamara, J., Carlson, D., and Ribbens, K., editors: The effects of surgical intervention on craniofacial growth, monograph no. 12, Ann Arbor, Mich., 1982, Center for Human Growth and Development, University of Michigan.

Epker, B.N.: Superior surgical repositioning of the maxilla: long-term results, J. Maxillofac. Surg. **9:**199, 1981.

Fish, L.C., and Epker, B.N.: Surgical-orthodontic cephalometric prediction tracing, J. Clin. Orthodont. **14**(1):36-52, 1980.

Fish, L.C., Wolford, L.M., and Epker, B.N.: Surgical-orthodontic correction of vertical maxillary excess, Am. J. Orthodont. **73:**241, 1978.

Forssell, K., Turvery, T.A., Phillips, C., and Proffit, W.R.: Superior repositioning of the maxilla combined with mandibular advancement: mandibular RIF improves stability. Am. J. Orthodont. Dentofac. Orthop. **102**(4):342, 1992.

Isaacson, J., et al.: Extreme variations in vertical facial growth and associated variations in skeletal and dental relations, Angle Orthodont. **41:**219, 1971.

LeBanc, J.P., Turvey, T.A., and Epker, B.N.: Result following simultaneous mobilization of the maxilla and mandible for the correction of dentofacial deformities: analysis of 100 consecutive patients, Oral Surg. **54:**607, 1982.

Nanda, R., et al.: Mandibular adaptations following total maxillary osteotomy in adolescent monkeys, Am. J. Orthodont. **83:**485, 1983.

O'Ryan, F., and Epker, B.N.: Deliberate surgical control of the mandibular growth: a biomechanical theory, J. Oral Surg. **53:**2, 1982.

O'Ryan, F., and Epker, B.N.: Surgical-orthodontics and the temporomandibular joint. I. Superior repositioning of the maxilla, Am. J. Orthod. **83:**407, 1983.

Rickets, R.M., et al.: Bioprogressive therapy, book 1, Denver, 1979, Rocky Mountain Orthodontics.

Saaouni, V., and Nanda, S.: Analysis of dentofacial vertical proportions, Am. J. Orthodont. **50:**801, 1964.

Savara, B.S., and Singh, I.J.: Norms of size and annual increments of seven anatomical measures of maxillae in boys from three to sixteen years of age, Angle Orthodont. **38:**104, 1968.

Schendel, S., et al.: The long face syndrome: vertical maxillary excess, Am. J. Orthodont. **70:**398, 1976.

Schendel, S. A., et al.: Superior repositioning of the maxilla: stability and soft tissue osseous relations, Am. J. Orthodont. **70:**663, 1976.

Seigel, M.L.: Mechanisms of early maxillary growth: implications for surgery, J. Oral Surg. **34:**106, 1976.

Sillman, J.H.: Dimensional changes in the dental arches: longitudinal study from birth to twenty-five years, Am. J. Orthodont. **50:**824, 1964.

Singh, I.J., and Savara, B.S.: Norms of size and annual increments of seven anatomical measures of maxillae in girls from three to seventeen years of age. Angle Orthodont. **36:**312, 1968.

Stoller, A.E.: The universal appliance, St. Louis, 1971, The C.V. Mosby Company.

Thurow, R.C.: Atlas of orthodontic principles, St. Louis, 1970, The C.V. Mosby Company.

Turvey, T.A., et al.: Surgical-orthodontic treatment planning for simultaneous mobilization of the maxilla and mandible in the correction of dentofacial deformities, Oral Surg. **54:**491, 1982.

Turvey, T.A., Journot, V., and Epker, B.N.: Correction of anterior open-bite deformity: a study of tongue function, speech changes and stability, J. Maxillofac. Surg. **4:**93, 1976.

CHAPTER 9

Class II dentofacial deformities with open bite

Introduction

The facial esthetics of the Class II open-bite deformity generally involve the same increased lower third face height, excessive interlabial distance, everted lower lip, and recessive chin found in the usual Class II vertical maxillary excess patient. However, unlike the routine Class II vertical maxillary excess patient, the open-bite variation has much less excessive exposure of the upper anterior teeth. In addition, the Class II deformity with open bite is most often a complex three-dimensional occlusal deformity consisting of (1) an anteroposterior Class II relation, (2) a vertical maxillary excess that is usually disproportionate, being greatest posteriorly, and (3) a transverse maxillary deficiency manifest as a posterior cross bite.

All aspects of the deformity may be corrected simultaneously by the appropriate surgery. The Class II occlusion is corrected by the superior and posterior repositioning of the maxilla accompanied by upward and forward rotation of the mandible. The open bite is corrected by segmentalization of the maxilla with more superior repositioning of the posterior than the anterior segment(s), and the cross bite is corrected by surgical expansion of the posterior and sometimes the anterior maxillary segments.

While nearly all aspects of these patients' facial appearance are routinely improved by superior repositioning of the maxilla, integration of pertinent clinical esthetic findings with a cephalometric prediction tracing is essential to decide whether isolated superior repositioning of the maxilla with or without genioplasty or simultaneous superior repositioning of the maxilla and mandibular advancement is indicated. Clinical esthetic findings including nasal anatomy, paranasal configuration, and nasolabial angle are studied along with a cephalometric prediction tracing using only superior repositioning of the maxilla and mandibular autorotation to correct both the Class II occlusion and the open bite. When this prediction is done, some posterior movement of the maxilla is almost always required. This posterior maxillary movement is usually small and produces either no visible effect or a positive change in most patients. Thus, with proper planning and execution of the presurgical orthodontic treatment, a majority of individuals with Class II open-bite deformity can be treated by isolated superior repositioning of the maxilla with or without advancement genioplasty.

Nevertheless, there exists a small patient population who have facial esthetic features that will be worsened by any posterior movement of the maxilla. When the prediction tracing shows that the maxilla will require several millimeters of posterior repositioning to correct the Class II occlusion *and* the individual in question has facial characteristics consistent with maxillary deficiency—a large nose, a concave paranasal configuration, and/or an obtuse nasolabial angle—facial esthetics will be worsened by isolated maxillary superior-posterior repositioning. The posterior maxillary movement in such an individual will make the nose appear more prominent, further flatten the paranasal area, and make the already obtuse nasolabial angle even more so. Accordingly, simultaneous superior repositioning of the maxilla and advancement of the mandible are preferred for such a patient.

Class II open-bite patients amenable to isolated superior repositioning of the maxilla with or without genioplasty are discussed in the first two sections of this chapter. The usual approach is to perform the maxillary surgery by a segmental LeFort I procedure. There are, however, several reasons for doing the superior repositioning by the segmental total subapical technique described as the first alternate approach. The few patients requiring simultaneous mandibular advancement are discussed as the second alternate approach in this chapter. An even rarer variation wherein mandibular advancement is the appropriate surgical approach to close an anterior open bite is presented as the third alternate approach in the last section of this chapter.

The usual orthodontic-surgical approach:

SEGMENTAL LE FORT I SUPERIOR REPOSITIONING OF THE MAXILLA WITH ADVANCEMENT GENIOPLASTY

Outline of treatment

Presurgical orthodontic treatment

1. Place lower appliances; align and level
2. Place upper appliances; align and level segments
3. Elastics as necessary to place lower incisors in optimal position
4. Coordinate upper segments with lower arch
5. Impressions for feasibility model surgery

Immediate presurgical planning

1. Surgical cephalometric prediction tracing
2. Model surgery
3. Splint construction

Orthognathic reconstructive surgery

1. Segmental LeFort I superior repositioning of the maxilla
2. Advancement genioplasty

Postsurgical orthodontic treatment

1. Check appliances; repair as necessary
2. Place coordinated archwires; stabilizing lingual arch(es)
3. Elastics as necessary
4. Routine finishing procedures
5. Retain

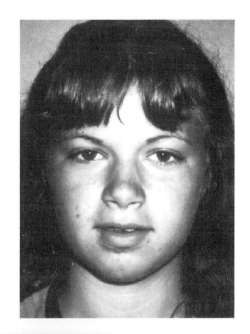

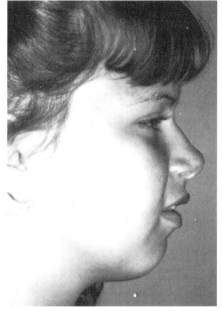

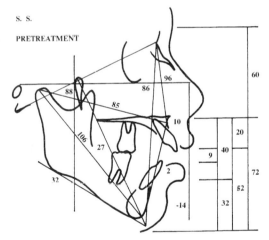

S. S.

PRETREATMENT

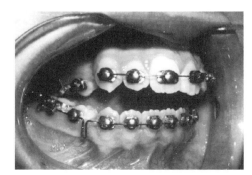

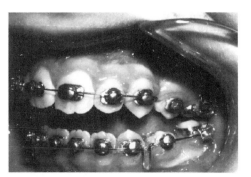

FIG. 9-1

Details of treatment

Presurgical orthodontic treatment

When maxillary segmentalization is indicated to correct the open bite and arch width, the presurgical orthodontic treatment is important with respect to facial esthetics, stability, and the need for simultaneous mobilization of the mandible. The presurgical orthodontic mechanics are not directed toward correcting the transverse or vertical problems, since they are most effectively corrected surgically. Rather, *the basic goal of the presurgical treatment is to place the lower dentition symmetrically in the proper anteroposterior and transverse position with respect to the mandible, such that when the maxilla is surgically repositioned, the maxillary teeth and their supporting bones will be in their proper anteroposterior, vertical, and transverse relations.*

Segmentalization of the maxilla can be done with or without extraction of teeth. Thus, the need for segmentalization to correct the vertical or transverse occlusal relations is not a factor in determining the need for extractions. There are two primary reasons to extract teeth in these patients: the dental movements necessary to place the lower incisors in their desired position, and the amount the maxillary molars must be moved posteriorly at surgery to correct the Class II occlusion.

The need for extractions in these patients is predicted to a major extent on the desired tooth movements as determined from an orthodontic-surgical prediction tracing (Chapter 2). In performing such a prediction tracing, particular attention is given to the anteroposterior movement of both the maxilla (paranasal support) and the maxillary teeth (nasolabial angle and upper lip support). When significant crowding exists in the lower arch such that nonextraction treatment could jeopardize the result by requiring excessive expansion that is frequently unstable and leads to periodontal complications, then extractions are the treatment of choice. When little or no crowding exists in the lower arch such that, independent of any other considerations, the lower arch can be treated without extractions, it is usually preferable to treat the lower arch nonextraction and add a larger genioplasty as opposed to retracting the lower incisors into the "normal" relation with the lower jaw (pogonion) and performing a simultaneous mandibular advancement since it simplifies the orthodontic treatment and avoids the need to simultaneously mobilize the mandible (Fig. 9-2).

When nonextraction treatment of the lower arch is possible, but so doing requires the maxillary posterior teeth to be moved farther posteriorly to achieve a Class I molar occlusion than the surgeon deems to be acceptable, two solutions are possible. The lower second premolars can be extracted and the lower molars advanced presurgically. (Care must be taken not to retract the lower incisors if doing so will create the need for two-jaw surgery.) This is then followed by extracting an upper premolar and producing a Class I molar relation at surgery. More commonly, the lower arch is still treated nonextraction, but an upper premolar is extracted at surgery to produce a Class II molar, Class I canine occlusion and eliminate the need to reposition the posterior maxillary segments posteriorly.

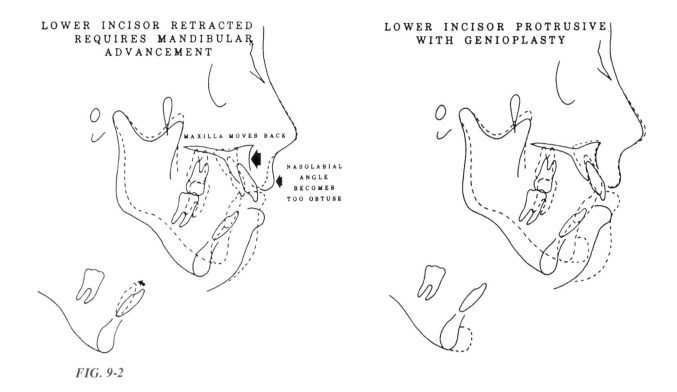

LOWER INCISOR RETRACTED
REQUIRES MANDIBULAR
ADVANCEMENT

LOWER INCISOR PROTRUSIVE
WITH GENIOPLASTY

MAXILLA MOVES BACK

NASOLABIAL
ANGLE
BECOMES
TOO OBTUSE

FIG. 9-2

The symmetry of the lower arch will ultimately dictate that of the upper arch.
Care must be taken during the presurgical orthodontic treatment of the lower arch
to ensure that the lower dental midline is coincident with the facial midline and
that the teeth in the mandibular buccal segments are placed symmetrically with
regard to their anteroposterior position before surgery.

Any orthodontic procedures that tend to open the bite must be done presurgically. Thus, molar uprighting and rotations are routinely treated presurgically
and the teeth are aligned so that no cross bites will need to be corrected following
surgery.

Tooth mass must be given special attention since it is desirable to place the
teeth not only in an ideal Class I canine relationship, but in the ideal overbite and
overjet relationship at surgery. Indeed, when an open-bite is present, it is preferable to produce a Class I canine relation *and* a slightly deep bite at surgery.
Achieving both is impossible when the lower anterior teeth are too wide relative
to the upper anterior teeth.

Any mechanics expressly intended to close the bite are avoided during the
presurgical orthodontic treatment. Vertical elastics, high-pull headgear with a
facebow, vertical-pull headgear to a chin cup, or any other device used in an attempt to close the bite is inadvisable. Conversely, further opening of the bite during the presurgical phase is considered to be positive and is of no concern (see
"Factors Affecting Stability").

Finally, when the maxilla must be expanded, it is preferable to effect such
expansion surgically, simultaneously with the superior repositioning of the maxilla. By so doing, the stability is improved.

With the aforementioned general principles in mind, and following appropriate notation on the patient's chart that combined orthodontic and surgical treatment is to be done, the actual presurgical orthodontic treatment can begin. The frequency of extraction versus nonextraction treatment for these patients is nearly equal and is decided on an individual basis. Herein, the principles of maxillary segmentalization are discussed with nonextraction treatment of the lower arch to avoid redundancy. The details of extraction treatment of the lower arch with maxillary segmentalization are described and illustrated in the next section of this chapter.

The lower appliances are usually placed first, since treatment of this arch takes longer than the upper arch. Bonded appliances are preferred, at least anteriorly, to allow any interproximal recontouring that may be needed to correct a minor tooth mass discrepancy. (Significant anterior tooth mass discrepancies may require extraction of one lower incisor.) When placing the lower anterior appliances in open-bite patients, it is best to place them slightly (0.5 to 1 mm) lower than usual so that the brackets do not interfere with the subsequent production of the desired overbite at surgery. The initial archwire selection depends on the irregularities of the lower arch and is most frequently an .014 nickel titanium, twist-o-flex, 16 × 22 multi-stranded, or other suitably flexible archwire. It is often helpful to place a lingual arch to avoid unwanted expansion of the lower posterior teeth.

The exact timing of the upper arch treatment will vary from patient to patient and is dependent on the crowding, alignment, and rotational movements that must be made. Generally, once the lower arch is almost aligned, the appliances and segmental archwires are placed in the upper arch. The objective is to complete idealization of the upper segments and the lower arch at approximately the same time. If extractions are to be done in the upper arch only, a decision must be made regarding the timing of same. When little crowding exists, it is often preferable to extract the premolar at the time of surgery as the extraction site becomes a large part of the required interdental osteotomy. However, when aligning the teeth without extraction requires sufficient labial movement of the teeth as to be inadvisable for periodontal reasons, the premolars are extracted before placing the appliances. It is particularly important that provision is made for using a removable lingual arch by attaching a lingual sheath to the upper molars (Fig. 9-3). Presurgically the lingual arch is effective in rotating and torquing the upper molars when this is de-

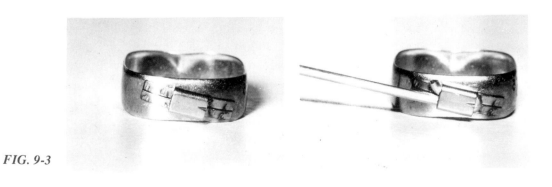

FIG. 9-3

sired. More importantly it is an effective method of stabilizing any surgically produced maxillary expansion, effecting torque control in the buccal segments, and producing cross-arch stability during the postsurgical orthodontic treatment.

Segmental mechanics are used in the upper arch to maintain the dual occlusal plane usually found in the Class II dentofacial deformity with open bite and/or to prevent undesirable orthodontic expansion of the maxilla (Fig. 9-4). Segmental mechanics virtually eliminate both the possibility of producing extrusive forces on the anterior teeth or intrusive force in the canine-premolar area and the possibility of producing undesired orthodontic expansion. Thus, there are two posterior segmental archwires incorporating the premolars and the molars on each side and an anterior segmental archwire from canine to canine.

DUAL OCCLUSAL PLANES

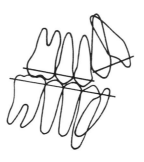

FIG. 9-4   typical of the Class II openbite

When the upper canines are excessively constricted relative to the lower canines and premolars, it is often desirable to split the anterior segment into two segments (Fig. 9-5) and to produce the desired canine expansion surgically. So doing will widen both the teeth and their supporting bone, thus, reducing the risk of periodontal problems and the potential relapse frequently encountered when the canines are expanded by orthodontic means alone. This decision is predicted on the amount of expansion required, whether such expansion will be produced by tipping as opposed to bodily movement, and the status of the periodontal tissues in the upper canine regions. Orthodontic correction is usually feasible when sufficient attached gingiva exists over the upper canines and less than 4 mm of canine widening is to be produced by tipping the crowns labially.

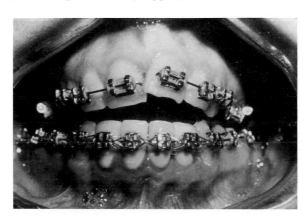

FIG. 9-5

The initial sectional archwires are generally light round wires to initiate bracket alignment. These wires are replaced (or not used at all when bracket alignment permits) by looped or plain square or rectangular wires as soon as possible. Round wires can never produce the desired results because they turn in the brackets and cannot produce control of the torque throughout the segments. Seldom is it necessary to use a wire larger than 16 × 22 in a .018 bracket slot to produce all the torque control necessary, although larger wires may be desired in some instances. The objective is to produce three or four maxillary dentoosseous segments that will fit the lower arch when surgically repositioned. As such, it is of little consequence how the maxillary segments are related to one another presurgically but only that the teeth within each segment are properly related to one another in all three planes of space.

One exception to this general rule may exist, particularly in the patient with an open bite who will have nonextraction treatment. There must be sufficient room between the roots of the canines and first premolar teeth for the osteotomies to be made between them. Some appliance systems possess enough tip-back in the canine bracket to produce significant interferences with these osteotomies near the apices of the teeth. In these instances, this tip-back must be eliminated before surgery to leave sufficient room between the premolars and canines for the osteotomies. This is easily done by placing a gable bend in the anterior segmental archwire to tip the canine roots mesially or by using canine brackets before surgery that do not have this tip-back. If necessary, the first premolar roots are tipped distally in a similar manner. The presence of sufficient space for the interdental osteotomies (ostectomies) is confirmed with periapical radiographs before surgery.

The surgery then places the segments into their normal relation to the lower arch, and by so doing, the upper teeth automatically assume the proper relation to one another and their axial inclinations become more normal (Fig. 9-6). If the canine tip-backs have been overridden during the presurgical orthodontic treatment and/or the premolars tipped distally, these teeth will require root paralleling during the postsurgical treatment.

FIG. 9-6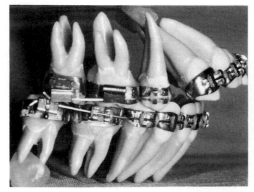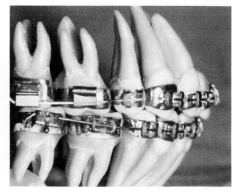

Once the lower teeth are aligned, a continuous 16 × 16 or larger lower arch-wire is placed. Note that since the canine and incisor brackets were intentionally placed gingivally, step-downs are necessary to produce a level lower arch rather than one with a slightly increased curve of Spee (Fig. 9-7).

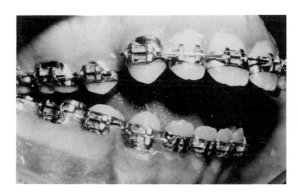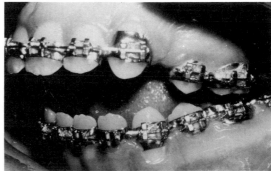

FIG. 9-7

The final archwires placed before surgery are generally 16 × 22. It is important that the upper sectional archwires be coordinated with the lower archwire. This is ensured by producing upper and lower continuous, coordinated archwires and then segmentalizing the upper archwire as necessary (Fig. 9-8). Again, proper step-downs are incorporated into the lower archwire as necessary. Care is taken so that the general shape and width of the lower arch has been maintained and particularly that the lower canines have not been overexpanded (see "Factors Affecting Stability".

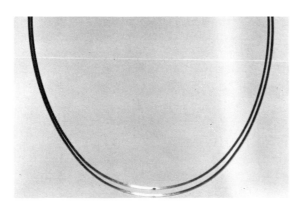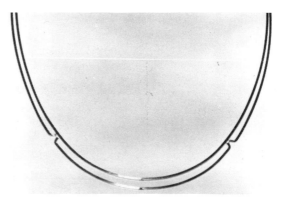

FIG. 9-8

Once these archwires have become passive, impressions are made and feasibility model surgery is done by the surgeon and approved by the orthodontist. The single most common problem encountered at this time is the existence of a small, previously undetected, tooth mass discrepancy that precludes the simultaneous production of a good Class I canine relationship and the desired amount of overbite. When this exists it can usually be corrected by interproximal recontouring of the lower incisors or opening small spaces distal to the upper lateral incisors. A second potential problem is insufficient space through which to do the surgical ostectomies. This may be particularly troublesome where the orthodontic appliance has a built-in tip-back for the canines. It may be necessary for the orthodontist deliberately to tip the canine root mesially and the premolar root distally to provide surgical access. The surgeon should advise if such movements are necessary. When any problem is noted in the feasibility model surgery, appropriate corrections are made by the orthodontist and the feasibility model surgery is redone to confirm the successful resolution of the problem before surgery. When such model surgery produces the desired result, the archwires are tied with ligature wires to prevent inadvertent disengagement at surgery, elastic hooks are placed where desired (usually the upper and lower canines), and the patient is referred for surgery.

Immediate presurgical planning
SURGICAL CEPHALOMETRIC PREDICTION TRACING

Unlike the combined orthodontic-surgical prediction tracings discussed in Chapter 2, the surgeon is bound by the position of the teeth that has been produced by the presurgical orthodontic treatment. As such, the surgical cephalometric prediction tracings are more simply and directly done. These prediction tracings provide much of the essential information required to perform the surgery properly. Furthermore, by superimposing the prediction tracing on the cephalometric radiograph obtained immediately following surgery, the accuracy of the surgical changes can be studied. Significant discrepancies between the predicted and actual result may warrant additional surgical intervention before the patient leaves the hospital (Chapter 5).

The surgery is to correct a Class II open-bite deformity by a three-piece superior repositioning of the maxilla, with more superior movement of the posterior segments than the anterior segment to close the open bite and normalize the upper tooth-to-lip relationship. In addition, a determination is made regarding the need for and the magnitude of an advancement genioplasty.

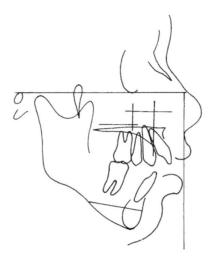

FIG. 9-9

All usual structures are traced from the presurgical cephalometric radiograph. Frankfort horizontal and subnasale perpendicular are constructed on this tracing for purposes of determining the need for and magnitude of a genioplasty. A maxillary reference line is constructed on this tracing that closely approximates the planned ostectomy. The anterior component of this line (*A*) is 35 mm above the cusp tip of the maxillary canine (occlusal plane) and the posterior component (*B*) is 25 mm above the cusp tips of the maxillary first molar. These lines are made parallel to the maxillary occlusal plane and are joined by a vertical line (*C*) perpendicular to the occlusal plane and just mesial to the first molar. An anterior vertical reference line (*D*) is placed perpendicular to the maxillary occlusal plane approximately at the position of the cusp tip of the maxillary canine. When an advancement genioplasty is anticipated, an additional reference line (*E*) is constructed on this tracing to correspond to the location of the horizontal osteotomy for the genioplasty (see Chapter 6 for detailed description of the genioplasty technique). This is referred to as the ***tracing*** (black line).

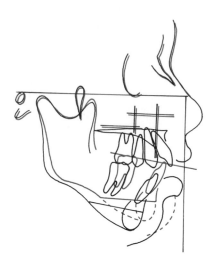

FIG. 9-10

The ***prediction*** (red line) is begun as described in Chapter 7. The mandible is traced, the mandibular occlusal plane is rotated to its appropriate position relative to the upper lip and the stable structures are traced. (Note: In all instances when lines are being traced from the ***tracing*** to the ***prediction***, superimpositions are shown slightly offset to better show which lines are being traced.)

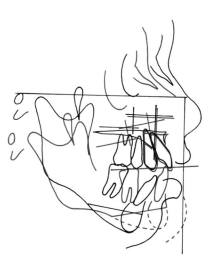

FIG. 9-11

The maxillary segments are now placed into their appropriate positions in two pieces—an anterior segment consisting of the bone and teeth approximating the anterior segment, and a posterior segment consisting of the bone and teeth of the posterior segments. The anterior piece is placed first. To accomplish this the ***prediction*** is placed on the ***tracing*** and rotated such that the upper incisors are in their ideal overbite and overjet relation *and* the occlusal plane of the anterior teeth parallels that of the mandibular dentition. While holding this superimposition, the maxillary incisor, canine, anterior maxillary bone, and anterior reference line are traced.

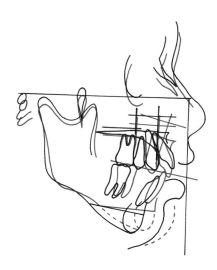

FIG. 9-12

Next, the posterior segment—second premolar and molars—is placed into its ideal occlusal relation. The teeth and bone corresponding to this segment are traced in this position. The reference marks located on this segment are likewise transferred to the ***prediction***. The changes in the skeletal references indicate the size of the lateral wall ostectomy (horizontal references) and the required antero-posterior repositioning of the maxilla (vertical references) that is to be achieved at surgery. In cases of segmentalization or asymmetry, experience has shown that the references taken from the definitive model surgery, described later in this chapter, are more precise because three-dimensional movements not perceived in the cephalometric prediction tracing are being done. Furthermore, because of the geometry of the anterior segment (a small base from central incisor to canine and a much larger dimension from the occlusal plane to the reference mark), any error in determining or repositioning the occlusal plane of the segment is greatly magnified at the level of the reference mark.

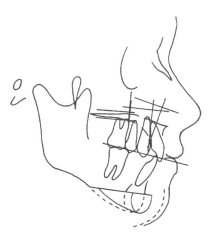

FIG. 9-13

The position of soft-tissue and bony pogonion is finally evaluated. If a genioplasty is necessary, it is added as described in Chapter 6 and the soft tissues are traced as described in Chapter 2. The completed prediction tracing is illustrated.

MODEL SURGERY FOR SUPERIOR REPOSITIONING OF THE MAXILLA
WITH SEGMENTALIZATION

The definitive model surgery for maxillary superior repositioning with segmentalization is described. When segmentalized maxillary surgery is performed, it is recommended that the models be mounted on a semiadjustable anatomic articulator using a face-bow transfer. This is necessary because the three-dimensional changes that occur during segmentalization are not well illustrated by prediction tracing.

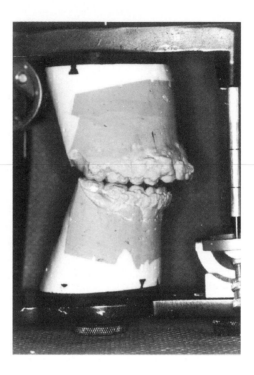

FIG. 9-14

Step 1. The models are mounted on a semiadjustable anatomic articulator by a face-bow transfer. The mounted models are trimmed to simulate the skeletal anatomy of the maxilla and mandible.

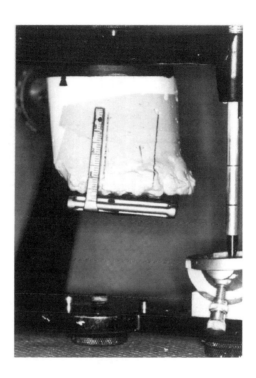

FIG. 9-15

Step 2. The models are marked as follows:

a. Vertical reference lines (perpendicular to the occlusal plane) are drawn from the mounting ring of the maxillary model to the first molar and canine teeth bilaterally using the maxillary reference device.* These vertical maxillary reference lines are then extended inferiorly onto the mandibular cast.

---

*Walter Lorenz Instrument Company, Jacksonville, FL

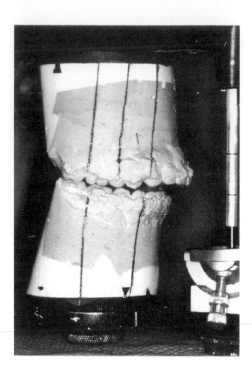

FIG. 9-16

b. An additional vertical reference line is drawn using the maxillary reference device in the premolar area just posterior to the proposed interdental osteotomy or ostectomy.

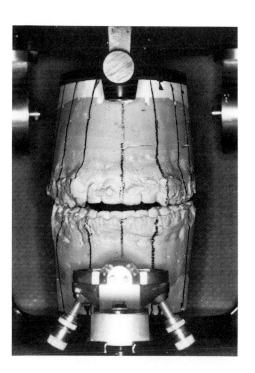

FIG. 9-17

c. The facial midline is drawn on the maxillary cast. This line is extended onto the mandibular dentition and down through the mandibular symphysis.

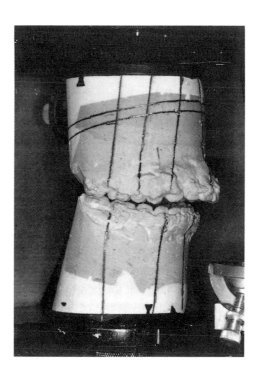

FIG. 9-18

    d. A horizontal line is drawn on the models beginning approximately 35 mm above the maxillary canine cusp tip and tapering posteriorly to 25 mm above the maxillary first molar cusp tips. This line marks the point at which the saw cut is made to section the maxillary model from its base and simulates the location of the most inferior aspect of the lateral maxillary wall ostectomy to be made at surgery. A second horizontal line is drawn on the maxillary model 2 to 3 mm farther above the first line than the anticipated vertical movement as determined from the prediction tracing (i.e., if 5 mm of superior movement is anticipated, this line is 7 to 8 mm above the first line). This line approximates the superior extent of plaster removal for the model surgery.

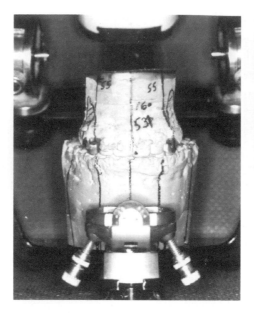
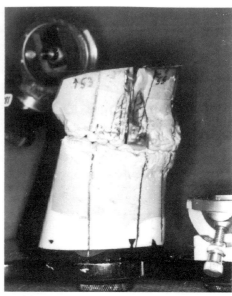

FIG. 9-26

Step 6. The anterior maxillary segment(s) is placed into its optimal occlusal relation with the mandibular teeth and lightly sticky waxed to the lower teeth in this position. In open-bite cases maximal overbite is desired. The posterior maxillary segments are then positioned to achieve the best possible occlusion. Doing so may require removal of some additional interdental plaster, however the clinician must be mindful of the position of the "roots" and interproximal contact areas such that they are not cut through. Once the desired occlusion has been achieved, the segmentalized maxilla is consolidated by a heavy application of sticky wax.

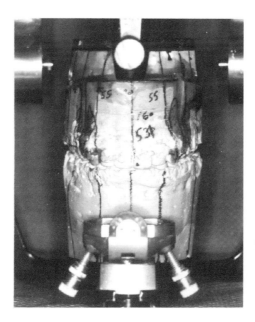
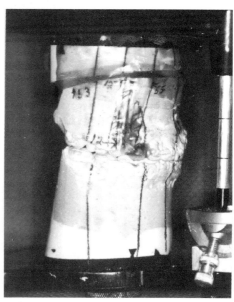

FIG. 9-27

Step 7. The consolidated maxilla is now autorotated into its desired position. This is done by loosening the set screw of the incisal guide pin and permitting the upper component of the articulator with the attached mounting ring to rotate inferiorly. As the upper component rotates inferiorly, the distance between the mounting ring and the upper central incisor edges is decreased. Some additional plaster may need to be removed from the base attached to the mounting ring to allow the upper component to close to the desired position. Once the proper vertical position of the incisors is reached—the distance from mounting ring to central incisor has decreased by the amount the upper incisor is to be superiorly repositioned—the set screw on the incisal guide pin is tightened.

Step 8. Once the maxilla is properly positioned to achieve both the best possible occlusion and the indicated amount of superior repositioning, it is secured rigidly to the superior base with a heavy application of sticky wax. The completed models are now measured as described below to determine the magnitude of the skeletal changes that must be duplicated at surgery and are subsequently used to fabricate the splint that will be used at surgery to produce accurate reapproximation of the dentoosseous segments.

The amount of the anteroposterior movements of the segments at the level of the LeFort I ostectomy are noted from the changes in the vertical reference lines. The vertical distances from the canine and molar cusps to the maxillary mounting ring are measured parallel to the vertical reference lines on the models. The vertical changes are calculated in the molar and canine areas by subtracting these values from those made and recorded prior to doing the surgery on the models. These changes are recorded for use at surgery.

The magnitude of superior repositioning in the incisor area, canine and first molar areas are almost always different and are best determined by carefully done model surgery. These measurements should closely approximate those obtained from the cephalometric prediction tracing but may not be exactly the same for segmental surgery. When there is *significant* disparity between these two treatment planning methods, it is important to determine precisely why.

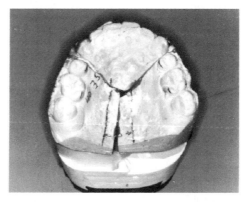

FIG. 9-28

The intermolar, interpremolar, and intercanine distances are measured and the changes in these dimensions are recorded. The distance between the two parallel lines on the palatal vault is measured. The change in this dimension illustrates the magnitude of widening or constriction at the level of the palatal plane and is important since the amount and direction of change determine the need for palatal soft-tissue relaxing incisions (expansion of more than 4 to 5 mm), or rarely a midpalatal ostectomy for constriction.

SPLINT CONSTRUCTION

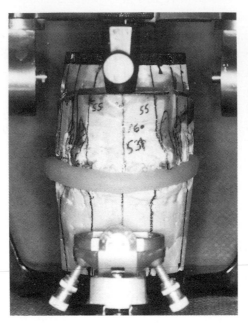 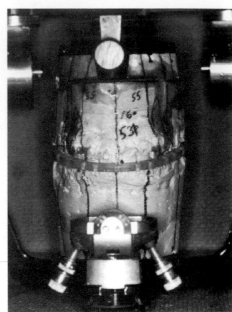

FIG. 9-29

The acrylic surgical occlusal splint with a palatal bar is now constructed on the maxillary model. To fabricate such a splint, the occlusal portion is first completed by coating the occlusal surfaces of the models with a separating medium and using self-curing acrylic rolled into a cylinder and placed between the maxillary and mandibular models. The models are closed into the soft-acrylic and gently opened and closed while the acrylic cures to prevent it from becoming locked into any undercuts in the models. After the acrylic fully cures, the splint is trimmed such that the maxillary dentition is maximally interdigitated into the splint to allow positive seating of the maxillary segments into the splint at the time of surgery. When these interdigitations are not discrete, there is a tendency for the segments to be arbitrarily tipped buccally or palatally at the actual time of surgery. The splint does not extend past the terminal molars. The mandibular occlusal interdigitations are definite but shallow, to preclude occlusal interferences when the intermaxillary fixation is released, and the patient begins to initiate jaw function (physiotherapy) with the splint left attached to the maxillary dentition. Importantly, this is not to be a functional splint from the standpoint that the patient can masticate with it in place. Rather, it is to permit hinge-axis closure of the mandible so that the patient's occlusion can be checked periodically after release of intermaxillary fixation to make certain the surgical result is stable.

After the splint is properly trimmed, holes are drilled just lateral to each interproximal space. The occlusal portion is now polished.

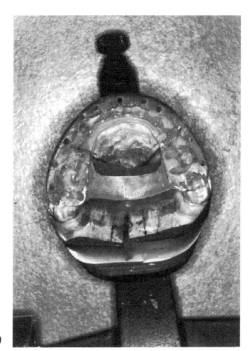 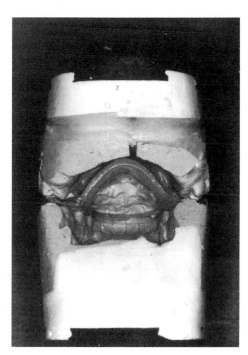

FIG. 9-30

Once the occlusal portion of the splint has been completed, it is lightly sticky waxed to the maxillary model and one layer of thin pink base plate wax is applied to the palatal vault between the maxillary first molars to provide relief for the palatal bar. A strip of acrylic approximately 2 to 3 mm thick and 10 mm wide is placed on the wax relief and is connected to the splint in the area of the maxillary first molar with a thin mixture of acrylic.

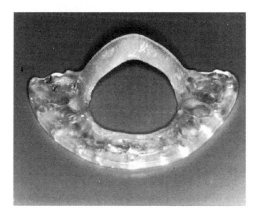

FIG. 9-31

After the palatal bar has been completed, the splint is polished. The completed splint is shown above.

Orthognathic reconstructive surgery

When simultaneously performing segmental LeFort I superior repositioning of the maxilla and advancement genioplasty, the surgical sequence preferred is completion of the genioplasty, followed by the LeFort I technique. This sequence is best because it reduces the amount of manipulation of the LeFort I segment(s) at the close of the procedure. If the genioplasty is performed last, the surgical manipulations of the mandible may cause sufficient loading of the maxilla to loosen bone plates and/or displace it from its surgically attained position. The next section discusses the surgical procedure for segmentalization of the maxilla during a LeFort I ostectomy for superior repositioning. In addition, the technique for augmentation-widening genioplasty is outlined. The technique for a standard advancement genioplasty is presented in Chapter 6.

The initial dissection and placement of reference markings for the segmentalized LeFort I are identical to those described in Chapter 7. Only the part of the orthognathic surgery pertaining to the segmentalization of the LeFort I is described herein.

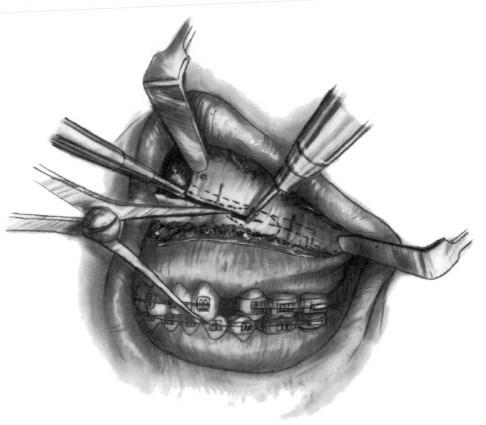

FIG. 9-32

The segmentalization of the maxilla is begun after completing the horizontal ostectomy of the maxilla but before down-fracturing. It may be accomplished by interdental osteotomies or by interdental ostectomies depending on the occlusal requirements of the patient. The amount and geometry of the interdental osteotomy or ostectomy are known from the definitive model surgery.

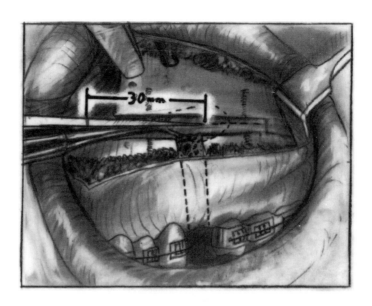

FIG. 9-33

The alveolar portion of the ostectomy is completed first, with no attempt to complete the transpalatal ostectomy. This is accomplished in two parts, a superior portion above the level of the attached gingiva, and an inferior portion from that point to the alveolar crest. The superior portion is completed first using a 703 bur on a rotary handpiece. It is best to remove approximately 20% less bone than is shown to be necessary on the model surgery since bone has some compressibility and if too much interproximal bone is removed, a severe periodontal defect may result.

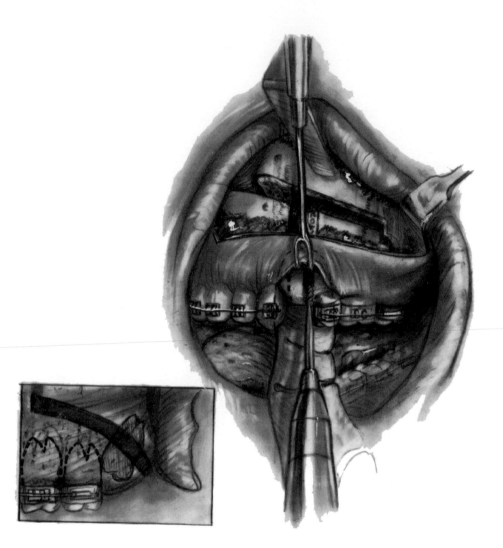

FIG. 9-34

Next, the inferior position of the alveolus is approached through a small crestal incision with judicious undermining of the buccal-palatal mucoperiosteum. This dual approach, from above and below, requires less detachment of and injury to the buccal and palatal soft tissue, allows bone removal under direct visualization, and permits the preservation of adequate alveolar crestal bone adjacent to each tooth. As was the case for the superior part of the interdental ostectomy, it is best to remove approximately *20% less* interproximal bone than indicated by the model surgery because the alveolar bone is compressible to some degree and the consequence of removing too much interproximal bone is the formation of a nonrestorable periodontal defect. The final refinements of all interproximal osteotomies and ostectomies are done as the maxillary segments are being placed into the occlusal splint. When a tooth is removed at the time of surgery, the same approach is used but no crestal incision is needed.

Similar soft-tissue incisions, subperiosteal dissection, osteotomies, and ostectomies are now completed on the opposite side. The exact geometry of the osteotomies and ostectomies may differ from side to side depending on the occlusal demands as determined from definitive model surgery.

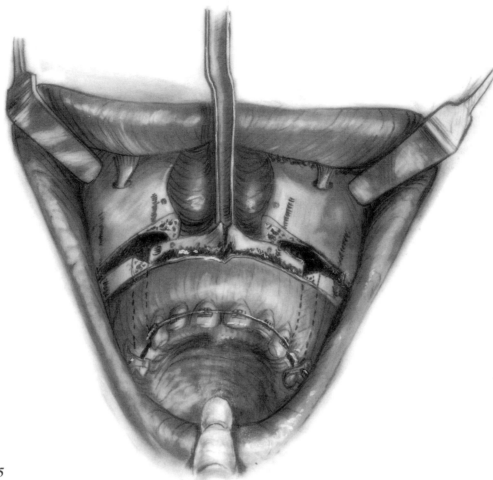

FIG. 9-35

After completing the lateral and alveolar portion of the osteotomies and ostectomies, the nasal septum is separated from the maxilla and the maxilla is downfractured, mobilized, and interferences to superior repositioning are removed as described in Chapter 7.

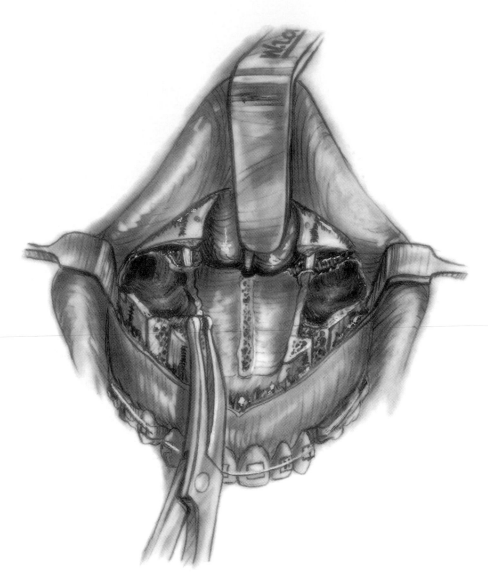

FIG. 9-36

After complete mobilization of the maxilla, segmentalization is easily completed under direct visualization. The lateral nasal walls are reduced using a rongeur. Care is taken not to cut or crush the greater palatine neurovascular bundle, which lies just below the lateral nasal wall.

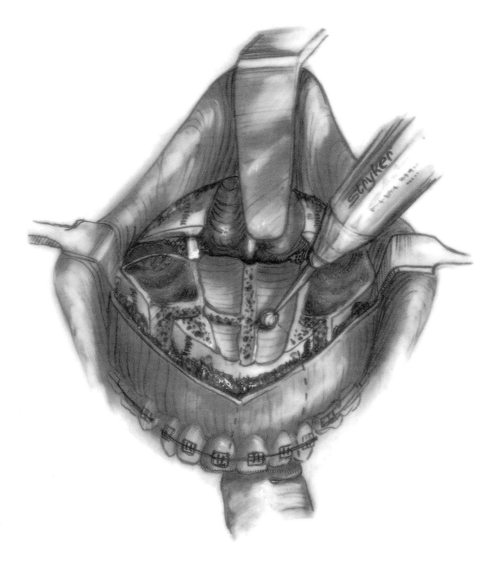

FIG. 9-37

The transpalatal osteotomy or ostectomy that joins one alveolar cut with the other is completed first. It is begun with a large round bur. After the transpalatal ostectomy is well initiated with the bur, an osteotome is malleted transpalatally until the anterior maxilla can be independently down-fractured. Great care must be taken in making this osteotomy (ostectomy) deep enough to permit the anterior portion of the maxilla to be down-fractured, but not so deep as to injure the palatal mucoperiosteum. *Avoiding injury to the palatal soft tissue is critical as it provides the primary blood supply to the anterior maxillary segment(s).* Transection or maceration of this tissue may result in loss of the anterior segment due to avascular necrosis.

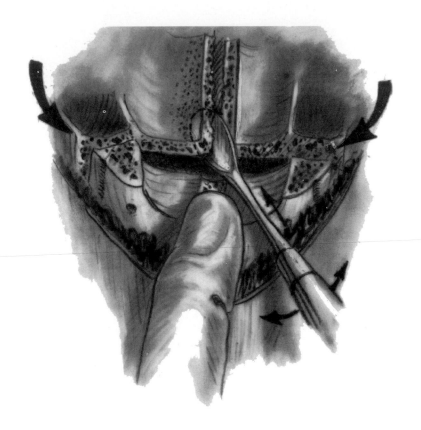

FIG. 9-38

Next, the posterior midpalatal osteotomy is completed. Midpalatal separation is achieved by manual pressure applied to the dentoalveolus with the thumb and index finger bilaterally to pinch the posterior segments palatally. When either minor expansion (less than 4 to 5 mm) or narrowing is indicated, the palatal mucoperiosteum is elevated bilaterally with a periosteal elevator through the midpalatal fracture.

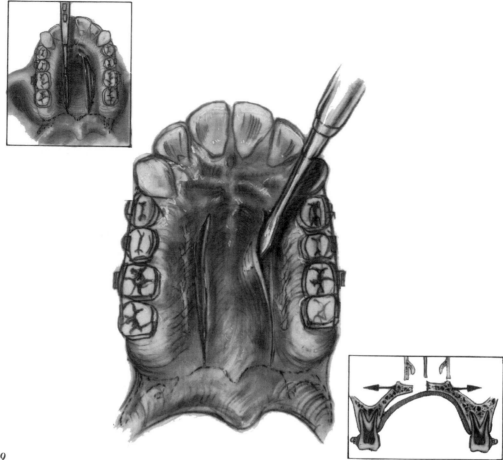

FIG. 9-39

When expansion of more than 4 to 5 mm is required, two lateral palatal soft-tissue relaxing incisions are required. These incisions are made just medial to the greater palatine neurovascular bundles from the posterior edge of the hard palate anteriorly to the premolar region. No local anesthetic is injected palatally. The mucoperiosteum between the two incisions is completely undermined subperiosteally. This flap is generally about 12 to 15 mm wide. Care is exercised not to tear either end of the flap, especially the posterior, because this will compromise its primary vascular source. This flap permits the maxilla to be surgically expanded without resistance from the palatal mucoperiosteum, and prevents both a midline palatal mucosal tear and/or stripping of the important palatal pedicles (blood supply) from the lateral maxillary segments during expansion.

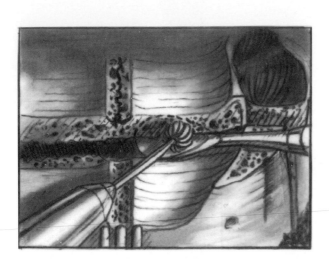

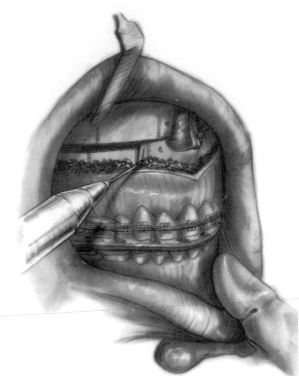

FIG. 9-40

The maxillary segments are now consolidated into the surgical occlusal splint. This is achieved by sequentially wiring them into the splint, beginning with a posterior segment. Any bony interferences that may exist palatally or in the interdental osteotomy or ostectomy sites are removed as each segment is placed. It is important that the original alveolar or interdental ostectomies are not more excessive than is required to close the spaces. Excessive ostectomies produce bone defects that impair healing and result in periodontal defects and/or fibrous or fibrocartilaginous unions. These untoward sequelae make subsequent orthodontic tooth movement into these areas impossible. These problems are avoided if, as previously described, approximately 20% less interdental-alveolar bone is initially removed than was determined to be necessary from the definitive model surgery. These areas are now refined and bony interferences are removed as required with a 701 bur *while the segments are being placed into the surgical occlusal splint.*

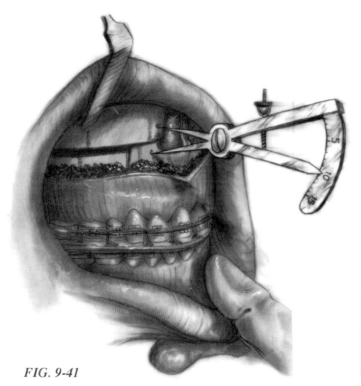

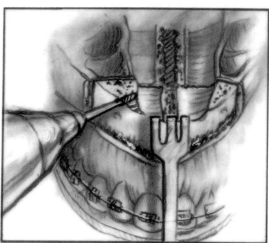

FIG. 9-41

After sequentially wiring the segments into the surgical occlusal splint to effect consolidation of the maxillary segments as a single unit, the superior repositioning of the "single-piece" maxilla is completed as described in Chapter 7. In summary, all internal and external references are checked to ensure accurate vertical positioning of the maxilla. Any interferences that prevent proper vertical positioning are removed with a 703 bur (Fig. 9-41, *inset*).

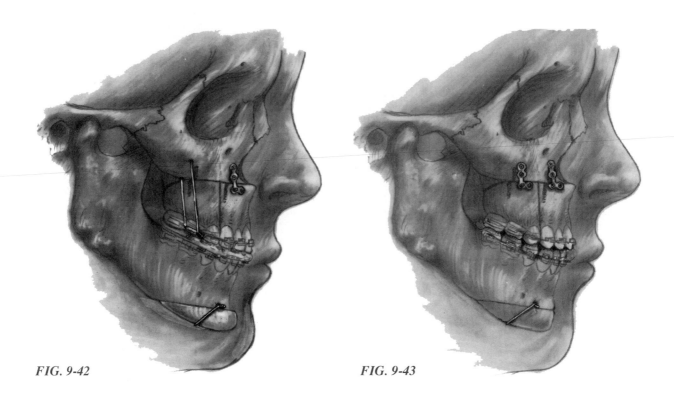

FIG. 9-42   *FIG. 9-43*

    Stabilization is routinely performed in a manner identical to that described in Chapter 7. It is emphasized that careful checking of the occlusion *before* finalizing the anterior bone plate stabilization is helpful.

An additional stabilization option is infraorbital skeletal suspension wires. This technique, described below, is fast and inexpensive. Furthermore, infraorbital suspension of the segmentalized maxilla provides some advantages with respect to the postsurgical orthodontic treatment. It allows postsurgical refinement of the occlusion by dental/orthopedic movement of entire dentoosseous segments rather than by dental compensatory movement within a "fixed" segment, as is seen subsequent to bone plate stabilization.

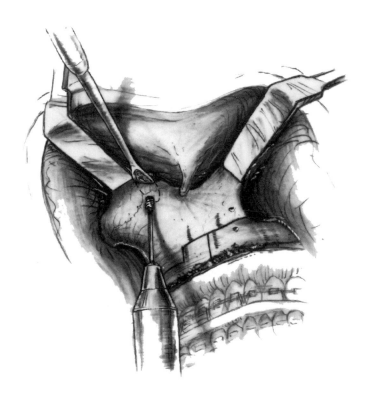

FIG. 9-44

When it is determined that the maxilla can be properly repositioned, bilateral 22-gauge infraorbital suspension wires are passed. The placement of these wires is technique sensitive. Once the technique is mastered, infraorbital wires may be passed quite rapidly. A periosteal elevator is used to dissect the periosteum up to and off of the infraorbital rim lateral to the infraorbital nerve. This periosteal elevator is then replaced by an "old" periosteal elevator that was previously used to protect soft tissues from injury by a bur on a rotary handpiece. A 703 bur is then used to drill a hole tangentially through the infraorbital rim, lateral to the infraorbital nerve. The drill is advanced until it contacts the periosteal elevator.

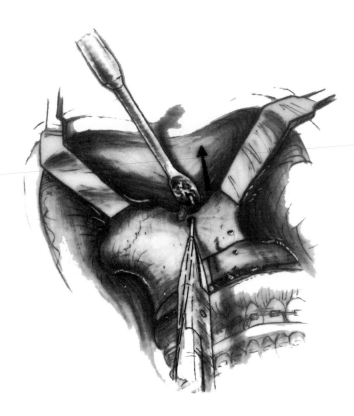

FIG. 9-45

The periosteal elevator is now used to lift the infraorbital rim periosteum superiorly and a 22-gauge stainless steel wire with a slight curve placed on the end is directed into the bur hole until it contacts the periosteal elevator.

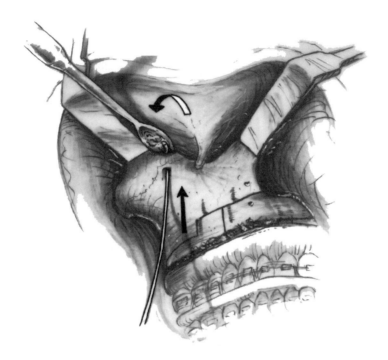

FIG. 9-46

The wire is advanced such that it remains in contact with the periosteal elevator as it is slowly pulled from beneath the orbit. When done properly, the periosteal elevator will deflect the wire anteriorly as it is withdrawn until the end of the wire can be grasped and pulled inferiorly. These infraorbital skeletal suspension wires are twisted in the maxillary vestibule to form loops from which two 24-gauge wires are passed loosely through the splint.

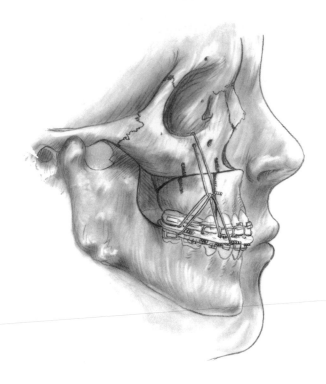

FIG. 9-47

One 24-gauge wire is passed distal to the canine and the second is passed distal to the first molar bilaterally. The oral cavity and surgical sites are irrigated and suctioned free of debris. The anterior suspension wires are tightened first to produce a superoposterior vector on the maxilla. The right and left wires are tightened simultaneously to prevent rotation of the maxilla. As the wires are being tightened, the lateral-wall reference lines are observed to ascertain the correctness of maxillary repositioning. The posterior suspension wires are then tightened, but more passively than the anterior wires. If bone interfaces are adequate and secure, intermaxillary fixation may be released at this time, providing the criteria previously noted in Chapter 2 (Step 4: Developing the Definitive Treatment Plan, Orthognathic Surgery, Type of Fixation) are met. After achieving stabilization, the position of the cartilaginous nasal septum is addressed and the maxillary soft tissue incisions are closed according to those principles described in Chapter 7.

The last incision closed is the genioplasty incision. The mentalis muscle and mucoperiosteum are not closed until the end of the surgery so the magnitude and symmetry of the chin advancement can be reevaluated following the maxillary surgery.

If intermaxillary fixation is used, it is maintained for 3 to 4 weeks. The exact time depends on the degree to which bone contact exists between the segments at the completion of surgery. With excellent contact, 3 weeks of fixation is generally adequate.

On removal of fixation, the splint is left wired to the maxillary teeth and the suspension wires are left in place. The patient's ability to occlude ideally into the splint is carefully checked periodically. This will be ideal in most cases, and the patient is instructed to exercise the mandible, to avoid mastication, and to return in several days for reevaluation. The details of this regimen are discussed in Chapter 7. When mandibular movement returns to near normal, usually within 1 week, the occlusal splint and associated skeletal suspension wires are removed. On splint removal, the patient is to see the orthodontist to initiate finishing orthodontics within 48 hours.

Adjunctive esthetic procedures

Modifications of the standard advancement genioplasty technique are useful to achieve additional width and increased projection of the chin. When the patient possesses a tapered chin and/or prominent parasymphysis grooves, chin advancement by the usual horizontal osteotomy creates a more pointed chin, a witch's chin, and/or unesthetic "marionette grooves" by accentuating the continuation of the nasolabial folds that extend to the inferior mandibular borders. Two things can be done to improve the esthetic result for such a patient: (1) extend the lateral genioplasty flanges and perform lateral augmentation and/or (2) perform lateral parasymphysis augmentation. Some patients would optimally benefit from an advancement genioplasty that is larger than is possible to achieve by the usual method. When this is so, additional projection can be obtained by the "maximum advancement" genioplasty. These techniques are discussed on the following pages.

LATERAL AUGMENTATION GENIOPLASTY

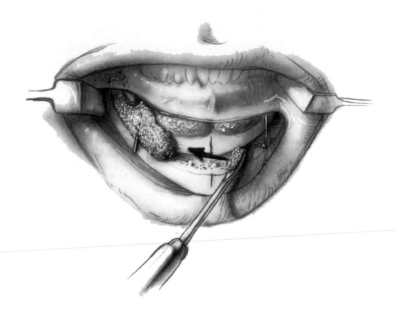

FIG. 9-48

Lateral alloplastic augmentation is routinely performed with a mixture of particulate hydroxylapatite and Helitene* mixed together with a few drops of sterile saline to form a doughy mixture that is placed in the parasymphysis areas over the lateral genioplasty flanges. This is extended posteriorly to the posteriormost edge of the genioplasty segment and is the reason it is so important to extend the osteotomy as far posteriorly as practical. It is relieved so it does not encroach on the mental neurovascular bundle (see Chapter 6).

---

*Integra LifeSciences Company, Plainsboro, N.J. 08536.

WIDENING GENIOPLASTY

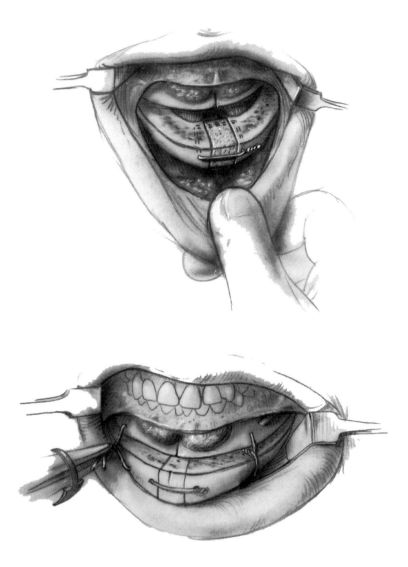

FIG. 9-49

In some patients, due to either the shape of the mandible itself and/or the magnitude of advancement, the lateral flanges of the advancement genioplasty are not extended sufficiently laterally to permit the optimal amount of lateral alloplastic augmentation. When this situation exists, a midline osteotomy of the mobilized chin segment is completed with the reciprocating saw and an interpositional graft is inserted and stabilized to widen the advanced chin segment. The interpositional graft material may be either bank bone or block hydroxylapatite.* When this procedure is done the remainder of the stabilization and lateral augmentation is identical to that previously described.

---

*Calcitek, Carlsbad, CA

MAXIMUM ADVANCEMENT GENIOPLASTY

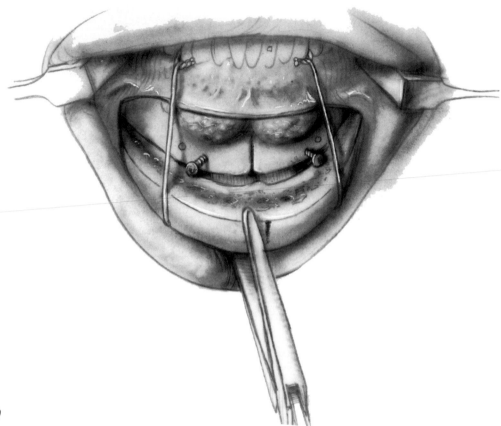

FIG. 9-50

When the preoperative cephalometric prediction tracing indicates that the patient would benefit from a chin advancement that *exceeds the thickness of the mandibular symphysis* in the region of the planned osteotomy (generally 10 to 12 mm), the following modification can be made to the usual genioplasty approach. After completion of the mobilization, two 2.7-mm screws are placed horizontally into the stable portion of the mandible just anterior and slightly inferior to the location of the mental foramina. The chin segment is then advanced and telescoped using these screws to prevent further superior displacement, which would result in compression neuropathy of the mental neurovascular bundles. While wiring as previously described and/or bone plating is possible to stabilize this advanced mandibular segment, stabilization of this segment is *best* achieved with two 22-gauge circummandibular wires, which are removed about 4 to 6 weeks postoperatively.

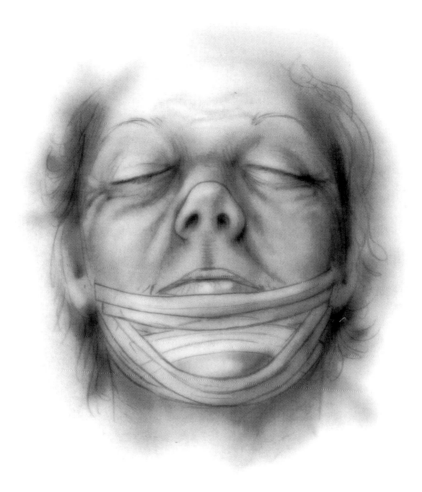

FIG. 9-51

In these instances both lateral and anterior hydroxylapatite-Helitene* augmentation is performed. When any of the aforementioned techniques are used, the soft tissues are closed in layers and pressure dressings are applied as described in Chapter 6.

---

*Integra LifeScience Company, Plainsboro, N.J. 08536.

Postsurgical orthodontic treatment

The use of rigid fixation for the postsurgical stabilization of the segmentalized maxilla has changed the postsurgical orthodontic treatment. Since not all patients will have rigid fixation, it becomes important that the surgeon communicate to the orthodontist specifically which of the three fixation techniques—total rigid fixation, anterior rigid fixation with posterior suspension wires, or infraorbital suspension wires only—has been used for the specific patient being treated. The postsurgical orthodontic treatment of patients stabilized by total rigid fixation or by anterior plates and posterior suspension wires is discussed here. Treatment of patients stabilized by infraorbital suspension wires is presented in the following section of this chapter.

TOTAL RIGID FIXATION (ANTERIOR AND POSTERIOR PLATES)

If all segments are stabilized with plates and screws there is little rush to see the patient after release from the surgeon's care. Indeed, the skeletal components are secured to such an extent that the postsurgical orthodontic treatment is just that—orthodontic. The orthodontist no longer has the ability to effect changes in the position of the segments, but can only move the teeth just as if no surgery had been done. It is still recommended that the patient be seen within a few days and that orthodontic refinement of the occlusion be done just as if no surgery had been done.

All archwires are removed at the first postsurgical visit and the orthodontic appliances are checked and repaired as necessary. The occlusion is documented with photographs so that postsurgical progress can be readily determined. If expansion was produced at surgery, a removable lingual arch is placed to maintain the arch width. Labial archwires are placed as if no surgery had been done, elastic therapy is begun when appropriate, and the patient is seen again in 1 to 2 weeks.

Progress is assessed at this appointment, and any appropriate mechanics changes are made. If loops were placed in the initial upper archwire, they may no longer be necessary and, if not, this wire may be replaced. Note that only dental movement is being done so any misalignment of the segments will require longer to correct than when stabilization is produced by infraorbital suspension wires. The need for continuing elastic therapy is noted and changed or discontinued as desirable. If there are no unanticipated problems, the patient is returned to the routine 4-week schedule for future adjustments. This rapid return to the usual schedule of appointments may seem to be beneficial; however, since all movements are effected by routine orthodontic methods, the postsurgical treatment, while less meticulous, will require a considerably longer time than when more rapid "orthopedic" movements of the segments are possible.

ANTERIOR RIGID FIXATION WITH POSTERIOR SUSPENSION WIRES

The more usual stabilization regimen for the segmentalized maxilla involves plate and screw fixation of the anterior segment and the use of skeletal suspension wires bilaterally for the posterior segments. When this technique is used, the posterior segments are more freely moved than the anterior segment for at least the first few weeks after the patient's return to the orthodontist. This fact is beneficial in that the teeth on either side of the osteotomy (ostectomy) can be rapidly leveled and aligned but *such is achieved primarily by movement of the posterior segment,* not the teeth in the anterior segment. If the teeth on either side of the osteotomy (ostectomy) site are not level, *these teeth will level by vertical movement of the posterior teeth.* When such leveling will elongate the premolars, it is best avoided during the first few weeks postsurgically, as the bite may be opened unless these teeth are not now in occlusion. If spaces exist at the osteotomy (ostectomy) site, these spaces will close rapidly *by forward movement of the posterior segments.* If an archwire is placed that is too wide, this increased width will rapidly be attained by the posterior segments. Each of these scenarios is somewhat opposite to the usual orthodontic situation, in which the posterior teeth are thought of as the anchor units used to produce movement of the anterior teeth. *Because of the "reverse anchorage" effect produced by this type of surgical stabilization, the orthodontist is cautioned to carefully consider the effect of any mechanics used during the first few weeks after the patient's return from surgery.* With the aforementioned general principles in mind, the following discussion will describe the usual postsurgical treatment for such a patient.

Treatment begins as soon as possible following the removal of the occlusal splint, preferably the same day and certainly within 48 hours following its removal. The ideal regimen is for the surgeon to remove the suspension wires, leave the splint wired to the maxillary teeth, and send the patient to the orthodontist's office. The orthodontist cuts the wires holding the splint, removes the splint, and proceeds with immediate orthodontic control of the maxillary dentition. This regimen is extremely beneficial, since the maxilla has been segmentalized at surgery, and when release of the suspension occurs 4 weeks postsurgically, the posterior segments are often still slightly mobile. When too much time elapses between removal of the splint and the first postsurgical orthodontic visit, such mobility can be detrimental. When no such time elapses, the posterior mobility can be effectively used by the orthodontist to effect rapid correction of minor arch shape or alignment problems *if the changes desired require movement of the posterior segments rather than movement of the anterior segment.*

After the splint is removed, the occlusion is documented with photographs. All archwires are removed, and the appliances are checked for damage. Any that are loose or bent are replaced. The lower archwire is checked for any crimps or bends and repaired or replaced as necessary. A continuous upper archwire, usually a 16 × 16 or 16 × 22 with T-loops at the osteotomy or ostectomy sites, is then made, coordinated with the lower archwire, and placed to effect leveling of the

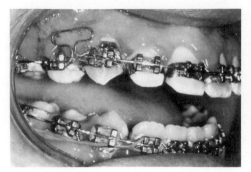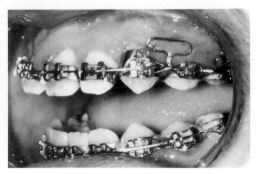

FIG. 9-52

teeth adjacent to the osteotomy (Fig. 9-52). Some clinicians may be tempted to use multistranded, nickel titanium or other flexible wire for their initial postsurgical archwire, but experience has shown that these are best avoided as they may produce considerable tipping of the teeth adjacent to the osteotomy or ostectomy. An alternative to using T-loops is to leave the presurgical segmental wires in place to preclude any tipping and tie a flexible archwire over them to produce alignment of the segments.

Leveling for this patient (anterior rigid fixation) will occur as the result of movement of the posterior segments. If the posterior segments are currently at their optimal vertical position, such that leveling would ideally be achieved by vertical movement of the tooth or teeth in the anterior segment, leveling is best delayed until osseous solidification of the posterior segments is complete (8 to 10 weeks postsurgically). At that time the anterior teeth can be intruded or extruded in the usual manner using the posterior teeth as anchorage.

Once the archwires are placed, wire ligatures are placed to tightly approximate the teeth on either side of the osteotomy or ostectomy sites (Fig. 9-52). These spaces will close by the forward movement of the mobile posterior segments in this patient. When this will tend to produce a Class II posterior occlusion, the spaces are "stabilized" by ligation of the adjacent teeth so that they cannot become larger and are closed by retracting the anterior teeth after the posterior segments have become solid.

When expansion of the maxilla has been performed, a lingual arch is placed to help stabilize this expansion (Fig. 9-53).

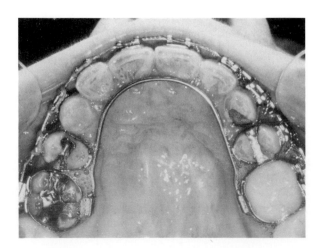

FIG. 9-53

The care necessary for making both the labial and lingual wires cannot be overstated. With segmentalization of the maxilla and mobility still present in the posterior segments, movement of these segments will be extremely rapid—a matter of hours rather than months. *Undesirable movements occur as rapidly as those that are desired.* Thus, the clinician must be certain that any movements that will take place are those intended.

The patient is instructed in the use of any elastics that are appropriate. Any type of elastics may be used, dependent only on the desired tooth movement. Note that elastics that attach to the "rigid" anterior segment (Class IIs to the canines) are capable of only orthodontic movement whereas those that attach to the posterior segments (Class III, cross bite) are capable of effecting movement of the entire posterior segment. When an elastic is used that produces an extrusive force on the posterior segments (such as Class III, or cross bite), this force must be balanced by light vertical elastics anteriorly. The patient is seen again in 2 to 3 days.

Progress is assessed at this appointment, and any appropriate mechanical changes are made. Usually the loops will no longer be necessary in the upper archwire, and this wire may be replaced unless leveling and/or space closure has been deferred for reasons previously discussed. The need for continuing elastic therapy is noted and changed or discontinued as desirable. Elastics are used as briefly as possible following surgery. Thus, elastics are worn at night only or discontinued altogether as soon as possible. The patient is seen again in 4 to 5 days.

Again, this appointment is to check progress. Minor adjustments in mechanics are made when desirable, and the patient is seen again in 1 week.

Further progress is closely observed. The next appointment is in 2 weeks and then, assuming the occlusion is progressing nicely, the patient is placed back on the routine 4-week adjustment schedule.

Finishing procedures are routine. There must be at least a 4-week period during which the occlusion remains stable with no elastic wear before the appliances are removed. Retention is done in the routine method with no special considerations being given to the fact that the patient had an open-bite before treatment.

Factors affecting stability of treatment
Orthodontic factors

Three orthodontic procedures have been noted as the most troublesome: (1) inappropriate use of vertical mechanics, (2) orthodontic maxillary expansion, and (3) failure to maintain lower arch width.

INAPPROPRIATE USE OF VERTICAL MECHANICS

The inappropriate use of vertical mechanics is almost exclusively related to attempted orthodontic closure of an open bite by extrusion of anterior teeth (Fig. 9-54). Such extrusion may be brought about in three ways: (1) leveling an exces-

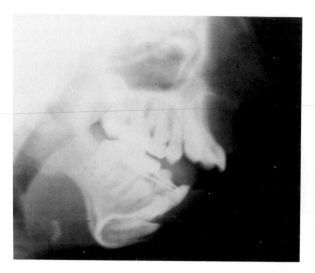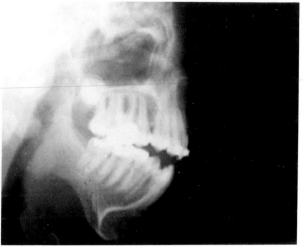

FIG. 9-54

sive maxillary curve of Spee by using continuous archwires from molar to molar, (2) leveling a reverse curve of Spee in the mandible in the same manner, or (3) using anterior vertical elastics. Regardless of how the anterior tooth extrusion is produced, it is unpredictably stable. Relapse of such extrusion postsurgically will result in recurrence of the open bite (Fig. 9-55).

PRESURGICAL ORTHO   SURGERY   ORTHO RELAPSE
                                           AFTER SURGERY

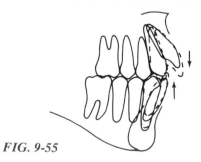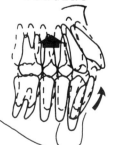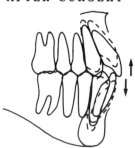

FIG. 9-55

To avoid this problem, segmental orthodontic treatment is recommended in any instance in which continuous archwires would tend to extrude anterior teeth. This does not mean that individual teeth within the segments cannot be leveled orthodontically but that this leveling is allowed to occur both by intrusion of teeth that are "too long" and by extrusion of teeth that are "too short," such that the teeth within a segment "seek their own level." By so doing, any tendency for relapse is greatly diminished. Ideally, intrusion of the incisors or maintaining their pretreatment level whenever possible is recommended. Doing so will often further open the bite orthodontically, but relapse of incisor intrusion following surgery will only serve to maintain the bite closed (Fig. 9-56).

PRESURGICAL ORTHO   **RELAPSE**

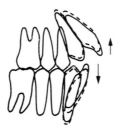 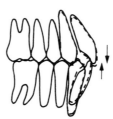

FIG. 9-56

ORTHODONTIC MAXILLARY EXPANSION

Maxillary expansion in individuals older than 16 to 18 years of age has been shown to be accomplished largely by dental tipping with little or no orthopedic movement. As such, this expansion is unstable in individuals who have a skeletal transverse maxillary deficiency. Surgical superior repositioning of the maxilla following orthodontic expansion does not increase the stability of this expansion. Relapse following orthodontic maxillary expansion, in addition to reestablishing a posterior cross bite, will tend to reopen the bite anteriorly by creating an increase in the effective posterior vertical dimension (that is, cusp-to-cusp instead of cusp-to-fossa occlusion or relative increase in the length of the teeth caused by the return to a more vertical position) (Fig. 9-57). Because of the problems associated with relapse of orthodontic maxillary expansion, it is recommended that this expansion be done surgically so that both the teeth and their supporting bone are repositioned. Although this does not preclude the possibility of relapse, with proper attention to technique, the potential for transverse relapse is greatly reduced.

EXPANSION   **RELAPSE**

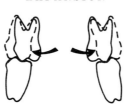 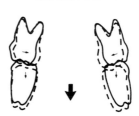

FIG. 9-57

The orthodontist cannot liberally expand the lower arch just because the maxilla will be expanded surgically. Indeed, the shape and width of the lower arch is maintained as close to the pretreatment condition as possible. The problems that have been experienced with maxillary narrowing following surgery have usually occurred in patients for whom the mandibular arch was excessively widened presurgically and subsequently retained by a fixed lower retainer.

Other orthodontic factors that are important in increasing stability are (1) effecting immediate orthodontic control following removal of the splint, (2) rapid reapproximation of teeth adjacent to osteotomies or ostectomies, and (3) judicious use of intermaxillary elastics. The first two of these are discussed in the postsurgical orthodontic treatment and will not be commented on further.

When both the presurgical orthodontic treatment and the surgical procedure have been well executed, there is little need for intermaxillary elastics. Usually brief wearing (2 to 4 weeks) of appropriate elastics immediately after removal of the splint will suffice to produce the desired occlusion. While movement is not so rapid with rigid fixation, when progress is slower than expected, it is important to determine carefully the reason why the occlusion is not being rapidly perfected (Chapter 5). Once a determination of etiology has been made, the possibility of correcting the problem orthodontically versus the need for reoperation must be carefully considered. As a general rule, *the more interarch elastics required and the longer the postsurgical orthodontic treatment, the more the tendency for relapse following the completion of treatment.*

One factor thought by some to be etiologically significant in both the creation of anterior open bite and the relapse of its treatment is the tongue. There is no scientific evidence to support this belief. Indeed, accumulating scientific and clinical evidence clearly indicates that the tongue is generally *not* contributory to either the original deformity or its relapse. The tongue is significant as an etiologic factor in the open-bite deformity only in the rare circumstances when the patient chronically or habitually postures the tongue anteriorly between the teeth, such that it actually hangs out of the mouth. In such an instance treatment by reduction glossectomy is considered (see "Tongue Evaluation," Chapter 1).

Surgical factors

When the Class II dentofacial deformity with open bite is corrected by segmental superior repositioning of the maxilla, there are generally anteroposterior, vertical, and transverse skeletal deformities that are simultaneously surgically corrected. Each of these has the potential for relapse and will be commented on sequentially.

ANTEROPOSTERIOR RELAPSE

When the Class II dentofacial deformity with open bite is corrected by isolated maxillary surgery, the maxilla will require both superior and posterior repositioning. To achieve these movements it is essential to remove bone posteriorly from the maxillary, palatine, and pterygoid bones (Fig. 9-58). Since this is technically the most difficult aspect of the operation, it is most apt to be incomplete.

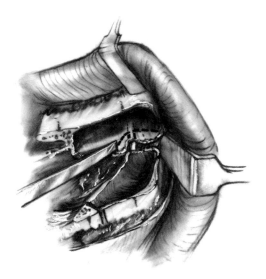

FIG. 9-58

When sufficient bone is not removed, the surgeon will, either unintentionally or in frustration, position the mandible forward a small amount at the time of surgery to place the teeth into occlusion. This results in an anterior and/or inferior displacement of the condyles from their fossas. Accordingly, during the period of intermaxillary fixation some skeletal relapse may occur, especially with dental fixation, at the expense of extrusion and tipping of the anterior teeth. However, on release of intermaxillary fixation, the mandible will acutely settle backward and a variable amount of Class II and/or open-bite malocclusion will reappear. Importantly, realization that the condyles have been displaced from their fossas is most often present at surgery and confirmed by the immediate postoperative radiographs. If left untreated, it becomes clinically manifest on release of fixation and the orthodontist must attempt, often unsuccessfully, to overcome the relapse.

Anteroposterior relapse can similarly result from basic errors in diagnosis and treatment planning. Failure to detect a centric occlusion–centric relation incompatibility or habitual occlusion during the diagnostic phase can result in errors in subsequent treatment planning that are then incorporated at surgery. Furthermore, if inaccurate surgical cephalometric prediction tracings or model surgery are done, the surgeon may believe that the maxilla is indeed properly positioned, despite the fact that it is not. A small error in each phase—diagnosis, treatment planning, and surgery—will generally compound rather than negate this problem.

VERTICAL RELAPSE

This results from a failure at surgery to establish a new maxillary occlusal plane that is compatible with the existing mandibular occlusal plane as the mandible autorotates upward and forward. This can result from inadequate superior repositioning of the posterior maxilla (inadequate posterior ostectomies), excessive superior repositioning of the anterior maxilla, or a combination of the two. In any instance the result is that the mandible will be forced upward anteriorly at surgery, using the posterior maxillary interferences as fulcrums, and displacing the condyles inferiorly from their fossas. When this occurs, the mandible will tend to resume its normal neuromuscular position both during fixation and on release of intermaxillary fixation. Relapse will be acutely or chronically manifest by an opening of the bite anteriorly. When inferior condylar displacement occurs in conjunction with an anterior displacement, as discussed in the preceding section, relapse occurs both vertically (open bite) and anteroposteriorly (Class II).

TRANSVERSE RELAPSE

Surgical expansion of the maxilla is possible to virtually any extent and can be stable if properly done. Presurgical knowledge of the amount the maxilla is to be expanded is necessary to prevent relapse. When greater than 3 to 4 mm of maxillary intermolar or premolar expansion is to be achieved at surgery, it is essential that (1) palatal soft-tissue-relaxing incisions are made, (2) the occlusal splint is constructed with a transpalatal bar to increase the transverse strength of the splint, and (3) the postsurgical orthodontic treatment deliberately retains the expansion for a few months after removal of the surgical occlusal splint to permit complete bone healing. In unusual cases requiring major expansion (greater than 10 mm), autogenous cancellous bone grafting of the lateral walls of the maxilla may be used to effect rapid bone union and promote transverse stability, especially when no palatal bone contact exists.

When transverse relapse occurs it is often manifest, at least in part, as an anterior opening of the bite. As the posterior teeth assume a cusp-to-cusp relationship, a downward and backward rotation of the mandible occurs and produces an anterior opening of the bite (see Fig. 9-57).

Age-related factors

The relationship of the age of the patient and the stability of treatment—specifically, at what age can the maxilla be successfully superiorly repositioned—has often been stated to be such that this surgery should be delayed until all facial growth is completed. This view is not supported by either the authors' experiences or the literature. Indeed, it is possible to successfully and stably superiorly reposition the maxilla once both the maxillary canines and second molars are sufficiently erupted to allow the surgery to be done (usually between 12 and 14 years).

To address the relationship of age, growth, and stability, two essential questions must be answered. First, what effect will maxillary superior repositioning have on subsequent facial growth? Second, what effect will this subsequent growth have on the result attained by the surgery?

EFFECT OF MAXILLARY SUPERIOR REPOSITIONING ON SUBSEQUENT FACIAL GROWTH

Considerable concern has been expressed about possible untoward effects of early maxillary surgery on subsequent maxillary growth. Specifically, it is known that early surgical resection of the nasal septum in animals can adversely influence subsequent maxillary growth. However, detailed experiments in primates have shown that (1) while septal resection does influence growth of the face, the effects depend on the amount of septum resected and the age at which resection occurs, and (2) some cartilaginous nasal septal resection can be accomplished without producing undesirable growth effects. Therefore, when considering superior repositioning of the maxilla during growth, the surgeon must consider performing the total subapical repositioning procedure, as described in the next section of this chapter, as opposed to the LeFort I procedure described herein, since the former involves minimal surgery on the nasal septum.

The growth of individuals following isolated superior repositioning of the maxilla has been studied. Observations have been made during postsurgical orthodontic treatment and retention for an average of 3 years and reveal that continued growth is expressed in a normal downward and forward direction for both maxilla and mandible. In general, the vector of growth is more favorable than would be predicted to occur in the Class II open bite patient without surgery. Specifically, facial growth is less vertical and more horizontal in nature. This altered vector of facial growth after surgery is, in part, the result of *reduced* vertical maxillary growth. Animal experiments have produced results that are almost identical to these.

In summary, early superior repositioning of the maxilla, especially by the total subapical technique, does not appear to produce detrimental effects on subsequent facial growth and may influence it favorably.

EFFECT OF SUBSEQUENT GROWTH ON THE SURGICAL RESULT

In addition to the fact that growth is observed to be essentially normal following superior repositioning of the maxilla, continued facial growth does not result in clinically significant effects on either the esthetic or occlusal result attained at surgery. During the postsurgical orthodontic treatment and retention, no more growth-related problems have been observed to occur in these patients than in the routine orthodontic population.

In summary, isolated superior maxillary repositioning during growth appears to produce a favorable effect on the subsequent vector of facial growth (relocation) and results in a stable occlusal result.

Results of treatment

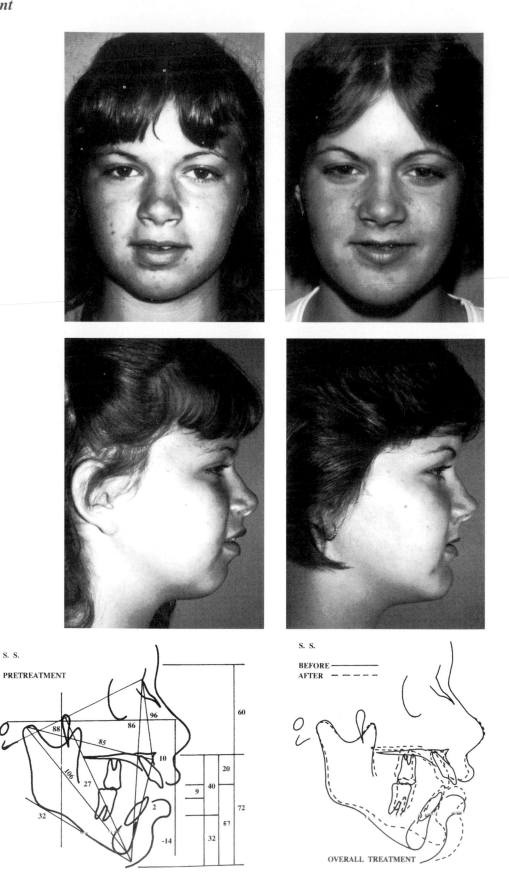

FIG. 9-59

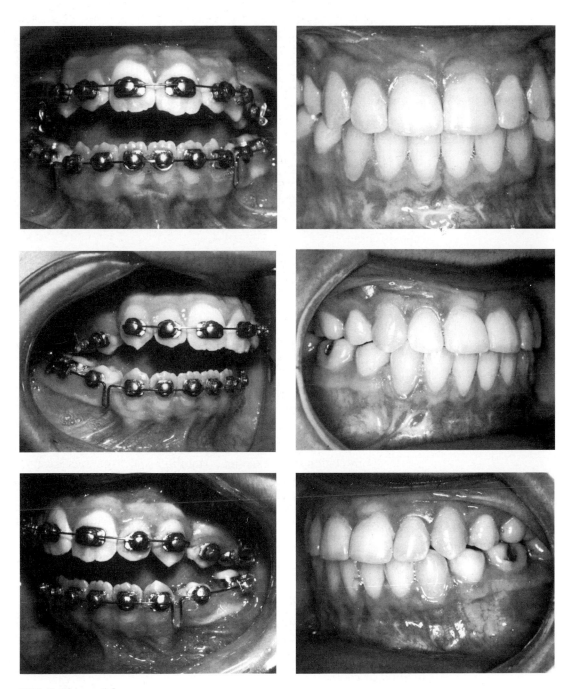

FIG. 9-59, cont'd

Alternate orthodontic-surgical approaches:
- *SEGMENTAL TOTAL SUBAPICAL SUPERIOR REPOSITIONING OF THE MAXILLA WITH ADVANCEMENT GENIOPLASTY*
- *SEGMENTAL SUPERIOR REPOSITIONING OF THE MAXILLA WITH MANDIBULAR ADVANCEMENT, ADVANCEMENT GENIOPLASTY, AND SUPRAHYOID MYOTOMIES*
- *MANDIBULAR ADVANCEMENT WITH ADVANCEMENT GENIOPLASTY AND SUPRAHYOID MYOTOMIES*

SEGMENTAL TOTAL SUBAPICAL SUPERIOR REPOSITIONING OF THE MAXILLA WITH ADVANCEMENT GENIOPLASTY

Contingency statement

When segmental superior repositioning of the maxilla is to be done, the surgeon must choose between performing the traditional LeFort I ostectomy or the total subapical superior repositioning of the maxilla, which leaves the nasal floor intact. The following are relative indications for total subapical superior maxillary repositioning.

1. More than about 6 mm of superior repositioning
2. Maxillary expansion, especially greater than 5 mm
3. Significant movement of multiple segments
4. Lateral maxillary walls more horizontal than usual

When these conditions exist, total subapical superior maxillary repositioning is preferred because:

1. It avoids decreased nasal airway function and avoids the necessity to perform turbinectomies.
2. It affords optimal bony contact or interfaces when the maxilla is expanded and thus eliminates the need for bone grafting while ensuring bony union and excellent stability since the increased bone contact minimizes the problems of "superior relapse" of the maxilla and nonunion (see Fig. 9-64).
3. It optimizes the vascular supply to the dentoalveolar segments.

The more severe the Class II vertical maxillary excess deformity with open bite the more complex the three-dimensional occlusal deformity—Class II relation, disproportionate vertical maxillary excess, and posterior cross bite. As the facial esthetic, skeletal, and occlusal discrepancies become more severe, it becomes increasingly likely that one or more of the indications for segmental total subapical superior repositioning of the maxilla exists. When several indications exist in the same patient, the total subapical procedure becomes the surgical method of choice.

As for the more usual segmental LeFort I procedure, the feasibility of correcting the existing deformity by isolated superior maxillary repositioning with or without advancement genioplasty, as opposed to simultaneous mandibular advancement, is predicted on facial esthetics, especially upper lip support. The details of orthodontic-surgical treatment are determined on an individual basis by carefully done orthodontic-surgical cephalometric prediction tracings (Chapter 2), which are correlated with the esthetic findings.

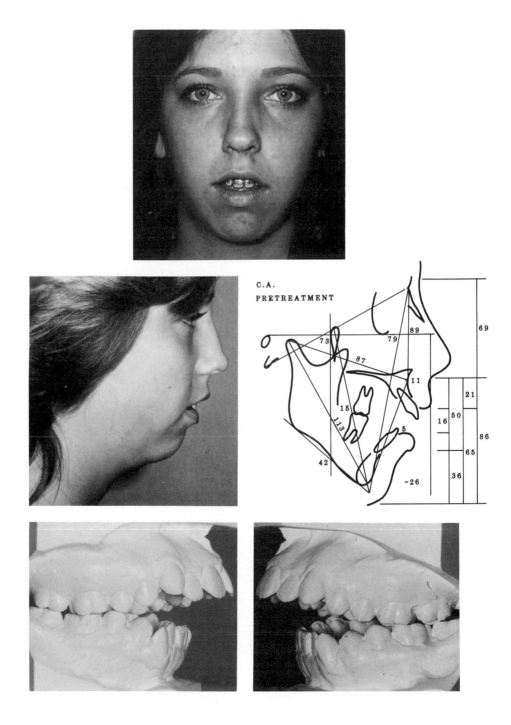

FIG. 9-60

Details of treatment

Presurgical orthodontic treatment

The presurgical orthodontic treatment for the patient with Class II deformity with open bite is extremely important with respect to facial esthetics, stability, and the need for simultaneous mandibular advancement. The presurgical orthodontic mechanics are not directed toward correcting the anteroposterior, transverse, or vertical problems, since they are most effectively corrected surgically. Rather, the basic goal of the presurgical treatment is to *symmetrically place the lower dentition in the proper anteroposterior, vertical, and transverse position with respect to the mandible such that when the maxilla is surgically repositioned, all the teeth will be in their proper position.* The symmetry of the lower arch will ultimately dictate that of the upper arch; thus, care must be taken during the presurgical orthodontic treatment of the lower arch to ensure that the lower midline is coincident with the facial midline and that the teeth in the buccal segments are placed properly with regard to their anteroposterior position. Any orthodontic procedures that tend to open the bite are best done presurgically. Thus, molar uprighting and rotation correction are routinely done presurgically, and the teeth are aligned so that no cross bites will need to be corrected following surgery. Finally, tooth mass must be given special attention, since it is desirable to place the teeth not only in an ideal Class I canine relationship, but in the ideal overbite and overjet relationship at surgery. Indeed, it is preferable to produce a slightly deep bite at surgery.

Any mechanics that are expressly intended to close the bite are avoided during the presurgical orthodontic treatment. As such, vertical elastics, high-pull headgear with a face bow, vertical pull headgear to a chin cup, or any other device used in an attempt to close the bite is inadvisable. Conversely, further opening of the bite during the presurgical phase is considered to be positive (see "Factors Affecting Stability").

Finally, when the maxilla must be expanded, it is preferable to effect such expansion as a part of the surgical procedure. By so doing, the stability is improved. Indeed, when expansion of the maxilla is necessary, the surgical procedure as described herein is actually simplified, by reducing the amount of bone that must be removed at the time of surgery (Fig. 9-61).

With the aforementioned general principles in mind and following appropriate notation on the patient's chart that combined orthodontic and surgical treatment is to be done, the actual presurgical orthodontic treatment can begin. Since the presurgical orthodontic treatment in the lower arch generally takes longer than that in the upper arch (12 to 18 months vs. 3 to 6 months) treatment is routinely begun in the lower arch.

Certainly not all patients will require extractions; the need for extraction is decided on an individual basis. When nonextraction treatment is desirable, it is done as described previously in this chapter. More commonly, extraction of upper and lower first premolars is necessary to treat the severe deformity described herein.

Following appropriate extractions in the lower arch, the lower appliances are placed. Bonded appliances are preferred, at least anteriorly, to allow any interproximal recontouring that may be needed to correct a minor tooth mass discrepancy. (Significant anterior tooth mass discrepancies may require extraction of one

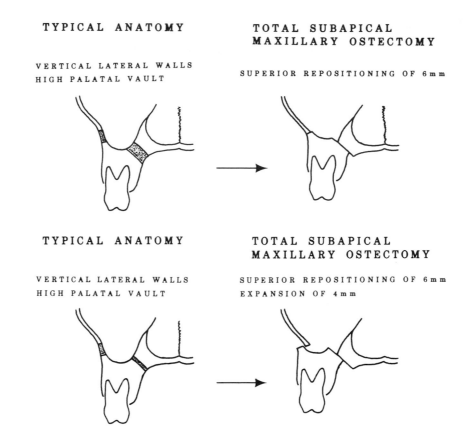

TYPICAL ANATOMY

VERTICAL LATERAL WALLS
HIGH PALATAL VAULT

TOTAL SUBAPICAL
MAXILLARY OSTECTOMY

SUPERIOR REPOSITIONING OF 6 mm

TYPICAL ANATOMY

VERTICAL LATERAL WALLS
HIGH PALATAL VAULT

TOTAL SUBAPICAL
MAXILLARY OSTECTOMY

SUPERIOR REPOSITIONING OF 6 mm
EXPANSION OF 4 mm

FIG. 9-61

lower incisor.) When placing the lower anterior appliances it is best to place them slightly (0.5 to 1 mm) lower than usual so that the brackets do not interfere with the production of the desired overbite at surgery. Although the initial archwire selection will depend on the anchorage requirements for the individual patient, most frequently a maximum anchorage situation exists in the lower arch and a stabilizing utility arch with retraction sectional arches to the lower canines is used. If the teeth in the buccal segments are poorly aligned, light flexible sectional archwires are used initially to produce alignment. When the lower canines are excessively labial, it is often helpful to place a lingual arch and use elastic thread from the lingual arch to the canines to supply a lingual vector during alignment and/or retraction to help move the canines out of the labial cortical plate thereby minimizing the strain on the anchorage (Fig. 9-62). When anchorage is critical, consideration can be given to banding the upper arch earlier than would otherwise be necessary and using Class III elastics to back up the lower anchorage.

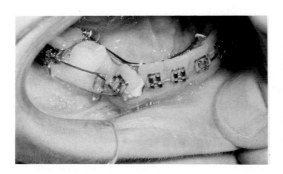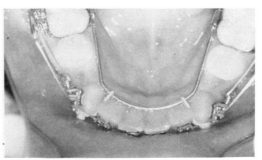

FIG. 9-62

Once the lower canines are fully retracted, 16 × 16 or 16 × 22 sectional arch-wires are placed to upright the canines as necessary and the lower incisor retraction is begun. When it is desirable to tip the lower incisors lingually (again most usual), this is most simply done with a boot hook utility arch made from .018 round wire and intraarch elastic traction (Fig. 9-63). This is an excellent time to take a progress lateral cephalometric radiograph to determine if retraction of the lower incisors will fulfill the pretreatment goals and if interarch elastics are necessary to supplement the anchorage.

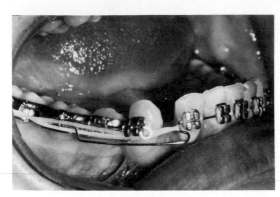 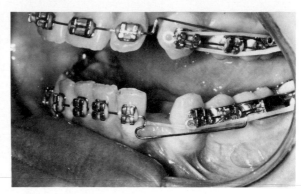

FIG. 9-63

Once the retraction of the lower incisors is begun, extractions are done in the upper arch. The exact timing of the upper arch treatment will vary from patient to patient and is dependent on the crowding, alignment, and rotational movements that must be made. The objective is to complete idealization of the upper segments and the lower arch at about the same time. Once the upper extractions are done, the appliances and segmental archwires are placed in the upper arch. It is particularly important that provision is made for using a removable lingual arch by attaching a lingual sheath to the upper molars (see Fig. 9-3). Presurgically, the lingual arch is effective in rotating and torquing the upper molars when this is desired. More importantly, it is an effective method of stabilizing any surgically produced expansion, effecting torque control in the buccal segments, and producing cross-arch stability during the postsurgical orthodontic treatment.

Sectional mechanics are used in the upper arch to maintain the dual occlusal plane usually found in the Class II open-bite dentofacial deformity and/or to prevent undesirable orthodontic expansion (see Fig. 9-4). Segmental mechanics virtually eliminate both the possibility of producing extrusive forces on the anterior teeth or intrusive force in the canine premolar area and the possibility of producing undesired orthodontic expansion. Thus, there are two posterior segmental archwires incorporating the second premolar and the first and second molars on each side and an anterior segmental archwire from canine to canine.

When the upper canines are excessively constricted relative to the lower canines and premolars, it is desirable to split the anterior segment into two segments (see Fig. 9-5) and to produce the desired canine expansion surgically, widening both the teeth and their supporting bone, rather than risk the periodontal problems and potential relapse frequently encountered when the canines are expanded by orthodontic means alone. This decision is predicated on the amount of expansion required and the status of the periodontal tissues in the upper canine regions. Orthodontic expansion is usually feasible when sufficient attached gingiva exists over the canines and less than 4 mm of canine expansion is to be produced primarily by tipping the crowns labially.

The initial sectional archwires are generally light, round wires to initiate bracket alignment. These wires are replaced (or not used at all when bracket alignment permits) by looped or plain rectangular archwires as soon as possible. Round wires can never produce the desired results because they turn in the brackets and cannot effect control of the torque throughout the segments. Seldom is it necessary to use a wire larger than 16×22 in an .018 bracket slot to produce all the torque control necessary, although larger wires may be desirable in some instances. The objective is to produce three or four segments that, when surgically repositioned, will fit the lower arch. As such, it is of no consequence how the segments are related to one another presurgically, but the teeth within each segment need to be properly related to one another in all three planes of space. The surgery then places the segments into their normal relation to the lower arch, and by so doing, the upper teeth automatically assume the proper relation to one another and their axial inclinations become normal (see Fig. 9-6).

Once the lower incisors have been retracted, a continuous 16×16 lower archwire is placed. It may be necessary to place loops mesial to the canines for vertical control of the incisors when changing from sectional wires to the continuous wires. (Loops are preferred to light flexible wires to effect this leveling as they do not produce the potentially adverse tipping of the teeth immediately adjacent to the vertical discrepancy.) Note that since the canine and incisor brackets were intentionally placed gingivally, step-downs are necessary to produce a level lower arch rather than one with a slightly increased curve of Spee (see Fig. 9-7).

The final archwires placed before surgery are generally 16×22. It is important that the upper sectional archwires are coordinated with the lower archwire. This is ensured by producing upper and lower continuous, coordinated archwires and then segmentalizing the upper archwires as necessary (see Fig. 9-8). Again, proper step downs are incorporated into the lower archwire as necessary. Care is taken that the general shape and width of the lower arch has been maintained and particularly that the lower canines have not been overexpanded (see "Factors Affecting Stability").

Once these archwires have become passive, impressions are made and feasibility model surgery is done by the surgeon and approved by the orthodontist. Perhaps the single most common problem encountered at this time is the existence of a small, previously undetected, tooth mass discrepancy that precludes the simultaneous production of a good Class I canine relationship and the desired amount of overbite. When this exists, it can usually be corrected by interproximal recontouring of the lower incisors or by opening spaces distal to the upper lateral incisors. A second potential problem is insufficient space through which to do the surgical ostectomies. This may be particularly troublesome where the orthodontic appliance has a built-in tip-back for the canines. It may be necessary for the orthodontist deliberately to tip the canine root mesially and the premolar root distally to provide surgical access. The surgeon should advise if such movements are necessary. When any problem is noted in the feasibility model surgery, appropriate corrections are made by the orthodontist and the feasibility model surgery is redone to confirm the successful resolution of the problem before surgery. When such model surgery produces the desired result, the archwires are tied with ligature wires to prevent inadvertent disengagement at surgery, appropriate hooks are placed where desired (usually on the canines), and the patient is referred for surgery.

Immediate presurgical planning

SURGICAL CEPHALOMETRIC PREDICTION TRACING

The surgical cephalometric prediction tracing for segmental total subapical superior maxillary repositioning with autorotation of mandible and advancement genioplasty is identical to that described in the previous section of this chapter except that the posterior portion of the bony palate is traced as a fixed structure after the mandible is rotated superiorly since it is not moved as part of this surgical procedure.

MODEL SURGERY FOR SEGMENTAL TOTAL SUBAPICAL MAXILLARY SUPERIOR REPOSITIONING

The definitive model surgery for total subapical superior maxillary repositioning with autorotation of the mandible and advancement genioplasty is identical to that described in preceding section of this chapter.

OCCLUSAL SPLINT CONSTRUCTION

The occlusal splint construction for segmental total subapical superior maxillary repositioning is similar to that described for segmental LeFort I superior repositioning with one critical difference—the palatal level remains the same while the adjacent dental alveolus moves superiorly. This results in a significant *decrease in the height of the palatal vault,* which must be taken into consideration when fabricating a palatal bar of the surgical splint.

The initial occlusal portion of the splint is made as previously described. Before making the palatal bar, base-plate wax is placed in the palatal vault to decrease the depth of the vault by the amount of the planned vertical movement of the posterior segments at the molars. Thus, if the molars are to be moved superiorly 8 mm, 8 mm of wax is placed in the vault. Once this is done, one thickness of base-plate wax is placed on the model from molar to molar to provide slight extra relief and the palatal bar is fabricated as described in the first section of this chapter.

Orthognathic reconstructive surgery

The definitive immediate presurgical cephalometric prediction tracing, model surgery, and splint construction are done shortly before surgery. The details obtained from these essential treatment planning aids are critical in determining the precise nature of the surgery to be performed and ensuring the stability of results. When segmental superior repositioning of the maxilla is to be done, the surgeon must choose between performing the traditional LeFort I ostectomy and the total subapical superior repositioning of the maxilla, which leaves the nasal floor intact. The following are relative indications for total subapical superior maxillary repositioning.

1. More than about 6 mm of superior repositioning
2. Maxillary expansion, especially greater than 5 mm
3. Significant movement of multiple segments
4. Lateral maxillary walls more horizontal than usual

When these conditions exist, total subapical superior maxillary repositioning is preferred for the following reasons:

1. It avoids decreased nasal airway function and avoids the necessity to perform turbinectomies.
2. It affords optimal bony contact or interfaces when the maxilla is expanded and thus eliminates the need for bone grafting while ensuring bony union and excellent stability since the increased bone contact minimizes the problems of "superior relapse" of the maxilla and nonunion (Fig. 9-64).
3. It optimizes the vascular supply to the dentoalveolar segments.

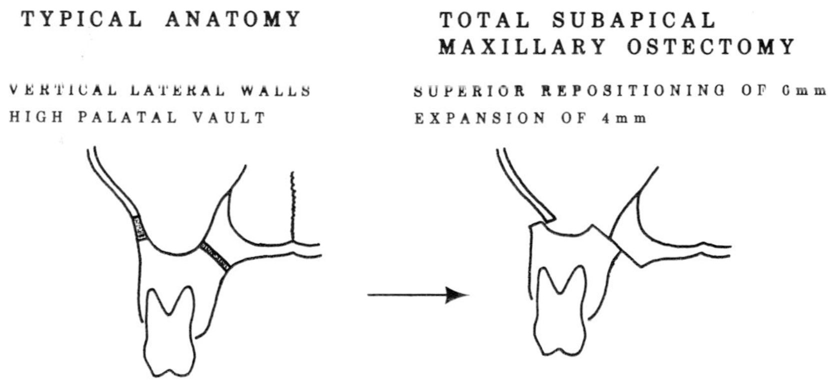

TYPICAL ANATOMY

VERTICAL LATERAL WALLS
HIGH PALATAL VAULT

TOTAL SUBAPICAL MAXILLARY OSTECTOMY

SUPERIOR REPOSITIONING OF 6mm
EXPANSION OF 4mm

FIG. 9-64

The surgical sequence preferred is first to complete the advancement and stabilization of the genioplasty. The mentalis muscle and mucoperiosteum are not closed until the end of the surgery so the magnitude and symmetry of the chin advancement can be reevaluated following the maxillary surgery. Second, a single midline palatal releasing incision is made. Third, the segmental total maxillary subapical ostectomy with superior repositioning is accomplished to completion and an alar-base-controlling suture is placed. Next, the maxillary vestibular incision is closed incorporating various extents of V-Y plasty depending upon the preoperative upper lip esthetics. Finally the layered closure of the chin incision is completed.

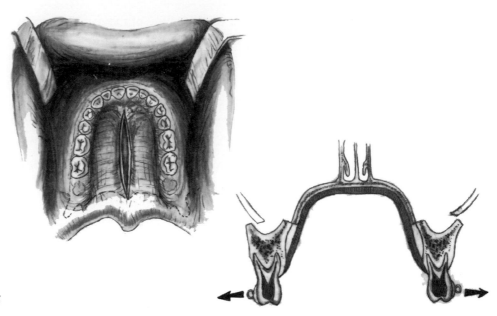

FIG. 9-65

The total maxillary subapical ostectomy with superior repositioning results in a decrease in the height of the palatal vault. This can potentially result in stripping the palatal soft tissues from the mobilized segments as they are moved superiorly. If this occurs it creates the potential for avascular necrosis due to significant reduction of the blood supply normally provided to the individual dentoalveolar segments by the attached palatal mucoperiosteum. To prevent this, a *midline* palatal-releasing incision is made from the posterior nasal spine anteriorly to the level of the second premolars and the palatal mucosa is undermined bilaterally about 5 mm. (It is subsequently completely removed from the stable palatal bone after down-fracturing; see Fig. 9-72.) Since this procedure maintains the bony nasal floor intact, the midline releasing incision will remain over well-vascularized bone and will heal by granulation after the maxilla has been repositioned.

About 5 to 10 minutes after injection of about 10 ml of 2% lidocaine with 1:100,000 epinephrine into the maxillary vestibule and posteriorly to effect second division anesthesia, an incision is made with a diathermy knife in the depth of the maxillary vestibule from the first molar area to the midline. The incision is stopped at the midline to preclude unnecessary bleeding on the opposite side while the ostectomies are being done on the first side. The subperiosteal dissection sequentially exposes the infraorbital nerve, the infraorbital rim lateral to the nerve, the piriform aperture of the nose, and the retromolar area to the pterygoid plate. The mucoperiosteal tissues inferior to the incision are not reflected from the underlying bone.

Internal and external reference marks and measurements are made as described in Chapter 7.

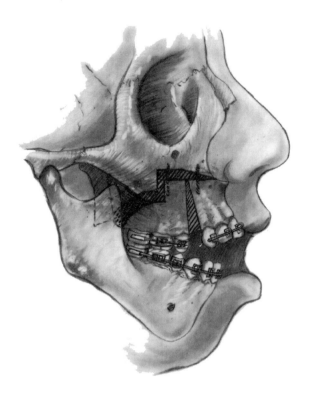

FIG. 9-66

The lateral wall ostectomy is begun anteriorly 35 mm above the canine cusp tip and is stepped inferiorly 10 mm at the first molar to a level 25 mm above the first molar cusps. As this ostectomy passes distal to the roots of the second molar tooth, it is tapered sharply inferiorly. If a maxillary third molar is present in this region, it is cut into or through, since it will be removed after the down-fracture. By directing the posterior ostectomy inferiorly, both the down-fracture and the subsequent removal of posterior bone are simplified.

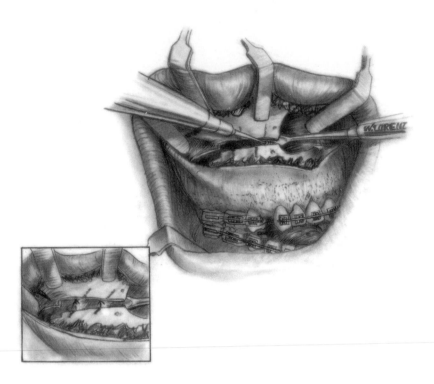

FIG. 9-67

The maxillary reference device used during the definitive model surgery is now interdigitated onto the maxillary dentition. Vertical reference lines are scored with a 701 bur on the lateral maxillary walls in positions similar to those made during the definitive model surgery—perpendicular to the occlusal plane in the area of the maxillary canine and first molar bilaterally.

Vertical reference lines made differently at surgery from those that were made on the model surgery will only serve to deceive the surgeon rather than aid him/her. A straight superior movement of the maxilla may appear as if the maxilla has been moved posteriorly as illustrated in the inset of Fig. 9-67. If the vertical reference lines were canted in the opposite direction, the maxilla would appear to have moved anteriorly with a straight superior movement.

The ostectomy of the lateral wall of the nose is completed about 10 to 15 mm posteriorly while a periosteal elevator is used to protect the nasal mucoperiosteum.

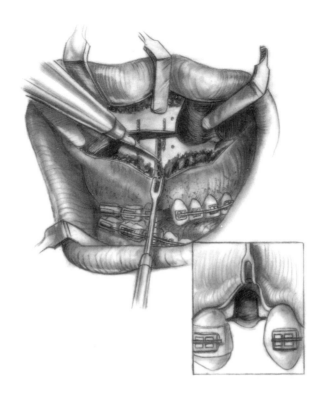

FIG. 9-68

In the Class II deformity with open bite, when a dual occlusal plane exists in the maxilla and segmental orthodontic treatment has been done, the interdental ostectomy is triangular in shape, being widest at the alveolar crest. In performing this ostectomy the outer cortex and its attached medullary bone is removed first through the vestibular incision so that the palatal cortex can be removed under direct visualization. While the palatal cortex is being removed, it is important to avoid direct injury to the major branches of the greater palatine artery lying beneath the periosteum. Moreover, while the palatal portion of this ostectomy is performed, care is taken not to elevate the palatal mucoperiosteum because it provides the primary blood supply, especially to the anterior maxillary segment(s). It is helpful to press a finger tightly against the palatal tissues to detect the bur as it just passes through the palatal bone. No attempt is made at this time to complete the transpalatal ostectomy, as this is more easily completed later (see Fig. 9-70).

The interdental ostectomy is continued by removing the necessary alveolar crestal bone through a soft-tissue crestal incision with limited subperiosteal dissection of the buccal attached gingiva. This permits direct visualization of the alveolar crestal bone during its removal and helps to avoid excessive removal of it or injury of the adjacent tooth roots. An adequate margin of alveolar crestal bone is always maintained adjacent to each tooth. At this time slightly less bone is removed than is thought to be necessary to avoid potentially creating a permanent periodontal defect. When the premolars are removed at the time of surgery, the same basic approach is used except that no crestal incision is required.

Similar soft-tissue incisions, subperiosteal dissection, and ostectomies are next completed on the opposite side.

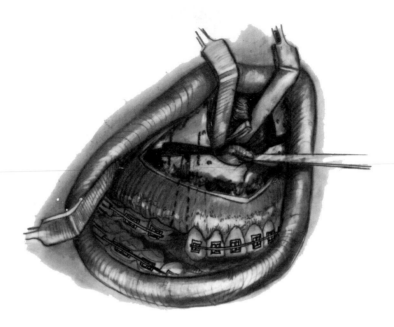

FIG. 9-69

The nasal mucoperiosteum is reflected from the anterior nasal floor about 15 mm posteriorly into the nose, and the cartilaginous nasal septum is reflected from the vomerian groove in the anterior nasal crest of the maxilla. The mucoperichondrium is reflected from the inferior aspect of the anterior cartilaginous nasal septum so that it can be removed later, if necessary, to avoid deviation of the nasal septum. The prominent anterior bony nasal crest of the maxilla is removed to provide improved access into the anterior nasal cavity for the transpalatal ostectomy and to prevent deviation of the cartilaginous nasal septum when the anterior maxilla is subsequently superiorly repositioned. After the nasal crest has been removed, it is smoothed with a mastoid bur and a groove is made to receive the cartilaginous nasal septum. When this phase of the surgery is performed, the nasopalatine vessels are transected and electrocoagulated if bleeding occurs. *The anterior nasal spine is not deliberately removed.*

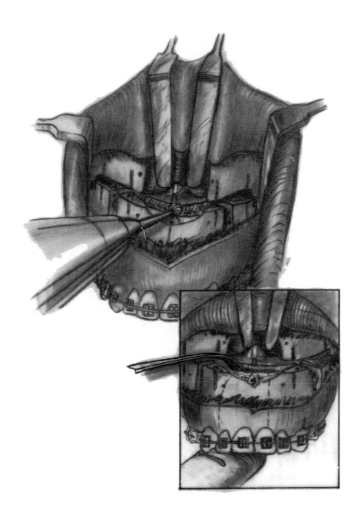

FIG. 9-70

The transpalatal ostectomy is now performed. A groove is made from the superior portion of the alveolar ostectomy on one side to that on the opposite side with a mastoid bur. The thickness of the palatal bone in this region is highly variable and can be estimated from the cephalometric radiograph. This groove is carried about 70% to 80% of the way through the palatal bone. Care is exercised not to make this initial portion of the ostectomy too deeply and transect the palatal mucoperiosteum and associated branches of the greater palatine vessels, since this will compromise the blood supply to the anterior maxillary segment and could result in its loss secondary to avascular necrosis.

No attempt is made to complete the transpalatal ostectomy with the mastoid bur. Rather, the osteotomy is completed with a small curved osteotome by sequentially malleting it along the groove (see Fig. 9-70, *inset*). While this is being done, a finger is maintained on the palatal tissues to detect the osteotome as it passes through the bone. Extreme care is exercised to avoid transection of the critical palatal mucoperiosteal vascular pedicle, which supplies the anterior segment(s).

On completion of the transpalatal osteotomy, the anterior maxillary segment is initially down-fractured either by manual pressure or by placing an osteotome in one of the alveolar osteotomies and prying it. *Completion of the down-fractur-*

ing and mobilization of the anterior segment is achieved only after both posterior segments are also initially down-fractured. Any attempt to complete the anterior down-fracture or to mobilize the anterior segment at this time will increase the possibility of compromising its critical palatal vascular pedicle.

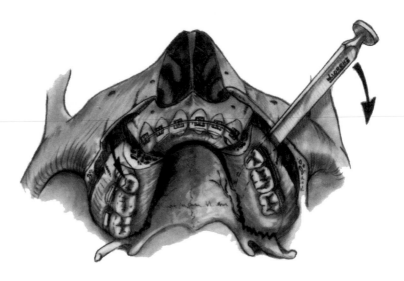

FIG. 9-71

A curved osteotome is now used to perform the transantral palatal osteotomies through the medialmost aspect of the maxillary sinus approximately where the vertical and horizontal components of the hard palate converge. This osteotomy is begun anteriorly and is progressively carried posteriorly to the region of the first molar tooth. After the osteotomy is completed to this point, the osteotome is left inserted into the palatal bone and the posterior maxillary segment is down-fractured by levering the osteotome inferiorly. This results in a posterior fracture that generally passes through the greater palatine foramen and preserves the associated neurovascular bundle. Posterior to the foramen the fracture extends predictably along the suture between the palatine-maxillary and pterygoid-maxillary bones. Neither extensive down-fracturing nor mobilization of the posterior segment is done at this time because doing so before reflecting the palatal mucoperiosteum from the stable horizontal portion of the palate can result in undesirable stripping of the palatal mucoperiosteal vascular pedicle from the alveolar segment (Fig. 9-71). The same procedure is now carried out on the opposite side.

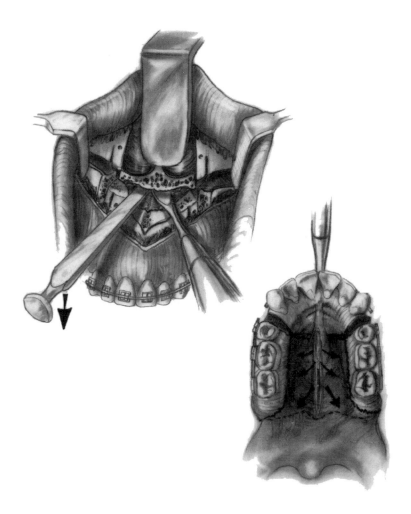

FIG. 9-72

After initial down-fracturing of the three maxillary segments has been achieved, the complete mobilization of the three segments is simultaneously achieved by *carefully reflecting the entire palatal mucoperiosteum from the stable horizontal portion of the palate through the transpalatal and transantral osteotomies.* During this dissection the greater palatine neurovascular bundles are readily observed just beneath the periosteum and preserved. On completion of elevation of the mucoperiosteum from the entire stable portion of the hard palate, the three maxillary segments become freely mobile.

The midline relaxing incision through the palatal mucoperiosteum previously described, permits unrestricted superior repositioning and expansion of the maxillary segments and avoids inadvertent stripping of the palatal mucoperiosteum from the *mobilized* segments as they are being superiorly and laterally repositioned. This incision results in exposure of the midpalatal bone after repositioning of the maxillary segments. This exposure is insignificant and will completely reepithelialize within 14 days.

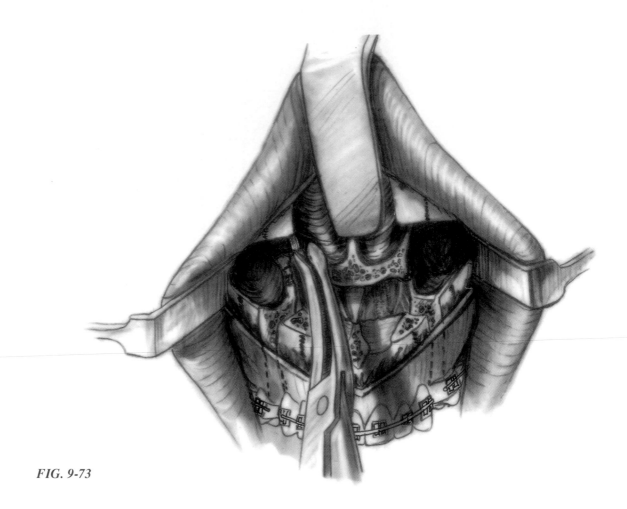

FIG. 9-73

On the basis of the planned direction and magnitude of movement of the segments, obvious areas of bone interference are removed at this time. These areas of interference vary depending on the details of the planned maxillary repositioning. If the maxilla is to be expanded and advanced with superior repositioning, generally no additional bone removal is required. When the maxilla is to be moved straight superiorly or superiorly and posteriorly without expansion, it is necessary to remove bone anteriorly and laterally from the stable portion of the palate and posteriorly from the retromolar areas. Anterior and lateral palatal bone is easily removed from the stable portion of the palate with a mastoid bur or rongeurs.

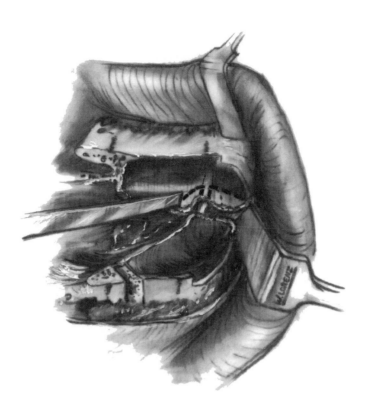

FIG. 9-74

When the maxilla is not being expanded or is being moved posteriorly, it is necessary to remove some bone medial and distal to the greater palatine neurovascular bundles. This is done with small curved or straight osteotomies while directly visualizing and preserving the neurovascular bundle. This decompresses the greater palatine neurovascular bundle and reduces the potential for both anesthesia and vascular compromise of the mobilized segments. Retromolar bone is readily removed from the mobilized segments by initiating an ostectomy with a bur and completing it with an osteotome. Often this will provide all the bone removal that is necessary, especially when the maxilla is being both expanded and minimally posteriorly repositioned. If the desired posterior repositioning cannot be achieved even after removing the maximum "safe" amount of retromolar bone, additional posterior bone is removed either by sectioning the pterygoid bone horizontally lateral to the neurovascular bundle, by sectioning the perpendicular portion of the palatine bone medially, or both. This is accomplished with an osteotome and the bone thus sectioned is depressed posteriorly.

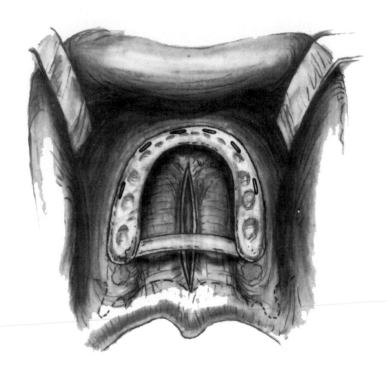

FIG. 9-75

After completion of these ostectomies, the segments are sequentially placed into the surgical splint. Wires are passed around the orthodontic brackets and through holes in the splint to secure the segments to the splint. When the segments are placed into the splint, there are often small areas of bony interference in the regions of the alveolar ostectomies. These interferences are judiciously removed with a 701 bur in a rotary handpiece as each segment is placed to avoid excessive removal of interdental bone that creates both periodontal defects and poor stability.

The surgical splint is constructed so that the maxillary teeth interdigitate maximally into it, thereby ensuring that the maxillary segments are optimally oriented as determined at the time of definitive model surgery. A heavy transpalatal acrylic bar is always incorporated into the splint to prevent bending of the splint with subsequent buccal tipping of the posterior segments when the maxilla is stabilized. The palatal bar also helps resist transverse relapse of any surgically produced expansion. This bar is constructed so that it will lie 2 to 3 mm away from the palatal soft tissues *after* superior repositioning of the maxillary dentoalveolus. Impingement of the transpalatal bar on the stable portion of the palate will both impair the vascular supply to the mobilized segments and preclude the desired amount of superior repositioning. The position of the transpalatal bar relative to the palate is always evaluated after the maxilla is stabilized.

After consolidating the maxillary segments sequentially into the surgical splint, the maxilla must now be able to be repositioned properly. This is checked by manually holding the maxilla into occlusion with the mandible and rotating the mandible-maxilla complex superiorly as a final check for possible bony interferences. While this is done, the condyles are carefully maintained within their fossas and the lateral maxillary wall reference lines are evaluated to make certain that they are related to one another as they were on the definitive model surgery. In order to ensure that the condyles are not displaced, the surgeon places his fingers directly on the gonial angles bilaterally and force is applied almost directly upward to effect the superior rotation of the maxillary-mandibular complex. Indiscriminately forcing the maxillary complex superiorly at this time without regard for maintaining the condyles "seated" in their fossa will result in either anterior or inferior condylar distraction. Any bony interferences that preclude the planned superior rotation with the condyles well seated must be detected and removed. Most often these will exist posteriorly.

Once the maxillary complex can be superiorly repositioned properly, the sinuses and oral cavity are irrigated and debris is suctioned. When adequate bone interfaces exist, the surgeon may choose from several stabilization techniques with equivocal results. Intermaxillary fixation is optional with any of the stabilization techniques outlined below. The criteria for skeletal suspension wiring verses rigid fixation are described in Chapter 2, "Step IV. Developing the Definitive Treatment Plan, Orthognathic Surgery, Type of Fixation."

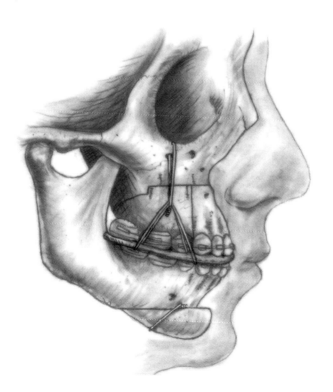

FIG. 9-76

The first and simplest option for maxillary stabilization is with infraorbital skeletal suspension wires. This technique is fast, inexpensive, and allows postsurgical orthodontic treatment to proceed quickly by permitting refinement of the occlusion by dental-orthopedic movement rather than by solely dental compensatory movement as seen with bone plate fixation. This stabilization technique is described on pages 501 to 504.

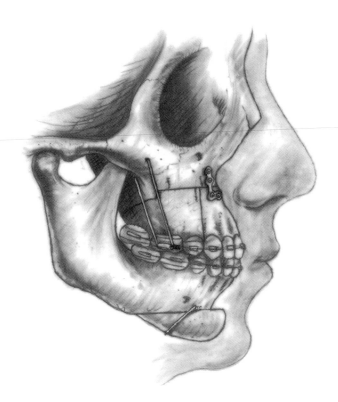

FIG. 9-77

The usual method used to stabilize the segmental total subapical maxillary ostectomy is with posterior buttress suspension wires and piriform rim bone plates. This technique is described in Chapter 7 and is not repeated here.

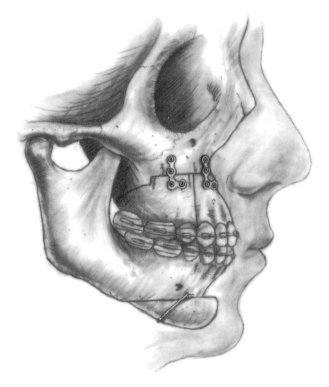

FIG. 9-78

If bone contact is inadequate or if the lateral maxillary walls are exceedingly thin, four bone plates may be used to stabilize the segmentalized maxilla.

After securing the maxilla, the cartilaginous nasal septum is inspected to make certain that it is in the midline and not deviated. If it is deviated because of inadequate removal of bone, a portion of the inferior aspect of the cartilaginous septum is removed until no deviation exists. This is done carefully to prevent excessive removal that will decrease nasal tip support and projection. The soft-tissue closure is variable and is predicted on control of nasal and upper lip esthetics. These factors are described and illustrated in Chapter 7.

Finally, if an advancement genioplasty was performed, the magnitude and symmetry of the advancement is checked to ensure that the chin is still accurately placed. If so, the chin is closed in a layered fashion.

If intermaxillary fixation is used, the fixation is released 2 to 3 weeks postsurgically by cutting the interdental wires. The occlusal splint remains attached to the maxillary teeth and any suspension wires. The patient is instructed to begin active jaw opening and protrusive exercises, but no chewing is permitted. The patient is to return for reevaluation in 24 to 72 hours. He/she is informed that during this time the teeth must continue to bite perfectly into the occlusal splint. No elastics are used because they will only mask relapse.

When the patient is observed to bite perfectly into the splint after the initial 24 to 72 hours, instructions are given to begin more vigorous isometric and isotonic exercises. This is to be done by the patient exercising four times daily as follows. First, the mouth is vigorously opened as widely as possible. Next, the patient is to bite into occlusion forcefully and then to protrude the lower jaw as far as possible. While performing these exercises, the patient is given visual objectives regarding the desired interincisal opening and protrusive movement consistent with the measurement of the presurgical range of jaw movement.

About 1 week later, when the patient has resumed essentially a normal range of jaw movement and the mandibular teeth continue to bite perfectly into the splint, the splint and suspension wires are removed under light sedation or local anesthesia. Before removal, the wires are carefully cleaned where they enter the mucosa and cut beneath the mucosa by forcing it down around the wire. This prevents possible infection and avoids the necessity to use antibiotics. The patient is to see the orthodontist within the next 48 hours to begin active postsurgical orthodontic treatment. A return to normal masticatory function is gradually and progressively resumed over the next 2 weeks.

If at any time after release of intermaxillary fixation the patient does not occlude properly, the specific reason(s) is identified and appropriately managed (Chapter 5).

Postsurgical orthodontic treatment

The advent of rigid fixation has changed the postsurgical orthodontic regimen; thus, it is important that the surgeon communicate to the orthodontist the specific fixation technique used for each individual patient. The discussion that follows pertains specifically to postsurgical treatment of the patient for whom the maxilla has been segmentalized and skeletal stabilization has been provided by *infraorbital suspension wires*. Postsurgical considerations for the patient whose maxilla has been segmentalized and for whom rigid fixation was used is described in the previous section of this chapter.

When infraorbital suspension wires have been used to provide skeletal stabilization, the postsurgical orthodontic treatment begins as soon as possible following the removal of the occlusal splint—preferably the same day and certainly within 48 hours following removal. The ideal situation is for the surgeon to remove the suspension wires, leave the splint wired to the maxillary teeth, and send the patient to the orthodontist's office. The orthodontist cuts the wires holding the splint, removes the splint, and proceeds with *immediate* orthodontic control of the maxillary dentition. This regimen is extremely beneficial, since when the maxilla has been segmentalized at surgery and release of the suspension occurs 4 weeks postsurgically, the segments are often still slightly mobile. When too much time elapses between removal of the splint and the first postsurgical orthodontic visit, such mobility can be detrimental because of unplanned movement of the dentoosseous segments. When no such time elapses, the mobility can be used by the orthodontist to effect rapid correction of minor arch shape or alignment problems.

After the splint is removed, the occlusion is documented with photographs. All archwires are removed, and the appliances are checked for damage. Any that are loose or bent are replaced. The lower archwire is checked for any crimps or bends and repaired or replaced as necessary. A continuous upper archwire, usually a 16 × 16 or 16 × 22 with T-loops at the osteotomy or ostectomy sites, is then made and carefully coordinated with the lower archwire (see Fig. 9-52). Some clinicians may be tempted to use multistranded, nickel titanium or other flexible wire for their initial postsurgical archwire, but experience has shown that these are best avoided as they may produce considerable tipping of the teeth adjacent to the osteotomy or ostectomy. An alternative to using T-loops is to leave the presurgical segmental wires in place to preclude any tipping and tie a flexible archwire over them to produce alignment of the segments.

When surgical expansion of the maxilla has been performed, a lingual arch is placed to help stabilize this expansion (see Fig. 9-53). The care necessary in making both the labial and lingual wires cannot be overstated. With segmentalization of the maxilla and mobility still present in the segments, movement of the segments is extremely rapid—a matter of hours rather than months. Undesirable movements occur as rapidly as those that are desired. Thus, *the clinician must be certain that any movements that will take place are those desired.*

Once the archwires are placed, ligature wires are placed to tightly approximate the teeth on either side of the osteotomy or ostectomy sites (see Fig. 9-52) and the patient is instructed in the use of any elastics that are appropriate. Note that any type of elastics may be used, depending only on the desired tooth movement. However, when an elastic is used that produces an extrusive force on the posterior teeth (such as Class II, Class III, or cross bite), this force must be balanced by light vertical elastics anteriorly. The patient is seen again in 2 to 3 days.

Progress is assessed at this appointment, and any appropriate mechanical changes are made. Usually the loops will no longer be necessary in the upper archwire, and this wire may be replaced. The need for continuing elastic therapy is noted and changed or discontinued as desirable. Elastics are used as briefly as possible following surgery. Thus, elastics are worn at night only or discontinued altogether as soon as possible. The patient is seen again in 4 to 5 days.

This appointment is again to check progress. Minor adjustments in mechanics are made when desirable, and the patient is seen again in 1 week.

Further progress is closely observed. The next appointment is in 2 weeks and then, assuming the occlusion is progressing nicely, the patient is placed back on the routine 4-week adjustment schedule. Finishing procedures are routine. There must be at least a 4-week period during which the occlusion remains stable with no elastic wear before the appliances are removed. Retention is accomplished routinely, with no special considerations being given to the fact that the patient had an open bite before treatment.

Factors affecting stability of treatment

The orthodontic, surgical, and age-related factors that affect the overall stability of results are the same as previously discussed in this chapter (pp. 514 to 519).

Details of treatment

Presurgical orthodontic treatment

The presurgical orthodontic treatment for these patients is the same as presented earlier in this chapter. The addition of a mandibular advancement and advancement genioplasty that requires the addition of suprahyoid myotomies to the surgical regimen in no way affects the presurgical orthodontic treatment objectives that are to place the teeth into their ideal anteroposterior and transverse relation and to eliminate crowding so that the teeth can be placed into a good Class I occlusion at surgery. A prediction tracing is necessary to determine the need for extractions and to plan the anchorage requirements. With the counterclockwise rotation of the distal mandible, the chin (pogonion) is advanced more than the teeth. Thus, the need for extractions and anchorage is generally less than for either isolated superior repositioning or mandibular advancement.

The reader is referred to the presurgical orthodontic discussions previously in this chapter for detailed explanation of this aspect of treatment when the maxilla is to be segmentalized. When nonsegmental maxillary superior repositioning is to be done, the discussions in Chapters 7 and 8 will provide the necessary information.

Orthognathic reconstructive surgery

The definitive surgical cephalometric prediction tracing, model surgery, and final and intermediate splint construction are done shortly before surgery as described previously in this chapter.

The sequencing of the surgery is as follows:

1. The genioplasty and suprahyoid myotomies are completed first and stabilized, but the incision is not closed.
2. The sagittal ramus osteotomies are completed and the splits initiated to assure that the desired split will occur, but the splits are not completed.
3. The maxillary surgery is completed. The maxilla is positioned with the aid of the intermediate splint and reference marks and is stabilized in its final position.
4. The sagittal splits are now completed, the mandible is mobilized, the teeth are wired into intermaxillary fixation, and the mandible is semi-rigidly (two screws) stabilized.
5. The skeletal suspension wires are completed from the piriform rims to the circummandibular wires.

Clinical evaluation of the patient and careful examination of the cephalometric prediction tracings are essential to determine the possible need for suprahyoid myotomies. If the patient can easily protrude the mandible into a Class III incisal relation with little palpable tension in the suprahyoid region, it is suggestive that the patient may not require a suprahyoid myotomy. However, when an anterior open bite is being corrected and an advancement genioplasty is also to be done, this clinical evaluation assumes less significance.

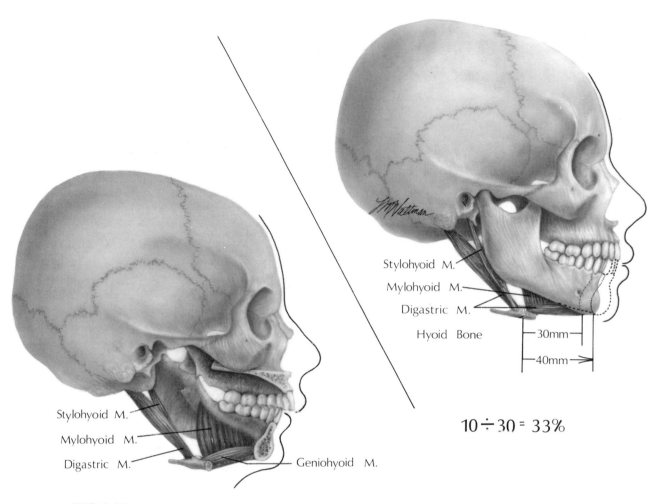

Stylohyoid M.

Mylohyoid M.

Digastric M.

Hyoid Bone

30mm

40mm

$$10 \div 30 = 33\%$$

Stylohyoid M.

Mylohyoid M.

Digastric M.

Geniohyoid M.

FIG. 9-81

In such instances measurements of the potential lengthening of the suprahyoid musculature is made from the completed cephalometric prediction tracing. If the suprahyoid musculature will lengthen more than 30%, a suprahyoid myotomy is planned (Fig. 9-81).

If suprahyoid myotomies are done in conjunction with the usual advancement genioplasty described in Chapter 6, this will result in a free bone graft of the chin segment that will subsequently undergo extensive resorption. Thus, *when suprahyoid myotomies are indicated, the genioplasty approach must be modified* as described next.

When advancement genioplasty, and suprahyoid myotomies are to be done simultaneously with other orthognathic surgical procedures, the genioplasty and suprahyoid myotomies are performed first. In addition, when circummandibular wires are to be used, they are best placed immediately *after* completion of the genioplasty.

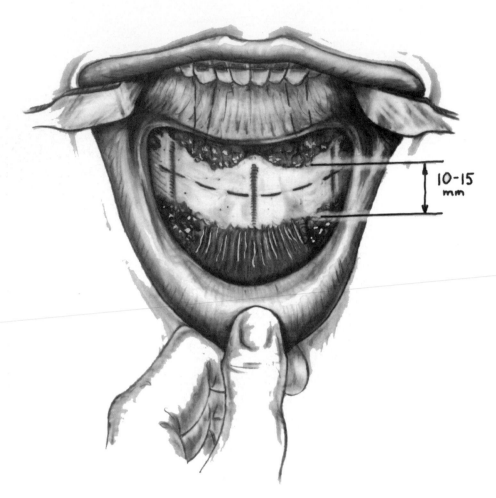

FIG. 9-82

The incision, soft-tissue dissection, and horizontal osteotomy for the genioplasty are performed *without degloving the symphysis* as described for the reduction genioplasty in Chapter 6. Care is taken to maintain maximal attachment of the labial and inferior border soft tissues to the chin segment that is to be advanced since, once the superhyoid myotomies are done, these soft-tissue attachments serve as the sole vascular predicle for the genioplasty segment.

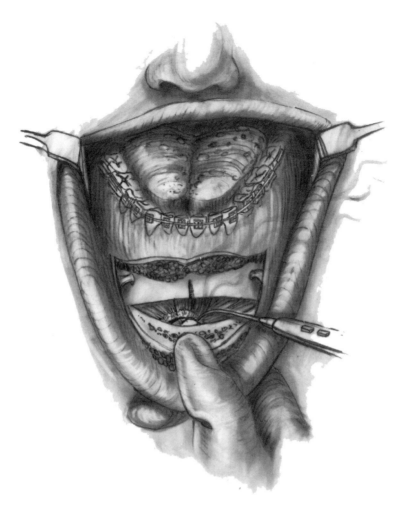

FIG. 9-83

On completion of the horizontal osteotomy, the genioplasty segment is mobilized inferiorly and the geniohyoid muscle and anterior bellies of the digastric muscles are removed from the mobilized segment by the lingual approach. The geniohyoid muscle is most readily removed with a diathermy knife; the digastric muscles are easily removed with a periosteal elevator.

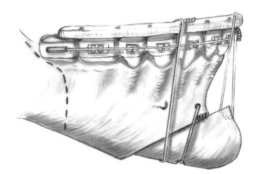

FIG. 9-84

On completion of the removal of the suprahyoid muscles, the chin is advanced and directly wired or plated as described in Chapter 6. A midline wire attached to the occlusal splint may be included to provide additional vertical stability.

After the genioplasty and suprahyoid myotomies are completed, the wound is packed with moist gauze sponges. The incision is left open until after completion of the maxillary superior repositioning and mandibular advancement to permit observation of the genioplasty surgical site to make certain that the genioplasty segment has not been inadvertently displaced during the subsequent orthognathic surgery.

The maxillary surgery is similar to that discussed previously in this chapter and the mandibular advancement is performed as described in Chapter 6. When correction of the Class II deformity with anterior open bite requires sufficient forward movement of pogonion to warrant suprahyoid myotomies, both the mobilization of the distal segment of the mandible and the method of stabilization are critical to avoid relapse.

Mobilization of the distal mandible is done in the same manner as described in Chapter 6. However, when the amount of correction is great, more time and effort must be expended in stretching the perimandibular soft tissues to ensure that the distal mandible can be placed into the desired occlusion *with little to no pressure*. It is also more difficult, yet more important, that the proximal segment be maintained in its original position while effecting this large mobilization to avoid potential injury to the temporomandibular joint.

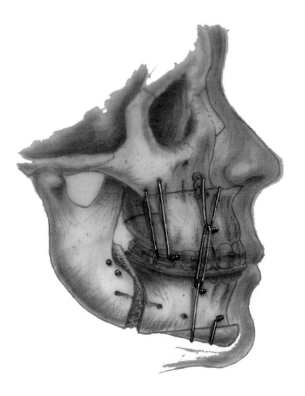

FIG. 9-85

Skeletal maxillomandibular intermaxillary fixation, as opposed to rigid fixation, is preferred when the pogonion is advanced 10 mm or more (including the genioplasty). When used, skeletal intermaxillary fixation is effected by placing 22-gauge intermediate wires between the piriform rim Wires and the circummandibular wires. This skeletal intermaxillary fixation is maintained for *at least*

6 weeks. In severe cases it is maintained for an additional 1 to 2 weeks, depending on the amount of pogonion advancement and open-bite correction. Following release of intermaxillary fixation, the same regimen of jaw physiotherapy and follow-up evaluation is followed as described for mandibular advancement in Chapter 6.

Postsurgical orthodontic treatment

The postsurgical orthodontic treatment is done as described previously in this chapter. The addition of a mandibular advancement does not affect the orthodontic mechanics necessary to finish the case in any manner except that this patient will be resuming orthodontic treatment about 10 weeks postsurgically, instead of 3 to 4 weeks, because of the need for a stable union of the sagittal advancement site. Thus, the maxillary segments exhibit little if any mobility, and the orthodontic movements, although still more rapid than if surgery had not been done, are considerably slower than when treatment is resumed with slightly mobile segments.

Factors affecting stability of treatment
Orthodontic factors

The factors affecting stability of orthodontic-surgical treatment of the Class II open bite by simultaneous superior repositioning of the maxilla and mandibular advancement are the total of those for superior repositioning of the maxilla and those for mandibular advancement:

1. Avoid inappropriate presurgical use of vertical mechanics
2. Maxillary expansion is to be done surgically
3. Make the occlusion more Class II before surgery
4. Properly manage tooth mass discrepancies before surgery
5. Adequately level the lower arch and upper segments
6. Adequately coordinate the lower arch and upper segments

The reader is directed to the factors affecting stability of treatment (usual treatment approach) in Chapters 6 and 7 for a complete discussion regarding these factors.

Surgical factors

Most surgically related relapse with superior maxillary repositioning and mandibular advancement surgery is directly related to surgical technique and occurs primarily during or immediately on release of intermaxillary fixation. The surgical factors that contribute to relapse have already been covered in Chapters 6 and 7 and include: (1) mobilization of the distal mandible, (2) distraction of the condyle from the fossa, and (3) method of intermaxillary fixation.

Results of treatment

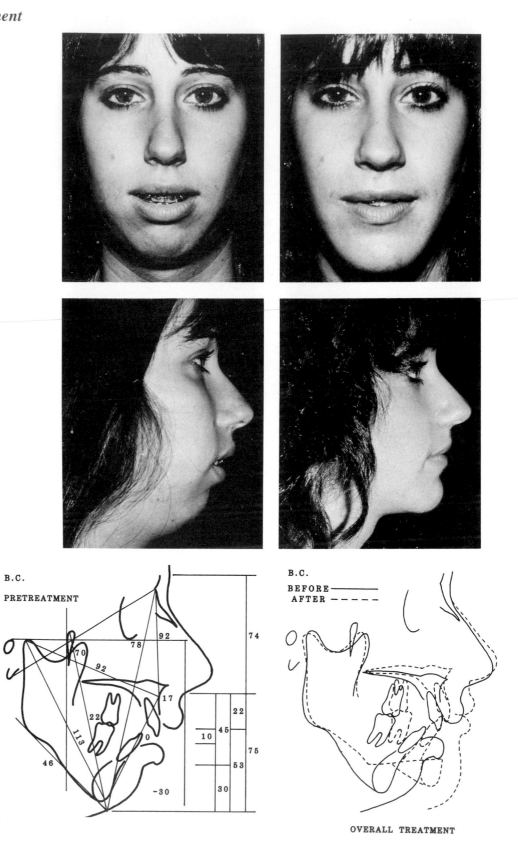

FIG. 9-86

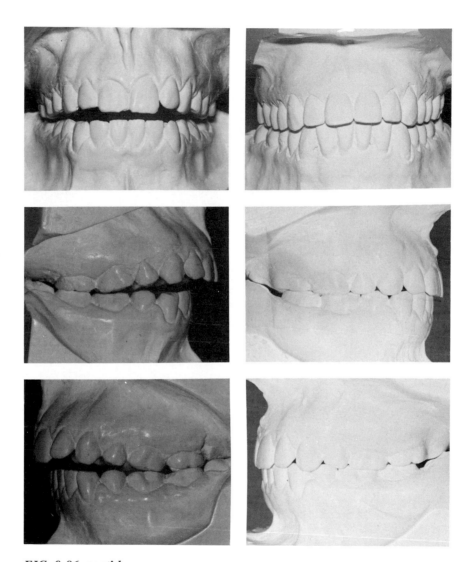

FIG. 9-86, cont'd

MANDIBULAR ADVANCEMENT WITH ADVANCEMENT GENIOPLASTY AND SUPRAHYOID MYOTOMIES

Contingency statement

A small percentage of patients with Class II dentofacial deformity and open bite do not have the typical facial, skeletal, or occlusal features associated with this deformity. Posterior vertical maxillary excess and transverse maxillary deficiency do not exist. Facially, these individuals have normal alar base width, nasal tip projection, upper lip support, and upper tooth-to-lip relations. They have a slightly increased lower face height, slightly excessive interlabial distance, and a recessive chin. Skeletally they are normal with the exception of a short ascending mandibular ramus height and an anteroposteriorly deficient mandible. The occlusion is Class II generally with an infantile type of open bite (only the terminal molars in occlusion). The occlusal planes are flat yet divergent, and normal transverse relations exist with minimal dental compensations. When these specific conditions are present, excellent facial esthetics and occlusion can be achieved by mandibular advancement surgery either with or without advancement genioplasty.

Pogonion will often be advanced a considerable distance for these patients. Accordingly, tension of the suprahyoid musculature may become considerable and exert additional forces that can contribute to relapse of the advanced mandible. Importantly, when a horizontal osteotomy for advancement genioplasty is also indicated, this will further increase the untoward effects of the suprahyoid musculature on stability. In such instances consideration must be given to performing suprahyoid myotomies.

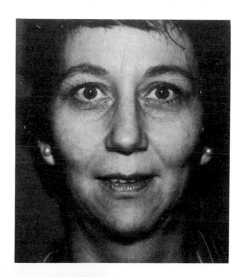

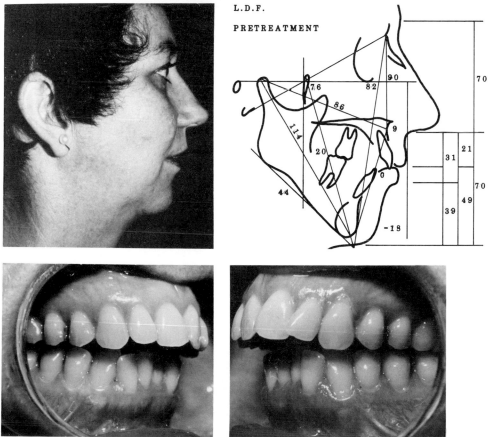

FIG. 9-87

Details of treatment

Presurgical orthodontic treatment

The objectives of the presurgical orthodontic treatment for these patients is to place the teeth into their ideal anteroposterior and transverse relation and to eliminate crowding so that the teeth can be placed into a good Class I occlusion at surgery and so that the chin will be in its ideal position or can be made so with an advancement genioplasty. A prediction tracing is necessary to determine the need for both a genioplasty and extractions and to plan the anchorage requirements. With the counterclockwise rotation of the distal mandible, the chin (pogonion) will be advanced more than the teeth. Thus, the need for extractions and anchorage is generally less than that encountered for the non-open bite dentofacial deformity, which requires mandibular advancement. Frequently, these patients do not require extractions. When this is so, the details of nonextraction treatment presented in Chapter 6 (second usual approach) are used. When extractions are necessary, the anchorage requirements must be determined from the prediction tracing and appropriate mechanics used to produce the desired presurgical result (first usual approach, Chapter 6).

Transversely there must be no more than 4 mm of total discrepancy at any given point with the models held in the desired Class I occlusal relation. When this is true, 1 mm of expansion on each side of the maxilla and 1 mm of constriction on each side of the mandible will eliminate the transverse problem and is within the range of stable orthodontic movement. When more transverse discrepancy exists and is not the result of dental tipping, combined orthodontic-surgical expansion of the maxilla as discussed in Chapter 6 is generally indicated for any patient over age 16 to 18 years, whereas orthopedic maxillary expansion can be used for the younger patient.

The use of vertical mechanics designed to close the bite (for example, vertical elastics, high-pull headgear, or chin cup) must not be used during the presurgical treatment because of the potential instability of these procedures. When a patient has had such procedures used (Fig. 9-88), it is recommended that all ver-

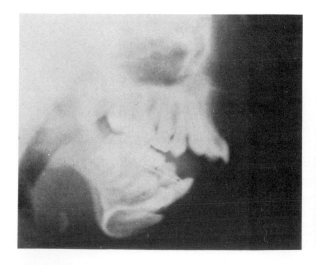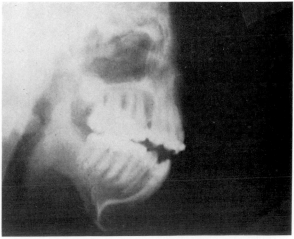

FIG. 9-88

tical mechanics be discontinued. Light (.012) sectional archwires are placed to hold alignment and rotations, and any vertical relapse is allowed to occur, until no further measurable opening of the bite occurs. At this time, the patient is reevaluated and treated as appropriate (that is, by the method described here, or by any of the methods described in Chapters 6 through 9) to correct the situation that exists after any vertical relapse has occurred.

With the above general principles in mind and after noting on the patient's chart that he/she will be treated by combined orthodontic and surgical procedures, the appliances are placed and initial leveling and aligning are done with flexible nickel titanium, braided round, or rectangular archwires. The bracket height is critical and must be carefully controlled so that a slight curve of Spee is produced with the lower second molar, lower canines, and incisors elevated above the functional occlusal plane by 0.5 to 1 mm while the upper arch is flat except for the second molars, which are elevated above the functional plane by 1 mm. Progressively larger archwires are placed, eventually reaching either 16 × 16 or 16 × 22 archwires for torque control and arch coordination.

Most commonly the upper and lower arches are treated independently. Class II or Class III elastics are avoided whenever possible because of the vertical component of their activity. (This is particularly pronounced in the patient with open bite, since the force cannot be directed close to parallel with the occlusal plane but will, of necessity, be more oblique.) Once ideal coordinated upper and lower archwires have been placed and have become passive, impressions are made for feasibility model surgery.

Unlike the routine Class II mandibular advancement, it is preferable that the occlusion produced by the feasibility model surgery be as nearly ideal as possible, especially with respect to vertical and transverse tooth positions. Tooth mass must be carefully observed and appropriate steps taken (that is, interproximal recontouring, opening upper spaces, or lower incisor extraction) to eliminate any discrepancy that precludes establishing adequate overbite and overjet. When there are obvious prematurities, these are eliminated by appropriate archwire adjustments or equilibration. Frequently, the upper and lower second molars will not be occlusion when the feasibility model surgery is done, and this is of little concern since they are easily brought into occlusion after surgery. *Ideally an occlusion is produced that will require as little orthodontic treatment as possible following surgery.* New models are made, the occlusion studied, and the archwires adjusted to detail the occlusion until the occlusion that will be produced at surgery is as nearly ideal as possible.

Once the orthodontist is pleased with the occlusion that can be produced surgically, all archwires are tied with ligature wires to prevent inadvertent disengagement at surgery, elastic hooks are placed as necessary, and the patient is referred for surgery.

Orthognathic reconstructive surgery

Clinical evaluation of the patient and the cephalometric prediction tracings are essential to determine if simultaneous advancement genioplasty and/or suprahyoid myotomies are indicated. If the patient is only going to undergo mandibular advancement and can easily protrude the mandible into a Class III incisal relation with little palpable tension in the suprahyoid region, it is suggestive that the patient may not require a suprahyoid myotomy. However, when advancement genioplasty is also to be done, this clinical evaluation assumes less significance. In such instances measurement of the proposed lengthening of the suprahyoid musculature is made from the surgical cephalometric prediction tracing *after both* the mandibular advancement and the advancement genioplasty are done. If the lengthening of the suprahyoid musculature exceeds 30% of their original length a suprahyoid myotomy is planned (see Fig. 9-81). If suprahyoid myotomies are done in conjunction with the usual advancement genioplasty, as described in Chapter 6, this will result in a free bone graft of the chin segment, which will subsequently undergo extensive resorption. Thus, when suprahyoid myotomies are indicated, the genioplasty approach must be modified as described in the preceding section of this chapter (see Figs. 9-82 through 9-84).

After the genioplasty is completed, heavy circummandibular wires (22-gauge) are passed bilaterally in the premolar-canine areas and help to hold the genioplasty segment in position. The circummandibular skeletal stabilization wires are passed over the occlusal splint and are placed more anteriorly than in the routine mandibular advancement to better resist the more dominant vertical relapse forces that exist with counterclockwise rotation of the distal segment as occurs in closure of an open bite with mandibular advancement.

The wound is packed with moist gauze sponges. The incision is left open until after completion of the mandibular advancement to permit observation of the genioplasty to make certain that it has not been inadvertently displaced during the sagittal split surgery.

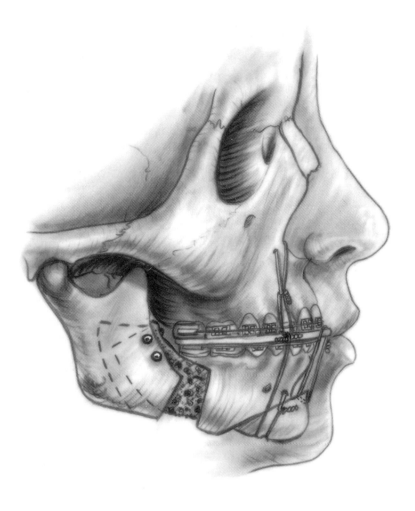

FIG. 9-89

The modified sagittal ramus splits are performed as described in detail in Chapter 6. However, because of the counterclockwise rotational effect of the distal segment in the Class II deformity with open bite, both the mobilization of the distal segment and the placement of intraosseous stabilization are critical to control the proximal segment and thereby avoid inadvertent distraction of the condyles from their fossa. Because of the magnitude and vector of advancement, it is preferred to use skeletal maxillomandibular fixation for 4 weeks. Two or three 2.0-mm screws may be used to secure the proximal to the distal segment. The screw placement necessary to achieve the desired relation of the proximal and distal segments of the mandible is determined in each case from the definitive surgical cephalometric prediction tracings as described previously.

Following release of intermaxillary fixation, the same regimen of jaw physiotherapy and follow-up evaluation is followed as discussed in detail in Chapter 4.

Postsurgical orthodontic treatment

The first postsurgical orthodontic appointment is within 48 hours of removal of the occlusal splint. At this time the archwires are removed, any damaged or loose appliances are replaced, the archwires are checked for coordination and fit and are repaired or replaced as necessary, and the patient is instructed in the use of any elastics that are indicated. Any mechanics that will tend to open the bite are carefully avoided. The patient is seen again in 2 to 3 days.

At the second postsurgical visit the occlusion is carefully studied. Appropriate adjustments are made in the archwires and elastic therapy. It is preferable to use elastics for as short a time as possible following surgery. Consequently, the elastics are discontinued as soon as the occlusion is acceptable, and the patient is informed that use of the elastics may or may not be resumed depending on any subsequent changes in the occlusion. If elastics are discontinued, archwire adjustments are made, or if it is anticipated that elastics can soon be discontinued, the patient is seen again in 1 week. When no archwire adjustments or change in elastic therapy have been made, the patient is seen again in 2 weeks.

The routine 4-week adjustment schedule is resumed once the clinician is certain that stability is good and that any subsequent mechanics will not adversely affect the stability. Finishing and retention procedures are routine.

Factors affecting stability
Orthodontic factors

This orthodontic-surgical treatment is relatively rare and no specific studies on its stability have been conducted. The following factors are those that logically would contribute to the stability of this treatment. Each of these factors is discussed and illustrated in Chapter 6.

1. Eliminate dental compensations.
2. Properly manage tooth mass discrepancies before surgery.
3. Appropriately level both upper and lower arches.
4. Properly manage any transverse discrepancy.

Surgical factors

Most surgically related relapse with mandibular advancement surgery is directly related to surgical technique and occurs primarily during or immediately on release of intermaxillary fixation. The following factors have been identified as being most important and have been previously discussed in detail.

1. Mobilization of the distal mandible.
2. Distraction of the condyle from the fossa.
3. Method of intermaxillary fixation.

Age-related factors

No studies have been reported in the literature regarding the stability of correction of the Class II open bite by mandibular advancement before the completion of facial growth. Other studies have shown that the patient who is retrognathic at 6 years of age will remain retrognathic and the degree of the Class II occlusion will remain essentially unchanged because of a proportionality of growth between the maxilla and mandible after age 6 years. It is reasonable to assume that the Class II dentofacial deformity with open bite *but without vertical maxillary excess* "grows" essentially the same as the Class II deformity without open bite after age 12 years and that the same factors affecting the stability of mandibular advancement during growth are operable in both deformities.

Results of treatment

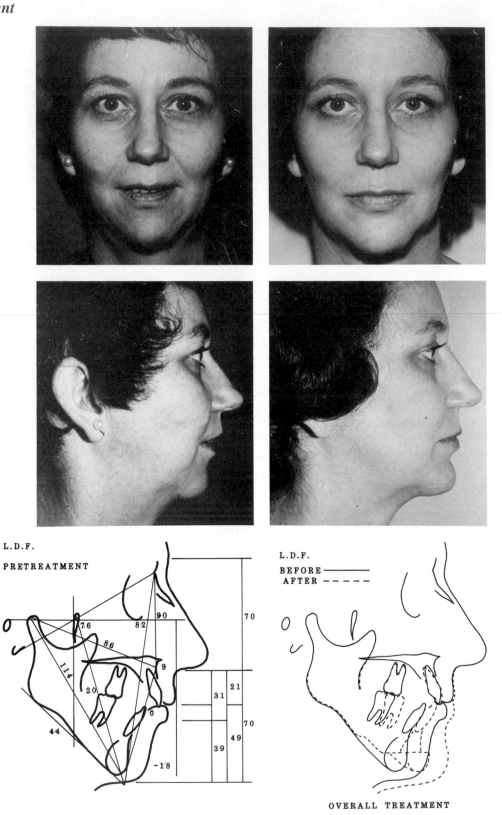

FIG. 9-90

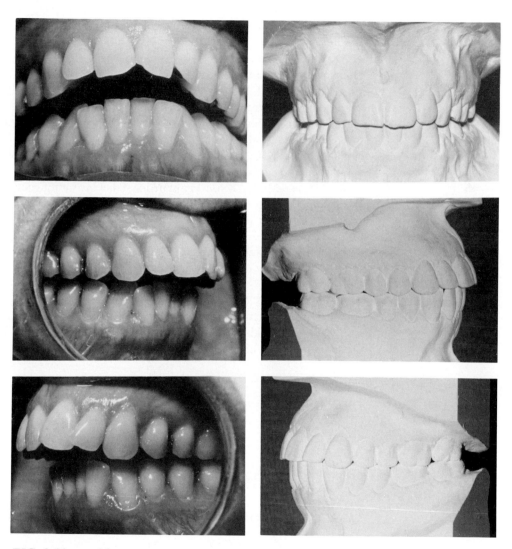

FIG. 9-90, cont'd

REFERENCES

Ackerman, R.I., and Klapper, L.: Tongue position and open bite: the key roles in growth and nasopharyngeal airway, J. Dent. Child. **48:**339, 1981.

Carlson, D.S., Ellis, E., and Dechow, P.C.: Adaptation of the suprahyoid muscle complex to mandibular advancement surgery, Am. J. Orthodont. Dentofac. Orthop. **92:**134, 1987.

Epker, B.N., and Fish, L.C.: Surgical-orthodontic correction of open bite deformity, Am. J. Orthodont. **71:**278, 1977.

Epker, B.N., Schendel, S.A., and Washburn, M.: Effects of early surgical superior repositioning of the maxilla on subsequent growth. III. Biomechanical considerations. In Mc Namara, J., Carlson, D., and Ribbens, K., editors: The effects of surgical intervention on craniofacial growth, monograph no. 12, Ann Arbor, Michigan, 1982, Center for Human Growth and Development, University of Michigan.

Fletcher, S.G., Casteel, R.L., and Bradley, D.P.: Tongue-thrust swallow, speech articulation and age, J. Speech Hear. Dis. **26:**201, 1961.

Isaacson, R.J., et al.: Extreme variations in vertical facial growth and associated variations in skeletal and dental relations, Angle Orthodont. **41:**219, 1971.

Krekmanov, L., and Kahnberg, K.E.: Soft tissue response to genioplasty procedures, Br. J. Oral Maxillofac. Surg. **30**(2):87, 1992.

Proffit, W.R., and Mason, R.M.: Myofunctional therapy for tongue-thrusting: background and recommendations, J. Am. Dent. Assoc. **90:**403, 1975.

Ricketts, R.M., et al.: Bioprogressive therapy, book 1, Denver, 1979, Rocky Mountain Orthodontics.

Stoller, A.E.: The universal appliance, St. Louis, 1971, The C.V. Mosby Company.

Thurow, R.C.: Atlas of orthodontic principles, St. Louis, 1970, The C.V. Mosby Company.

Turvey, T.A., Journot, V., and Epker, B.N.: Correction of anterior open-bite deformity: a study of tongue function, speech changes and stability, J. Maxillofac. Surg. **4:**93, 1976.

Wertz, R., and Dreskin, M.: Midpalatal suture opening, a normative study, Am. J. Orthodont. **71:**367, 1977.

Index

Posterior midpalatal osteotomy, 496
Posteroanterior cephalometric radiograph, 55-58
Pressure dressing, 159
  in mandibular advancement for Class II, division 2
      deformity, 269, 273
  in segmental LeFort I superior repositioning of
      maxilla with advancement genioplasty, 509
Profile analysis, 23-28
  lower third face, 27-28
  middle third face, 24-26
  upper third face, 23-24
Progressive records, 154-155, 163-170
Progressive monitoring, 151-170
  orthodontic considerations and
      postsurgical, 155-157
      presurgical, 151-155
  recordkeeping in, 163-170
  surgical care and, 157-163
Proximal segment position, 179-180
Psychologic evaluation of patient, 6-8, 51

R

Radiograph
  cephalometric, 29-41, 165-166, 178-180
    lateral rest-position, 54
    posteroanterior, 55-58
  panoramic, 42-43, 166, 168, 180-181
  of tongue posture, 62-63
Radionucleotide scans, 59-60
Reconstruction by three-dimensional computed tomo-
    graphy, 59
Recurrent complications, 186
Reduction genioplasty, mandibular advancement with,
    276-287
Release-of-fixation records, 168-170
Round wire, 239, 321

S

Sagittal ramus ostectomy, 313
  with advancement genioplasty, 251-259
  mandibular advancement and, 209-225
Sagittal ramus osteotomy, 213, 219, 358, 450,
    550
Segmental LeFort I superior repositioning of maxilla
    with advancement genioplasty, 392
  adjunctive esthetic procedures in
    lateral advancement genioplasty, 506
    maximum advancement genioplasty, 508-509
    widening genioplasty, 507
  and factors affecting stability of, 514-519
  orthognathic reconstructive surgery in, 490-509
  outline of treatment for, 466

Segmental Le Fort I superior repositioning of maxilla
    with advancement genioplasty—cont'd
  postsurgical orthodontics in
    anterior rigid fixation with posterior suspension
      wires and, 511-513
    total rigid fixation and, 510
  presurgical orthodontics in, 468-489
  results of, 520-521
Segmental maxillary feasibility model surgery, 96-98
Segmental superior repositioning of maxilla with
    mandibular advancement, advancement ge-
    nioplasty, and suprahyoid myotomies
  contingency statement for, 548
  and factors affecting stability of, 555
  orthognathic reconstructive surgery and, 550-555
  postsurgical orthondontics in, 555
  presurgical orthondontics in, 550
  results of, 556-557
Segmental total subapical superior repositioning of
    maxilla with advancement genioplasty
  contingency statement for, 522
  and factors affecting stability of, 545
  orthognathic reconstructive surgery in, 528-544
  postsurgical orthodontics in, 544-545
  presurgical orthondontics in, 524-528
  results of, 546-547
Segmentalization, 152-153
Simultaneous mobilization of both jaws, 358
Sinus series, 58
Skin, 21
SN-LLV:LLV-ME, 30
SN-ST, 30
SN-ST:ST-ME, 30
Social-psychologic evaluation, 6-8, 51
Speech evaluation, 62
Static evaluation, 44
Subapical ostectomy, 318
Submental
  and neck area, 20, 28
  photographic view of, 52
Subnasale perpendicular, 32, 202, 243, 377, 475
Subnasale to menton, 16-20
Subnasale-lower lip vermilion:lower lip vermilion-
    menton, 30
Subnasale-stomion:stomion menton, 30
Superior osteotomy, 216
Superior photographic view, 52
Superior repositioning of maxilla, 115-131, 132-135
  with advancement genioplasty
    adjunctive esthetic maxillofacial procedures in,
      404-417
      alar base width control and, 408
      buccal lipectomy and, 413-415

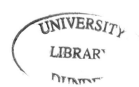